Men's Aesthetics

A Practical Guide to Minimally Invasive Treatment

First Edition

Jeremy A. Brauer, MD
Clinical Associate Professor
Ronald O. Perelman Department of Dermatology
New York University;
Founder and Director
Spectrum Skin and Laser
New York, New York, USA

204 images

Thieme
Stuttgart • New York • Delhi • Rio de Janeiro

Library of Congress Cataloging-in-Publication Data is available from the publisher.

Important note: Medicine is an ever-changing science undergoing continual development. Research and clinical experience are continually expanding our knowledge, in particular our knowledge of proper treatment and drug therapy. Insofar as this book mentions any dosage or application, readersmay rest assured that the authors, editors, and publishers have made every effort to ensure that such references are in accordance with **the state of knowledge at the time of production of the book.**

Nevertheless, this does not involve, imply, or express any guarantee or responsibility on the part of the publishers in respect to any dosage instructions and forms of applications stated in the book. **Every user is requested to examine carefully** the manufacturers' leaflets accompanying each drug and to check, if necessary in consultation with a physician or specialist, whether the dosage schedules mentioned therein or the contraindications stated by the manufacturers differ from the statements made in the present book. Such examination is particularly important with drugs that are either rarely used or have been newly released on the market. Every dosage schedule or every form of application used is and publishers request every user to report to the publishers any discrepancies or inaccuracies noticed. If errors in this work are found after publication, errata will be posted at www.thieme.com on the product description page.

Some of the product names, patents, and registered designs referred to in this book are in fact registered trademarks or proprietary names even though specific reference to this fact is not always made in the text. Therefore, the appearance of a name without designation as proprietary is not to be construed as a representation by the publisher that it is in the public domain.

Thieme addresses people of all gender identities equally. We encourage our authors to use gender-neutral or genderequal expressions wherever the context allows.

© 2024. Thieme. All rights reserved.

Georg Thieme Verlag KG
Rüdigerstrasse 14, 70469 Stuttgart, Germany
+49 [0]711 8931 421,
customerservice@thieme.de

Cover design and image: © Thieme
Cover image source: the cover image was
composed by Thieme using
images provided by Juan Venegas

Typesetting by TNQ Technologies, India

Printed in Germany by Beltz Grafische Betriebe GmbH   5 4 3 2 1

DOI: 10.1055/b000000260

ISBN: 978-3-13-242837-9

Also available as an e-book:
eISBN (PDF): 978-3-13-242838-6
eISBN (epub): 978-3-13-258266-8

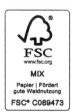

FSC
www.fsc.org
MIX
Papier | Fördert
gute Waldnutzung
FSC® C089473

To my wife, Anate, thank you for all of your support, in everything, always, and allowing me to pursue all of my personal and professional dreams. Thank you to our children, Maddie, Noa, and Sophie–the lights of our life, who continue to keep us young, smiling, and exhausted! To my mother, Bobbi–your unconditional love, guidance, and support have made me the person I am today. Lastly, I would like to thank Stephan Konnry, Lewis Enim, and the staff at Thieme for all of their efforts in bringing this book to life.

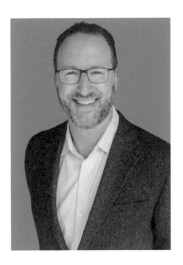

Contents

5   Following the Pattern: Hair Restoration   50

Nicole Rogers and Marisa Belaidi

6   Finding the Right Balance: Chemical Peels   64

Jeave Reserva, Rebecca Tung, and Seaver Soon

Contents

Foreword

Minimally invasive treatments made their debut with the development of the pulsed dye laser in the late 1980s. And, since then, there have been rapid and dramatic developments in this field including the development of selective pulsed lasers and lights for treating pigmented lesions, hair removal, treating wrinkles, removing excess fat and hair, growing hair, and the development of a variety of minimally invasive no-downtime procedures using neuromodulators and fillers. This revolution first took place in the female population, but men have slowly but surely joined the party. It is said that up to 10% of all cosmetic procedures performed yearly are done on male patients. And the number is on the upswing.

Perhaps, not surprisingly, it has taken this many years before a well-crafted volume on *Men's Aesthetics* has been prepared. Jeremy Brauer, a leader in the field, deserves a huge amount of credit for putting this wonderful text together. He has invited a group of exciting young experts from around the world to cover virtually all the topics in the field including aesthetic preferences of men, anatomical differences and changes in men as they age, and a variety of treatments and procedures from volumizing the face to the use of neuromodulators and fillers, chemical peels, lasers, lights and energy devices, skin tightening, and treating male pattern hair loss and hair restoration. He has rounded out the book with fine discussions of aesthetic concerns in men, men of color, and transgender patients.

Men's Aesthetics is not intended to serve as a reference textbook, it is rather a guide for practitioners interested in the spectrum of male aesthetic topics. It will be helpful both to novices but also to seasoned veterans in the aesthetic medicine field. The book is beautifully written, and I know you will enjoy it. Happy learning!

Jeffrey S. Dover MD, FRCOC
SkinCare Physicians, Chestnut Hill, Massachusetts

Preface

As greater awareness and acceptance of minimally invasive aesthetic procedures continues, individuals across all demographics are increasingly seeking out these treatments. It was with this in mind, along with a particular focus on the male aesthetic patient, that I set out to create this book. Fortunately, many great minds in the fields of dermatology and plastic surgery from around the world agreed to join me on the journey to bringing you the most comprehensive collective experience in the space of male aesthetics to date.

Our hope and expectation is that, if read carefully, this text will help you to better understand and convey to your patients the risks, benefits and alternatives to these treatments, while optimizing their outcomes. The intention is not to serve as a reference text per se, but instead as a resource for those interested in building, growing, and maintaining a well-rounded male aesthetic practice. The chapters were constructed to be easily accessible, so that you can identify and access the sections most appropriate for your practice and needs.

Across all chapters the reader will have an opportunity to appreciate the broad strokes of a topic of interest as well as glean specific tips or "pearls" regarding best practices. This will allow the practitioner to more readily digest important facts and nuances of the procedures while keeping the big picture in mind, and effectively apply them to their own patients. Utmost effort has been made by the chapter authors to include every minimally invasive procedure currently being performed.

The text opens with an overview of men's aesthetics and a targeted discussion of the male aesthetic patient. In this chapter, the authors discuss the most recent trends, as well as emphasize the importance of the similarities and differences from their female counterparts as it relates to anatomy and preferences. Perhaps most importantly, the chapter ends with how the patient experience begins–the consultation visit and the first steps toward the development of a strong physician-patient relationship. The importance of this initial visit cannot be overemphasized, as it is your opportunity to evaluate and assess the patient's goals and needs and develop an appropriate treatment plan.

The second chapter naturally builds off the first, providing a much more in-depth look at the anatomy and aging male face. Methodically working their way from the forehead and temples to the jawline and lower face, the authors provide incredible detail and insight into the structural changes observed over time. While doing so, they seamlessly integrate the identification of target areas for treatment, providing both options and guidance in best approach and practice.

From there, chapters three through nine are dedicated to the review of minimally invasive treatments in male patients. Chapter three seamlessly continues the developing conversation of chapters one and two, highlighting cutting edge techniques and utilization of various fillers to enhance features of the male face. Of significant importance is how well the authors present common adverse reactions and severe complications with filler injections. Avoiding and managing complications of these minimally invasive procedures is paramount to both the patient and physician.

By far the most popular minimally invasive treatment in men, neuromodulators, or botulinum toxins, are discussed in chapter four. The reader is presented with the opportunity to learn not only about best practices and techniques, but also how to optimally perform these procedures with the male perspective and anatomy in mind. Chapter five addresses all aspects of hair loss and restoration, beginning with diagnosis and identification of potential causes, as well as a complete presentation of non-surgical and surgical options. The remainder and majority of this chapter is dedicated to a detailed presentation of surgical options available to practitioners and patients for hair restoration. In chapter six, the reader is fortunate to learn about all aspects of chemical peels, generally, as well as detailed information specific to the male patient. The chapter methodically presents the authors approach, utilizing various peeling agents, but also going much further to include information on indications for treatment, best approaches to the pre-peel consultation and conditioning, as well as post treatment care.

For chapters seven through nine, the focus of the text shifts to treatments with laser, light, and energy-based devices. Considering the risks involved–as with all of the other treatments discussed in the book–it is of the utmost importance to understand and to know how to avoid, minimize, and treat complications associated with these procedures. Chapter seven introduces the topic, with an overview of anatomy and physiology, highlighting the different categories of lasers utilized in addressing the various aesthetic concerns of our male patients. Approaching the evaluation and treatment of unwanted fat with all currently available modalities is what one will gain from reading chapter eight. Then in chapter nine, skin tightening procedures, technologies, and techniques are emphasized to round out the discussion of body contouring.

The final three chapters of the book provide a synthesis of the information in the prior chapters, with an appreciation of the content through a specific lens. Chapters ten and eleven are integral to the conversation about minimally invasive aesthetic treatments in men, identifying the specific concerns of, as well as detailing an approach to, skin of color patients in chapter ten and transgender patients in chapter eleven. In chapter twelve, the reader will find a concise but thorough summary of all of the topics presented in the book, with additional insights as well and discussion of skin care options for our male patients.

It is my sincere hope that you enjoy reading this book and find its content informative and helpful in your own men's aesthetics practice at whatever stage in your career that may be! I have every expectation that this field will continue to rapidly evolve as more and newer treatments are perfected and performed, so please feel free to reach out with any comments or questions you may have.

Jeremy A. Brauer MD

Contributors

Shino Bay Aguilera, MD
Dermatologist
Shino Bay Cosmetic Dermatology & Laser
Institute;
Clinical Assistant Professor
NOVA South Eastern University
Fort Lauderdale, FL, United States

Murad Alam, MD, MSCI, MBA
Vice Chair Department of Dermatology
Chief of Cutaneous and Aesthetic Surgery
Professor of Dermatology (Cutaneous and Aesthetic
Surgery), Medical Social Sciences,
Otolaryngology - Head and Neck Surgery, and Surgery
(Organ Transplantation)
Northwestern University
Feinberg School of Medicine
Chicago, IL, United States

Andrew F. Alexis MD MPH
Professor of Clinical Dermatology
Vice Chair for Diversity and Inclusion
Department of Dermatology
Weill Cornell Medical College
New York, NY, United States

Marisa Belaidi, MD
Dermatologist
Hudson Dermatology
New York, NY, United States

Vince Bertucci, MD
Founder and Medical Director
Bertucci MedSpa
Woodbridge, ON, Canada;
Instructor
Division of Dermatology
University of Toronto
Toronto, ON, Canada

Merrick A. Brodsky, MD
Dermatologist
Department of Dermatology
Ohio State University
Columbus, OH, United States

Yunyoung C. Chang, MD
Dermatologist
UnionDerm
New York, NY, United States

Cameron Chesnut, MD, FAAD, FACMS, FASDS
Dermatologist
Clinic 5C
Spokane, WA, United States;
Clinical Assistant Professor
University of Washington School of Medicine
Seattle, WA, United States

Sebastian Cotofana, MD PhD, PhD
Associate Professor of Anatomy
Department of Clinical Anatomy
Mayo Clinic College of Medicine and Science
Rochester, MN, United States

Jonathan J. Dutton, MD
Professor Emeritus of Ophthalmic Plastic and
    Reconstructive Surgery and Ophthalmic Oncology
University of North Carolina
Chapel Hill, NC, United States

Andrés M. Erlendsson, MD
Department of Dermatology
Karolinska University Hospital
Stockholm, Sweden

Daniel P. Friedmann, MD, FAAD
Associate and Clinical Research Director
Westlake Dermatology & Cosmetic Surgery
Austin, TX, United States

Jeremy B. Green, MD
Dermatologist
Skin Associates of South Florida
Coral Gables, FL, United States

Edith A. Hanna, MD
Département de dermatologie
Centre Hospitalier Régional du Grand-Portage
CISSS du Bas-Saint-Laurent
Rivière du-Loup, QC, Canada

Michelle Henry, MD, FAAD
Dermatologist and Founder
Skin and Aesthetic Surgery of Manhattan;
Clinical Instructor of Dermatology
Weill Cornell Medical College
New York, NY, United States

Brian P. Hibler, MD
Dermatologist
Schweiger Dermatology Group
New York, NY, United States

Derek Hsu, MD
Dermatologist
Southern California Dermatology
Santa Ana, CA, United States

Terrence C. Keaney, MD, FAAD
Dermatologist and Founder
Skin DC
Washington DC, United States

Michael B. Lipp, DO, FAAD
Dermatologist
Skinaesthetica Medical Aesthetics
Redlands, CA, United States

Jennifer L. MacGregor, MD
Dermatologist
UnionDerm
New York, NY, United States

José R. Montes, MD FACS, FACCS
Professor
Department of Ophthalmology
University of Puerto Rico School of Medicine;
Medical Director
Jose Raul Montes Eyes and Facial Rejuvenation
San Juan, Puerto Rico

Gilly Munavalli, MD, MHS, FACMS
Medical Director and Founder
Dermatology, Laser, and Vein Specialists of the
  Carolinas
Charlotte, NC, United States;
Assistant Clinical Professor
Department of Dermatology
Wake Forest School of Medicine
Winston-Salem, NC, United States

Mildred Lopez Pineiro, MD
Medical and Cosmetic Dermatologist
Bellaire Dermatology
Bellaire, TX, United States

Deanne Mraz Robinson, MD, FAAD
Dermatologist
Modern Dermatology
Westport, CT, United States

Anthony M. Rossi, MD, FAAD, FACMS
Mohs Surgeon
Memorial Sloan Kettering Cancer Center
Weill Cornell Medical College
New York, NY, United States

Nicole E. Rogers MD, FAAD, FISHRS
Assistant Clinical Professor
Department of Dermatology
Tulane University
New Orleans, LA, United States;
Private Practice
Hair Restoration of the South
Metairie, LA, United States

Jeave Reserva, MD
Dermatologist
Springfield Clinic
Springfield, IL, United States

Nazanin Saedi, MD
Dermatologist
Dermatology Associates of Plymouth
Meeting
Plymouth Meeting, PA, United States;
Clinical Associate Professor
Department of Dermatology
Thomas Jefferson University
Philadelphia, PA, United States

Matthew K. Sandre, MD
Dermatologist
Bertucci MedSpa
Woodbridge, ON, Canada
Department of Dermatology
Sunnybrook Hospital
Toronto, ON, Canada

Seaver Soon, MD
Dermatologist
The Skin Clinic MD;
Scripps Green Hospital
San Diego, CA, United States

Luis Soro, MD
Dermatologist
Shino Bay Cosmetic Dermatology & Laser Institute
Fort Lauderdale, FL, United States

Rebecca Tung, MD
Mohs and Dermatologic Surgeon
Florida Dermatology and Skin Cancer Centers
Winter Haven, FL, United States;
Professor
Department of Medicine and Dermatology
University of Central Florida
Orlando, FL, United States

Jordan V. Wang, MD, MBE, MBA
Dermatologist
Laser & Skin Surgery Center of New York
New York, NY, United States

Yiping Xing, MD
Dermatologist
Hudson Dermatology
Tarrytown, NY, United States

1 The Male Aesthetic Patient: Preferences and Practice

Jeremy B. Green, Terrence C. Keaney, Sebastian Cotofana, and Mildred Lopez-Pineiro

Summary

This chapter focuses on describing the key differences in gender preferences regarding minimally invasive cosmetic procedures. With the surge in cosmetic procedures performed for men, it is important for clinicians to understand not only anatomic variations in males versus females but also their aging concerns and any possible barriers to treatment.

Keywords: male aesthetics, male cosmetics, gender differences, cosmetic preferences, masculine anatomy

1.1 Background

As minimally invasive cosmetic procedures requested by male patients continue to increase, there still remains a dearth of studies focusing on the specifics of male aesthetic preferences (▶ Table 1.1). According to recent statistics, the total number of minimally invasive procedures sought by men has increased by 72% since year 2000, with 1,092,103 reported cases.[1] The most common minimally invasive cosmetic procedures performed for men were botulinum toxin type A (BTX-A) and laser hair removal, followed by microdermabrasion, chemical peels, and soft-tissue fillers. Compared to statistics from the year 2000, the procedure with the most growth overall was neuromodulators (BTX-A), with a 381% increase. Interestingly, the three cosmetic procedures that demonstrated a growth pattern year over year (compared to 2017) were vein treatments

Table 1.1 Minimally invasive cosmetic procedures, 2018 (modified from the ASPS 2018 Annual Survey)

Procedure	Total males	Overall total
Botulinum toxin type A	452,812	7,437,378
Laser hair removal	184,668	1,077,490
Microdermabrasion	136, 885	709,413
Chemical peels	102,683	1,384,327
Soft tissue fillers	100,702	2,523,437
Laser skin resurfacing	75,584	594,266
Laser treatment of veins	29,505	217,836
Cellulite treatment	4,721	37,220
Sclerotherapy	5,543	323,234
Total	1,092,103	14,304,601

(including sclerotherapy and laser treatment), laser skin resurfacing, and soft-tissue fillers.[1] It is evident that with this advancing and evolving male interest, clinicians need to be more cognizant of men's anatomy, aging differences, and beauty preferences as compared to females in order to optimize outcomes and patient satisfaction.

1.2 Anatomy

Gender differences in male facial anatomy include increased skin thickness, higher muscle mass, higher number of terminal hairs as well as sebaceous glands, higher vascularity associated with pilosebaceous units, and different rates of fat and bone resorption with aging given hormonal variations.[2] Men have more strongly developed supraorbital ridges and flatter cheeks. They also have a larger glabella and frontal sinus, smaller orbits, and more acute glabellar angles. The mandible is larger and thicker, and the chin wider and square.[3] (▶ Fig. 1.1) The subcutaneous architecture in men is significantly different as men have a more developed superficial fascial system and the number of retinacula cutis per defined area is significantly increased compared to females. This implies that the containment forces of the skin to the underlying soft tissues are increased with a decreased probability for skin laxity in comparable female matching pairs.[4] In the perioral area, the amount and thickness of terminal hair increases the stability and adhesion forces between dermis and the lamina propria, resulting in the less frequently observed perioral lines ("barcode wrinkles") compared to females. These notable variations in skin quality and composition, as well as soft tissue and bony anatomy, are essential to understand and consider when planning facial rejuvenation or enhancement procedures. Additionally, one must also consider these differences when estimating the amount of product that will be required to achieve the desired outcome. Longitudinal changes in male anatomy compared to female aging anatomy are complex (▶ Fig. 1.2). With increasing age, males experience an increase in their forehead angle resulting in a steeper forehead, which resembles the female forehead outline.[5] The calvarial volume decreases with increasing age, and bone thickness of the skull (temple and forehead) becomes thinner, a trend that interestingly is not observed in females.[6]

1.3 Patient Preferences

There is one published study in the literature describing the male patient preferences in regard to cosmetic procedures. This cross-sectional online study focused on deciphering which facial areas men are more likely to treat

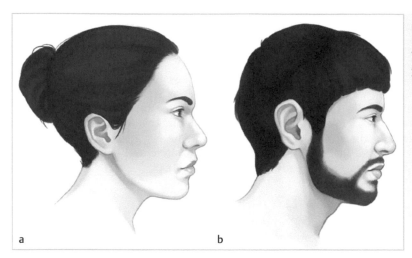

Fig. 1.1 Gender differences in facial anatomy, **(a)** female vs. **(b)** male. (Reproduced with permission from Steinbrech S, ed. Male Aesthetic Plastic Surgery. 1st Edition. New York: Thieme; 2020.)

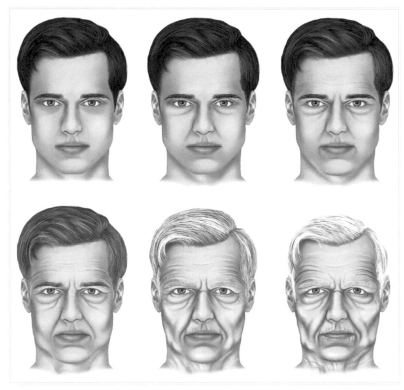

Fig. 1.2 Longitudinal changes in male facial anatomy. (Reproduced with permission from Steinbrech S, ed. Male Aesthetic Plastic Surgery. 1st Edition. New York: Thieme; 2020.)

first and the correlation with their areas of most concern, awareness to procedures, and their motivations to undergoing minimally invasive injectable treatment, specifically neuromodulators and soft-tissue fillers.[7] They enrolled a total of 600 injectable-naive men between the ages of 30 and 65 years who were "aesthetically oriented," aware of Botox cosmetic, and considering at least one facial cosmetic treatment within the next 2 years.

In this study, they found that most men were open to talking to their physicians about facial wrinkles (48%) and bags under the eyes (44%). Additionally, it was noted that

they were least likely to talk about red/vascular facial appearance (14%) and razor burn (16%). Overall awareness for all aesthetic procedures ranged from 2 to 6%. Specifically, for soft-tissue fillers the awareness was 39%, and for surgical procedures such as liposuction and hair transplant, it was greater than 90%. The two main motivators for undergoing cosmetic procedures were wanting to look good for their age (70%) and wanting to look more youthful (51%).[7]

On the other hand, the main barriers to treatment were not thinking they needed treatment yet (47%) and

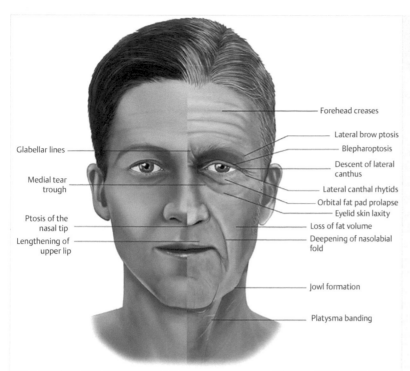

Fig. 1.3 Hallmarks of the aging male face. (Reproduced with permission from Leatherbarrow B, ed. Oculoplastic Surgery. 3rd Edition. New York: Thieme; 2019.)

Glabellar lines

Medial tear trough

Ptosis of the nasal tip

Lengthening of upper lip

Forehead creases

Lateral brow ptosis

Blepharoptosis

Descent of lateral canthus

Lateral canthal rhytids

Orbital fat pad prolapse

Eyelid skin laxity

Loss of fat volume

Deepening of nasolabial fold

Jowl formation

Platysma banding

concerns about safety or side effects (46%). The five areas of most aesthetic concern were hair loss (27%), double chin (22%), tear troughs (22%), crow's feet (18%), and forehead lines (15%). Not surprisingly, given what we know about men facial anatomy, perioral lines were the area of least concern (3%). Tear trough and crow's feet were the two areas that were prioritized in terms of receiving treatment (80%). Finally, they noted a strong correlation (r^2 = 0.81) between areas of most concern and areas with treatment priority.[7]

Of interest, aging concerns of men directly correlate with the expected anatomic changes based on gender (▶ Fig. 1.3). As men age, they are more preoccupied by upper facial lines as opposed to females who switch from being worried about upper facial lines to being more concerned with lower facial lines and perioral wrinkling.[8] These concerns likely stem from the expected age-related inversion of the triangle of youth where the cheeks flatten and jowls form, as well as the lack of terminal pilosebaceous units in the perioral skin of females. All these changes seem to be more accentuated in the female face given the drastic hormonal changes endured during menopause.

Moreover, one of the main barriers to treatment identified by this study was lack of knowledge of what minimally invasive cosmetic procedures entail, including risks, benefits, safety, and side effect profiles. This suggests that even "aesthetically oriented" male patients deserve and require a full cosmetic consultation with specific education about procedures that may fit their lifestyle and long-term aging goals. This pretreatment consult visit is a pivotal event in formulating a successful procedural treatment plan that will lead to a positive patient outcome.

Finally, it is important to reiterate that the two main reasons for men to proceed with a cosmetic procedure were to look good for their age and to appear more youthful. These two motivations have social implications in their lives as well, as being youthful gives males a more competitive appeal in the workplace, which can lead to a 5 to 10% higher salary.[9] In addition, two studies have demonstrated that cosmetic procedures, such as botulinum toxin neuromodulation, can lead to improved self-esteem and feelings of attractiveness that lead to a better quality of life.[10,11] All these represent psychosocial factors to be considered during the cosmetic consult.

1.4 Clinical Practice

The goal of the initial cosmetic visit, as with any patient encounter, is to establish a strong physician–patient relationship in order to prepare for the cosmetic procedure. The first step is to understand the reason for the visit. One must determine, for example, if the patient desires broad improvements such as overall rejuvenation or improvement in skin quality, or perhaps has specific goals such as erasing a few lines prior to an important event, or enhancing their natural bone structure. Given men's lack of awareness regarding the available aesthetic procedures and their indications, in general, it is not uncommon for male patients to present with vague cosmetic complaints. "I look tired" and "I am getting old" are common concerns that require the treating physician to ascertain what the patient wants. There are clues that a physician can use to identify a male patient's cosmetic concerns. For example, a male patient who is concerned about "looking tired" may be subconsciously bothered by periocular changes. Once concerns and goals are discussed and understood in detail, a thorough physical examination should be performed. This examination should include evaluation of static and dynamic lines, facial movement, muscle mass, bone structure, and skin quality (▶ Fig. 1.4). The physical examination will help the clinician to understand which products or devices are appropriate for the patient's skin. It will also serve as a guide in terms of approximating how much product or how many sessions will be required to achieve the discussed outcome. Once a plan is formulated by the physician, the patient should be educated on the possible cosmetic procedures that would best address their specific concerns. In addition to reviewing the risks, benefits, and alternatives, this detailed discussion should include the potential need for multiple sessions or retreatments, as well as anticipated downtime of the recommended procedures. This point is critical, as one of the easiest—and most avoidable—ways to lose a new male patient is an undesired and unanticipated outcome.

In our clinical experience, we have noticed a few key differences in how to approach the male's first cosmetic treatment session. First, it is important to note that men schedule a 2-week follow-up appointment for potential touch-up treatments after their first ever neuromodulator treatment. We have noticed that male patients are

less likely to follow up if they are unhappy versus females. Hence, having that 2-week follow-up appointment scheduled guarantees you can discuss what they liked and what they did not. Injectors can communicate to the patient that this will enable them to have a reproducible treatment plan for subsequent visits that will help ensure desired aesthetic outcome at subsequent visits. When it comes to neuromodulators, keep in mind males may take a 50% higher dose in order to achieve the same result you would expect in a female. This is because anatomically males tend to have a higher muscle bulk and stronger muscles. Males also have a flatter brow to begin with as compared to their female counterparts, and therefore it is acceptable to treat corrugator muscle to its lateral most aspect/insertion into the skin, even if it results in a flatter brow. Females would not be pleased with this result, as this approach may yield unappealing brow ptosis. Finally, the male forehead should be more superiorly than that of females given that they may have a receding hairline, and treating the inferior frontalis while ignoring the superior may result in the unnatural appearance of a "shower cap," where superior frontalis fibers continue to contract. Once the face is treated with neuromodulators, a map should be drawn or a picture should be taken demonstrating precise injection points in order to use this as a reproducible template for follow-up treatments. The authors have found this approach (immediately after injection photography) to be especially helpful in treating the forehead in men. Male patients tend to be very loyal, but they require proper treatment during their first visit. Hence, providers should make the 2-week follow-up after the first treatment session mandatory in order to ensure the patient is happy and you have a reproducible treatment template for future visits.

1.5 Conclusion

With the continued increase in minimally invasive cosmetic procedures pursued by males, it is important for clinicians to recognize the main anatomic and aesthetic differences in males versus females. Understanding these anatomic variances will lead to correct treatment dosing and placement of product, and therefore a pleased and loyal patient.

1.6 Pearls

- Gender differences in male facial anatomy include increased skin thickness, higher muscle mass, higher number of terminal hairs as well as sebaceous glands, higher vascularity associated with pilosebaceous units, and different rates of fat and bone resorption with aging given hormonal variations.
- The two main reasons for men to proceed with a cosmetic procedure were to look good for their age and to appear more youthful.

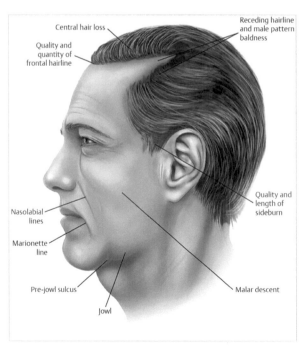

Fig. 1.4 Physical examination of the aesthetic male patient. (Reproduced with permission from Steinbrech S, ed. Male Aesthetic Plastic Surgery. 1st Edition. New York: Thieme; 2020.)

- One of the main barriers to treatment identified by this study was lack of knowledge of what minimally invasive cosmetic procedures entail, including risks, benefits, safety, and side effect profiles.
- Men are less likely to follow up if they are unhappy compared to female counterparts, therefore schedule a short-term (2–4 weeks), follow-up visit at the end of their treatment.

References

[1] ASPS 2018 Annual Survey. Available at: https://www.plasticsurgery.org/documents/News/Statistics/2018/cosmetic-procedures-men-2018.pdf. Accessed October 24, 2019

[2] Leong PL. Aging changes in the male face. Facial Plast Surg Clin North Am. 2008; 16(3):277–279, v

[3] Hage JJ, Becking AG, de Graaf FH, Tuinzing DB. Gender-confirming facial surgery: considerations on the masculinity and femininity of faces. Plast Reconstr Surg. 1997; 99(7):1799–1807

[4] Rudolph C, Hladik C, Hamade H, et al. Structural gender dimorphism and the biomechanics of the gluteal subcutaneous tissue: implications for the pathophysiology of cellulite. Plast Reconstr Surg. 2019; 143(4):1077–1086

[5] Frank K, Gotkin RH, Pavicic T, et al. Age and gender differences of the frontal bone: a computed tomographic (CT)-based study. Aesthet Surg J. 2019; 39(7):699–710

[6] Cotofana S, Gotkin RH, Morozov SP, et al. The relationship between bone remodeling and the clockwise rotation of the facial skeleton: a computed tomographic imaging-based evaluation. Plast Reconstr Surg. 2018; 142(6):1447–1454

[7] Jagdeo J, Keaney T, Narurkar V, Kolodziejczyk J, Gallagher CJ. Facial treatment preferences among aesthetically oriented men. Dermatol Surg. 2016; 42(10):1155–1163

[8] Narurkar V, Shamban A, Sissins P, Stonehouse A, Gallagher C. Facial treatment preferences in aesthetically aware women. Dermatol Surg. 2015; 41 Suppl 1:S153–S160

[9] Rieder EA, Mu EW, Brauer JA. Men and cosmetics: social and psychological trends of an emerging demographic. J Drugs Dermatol. 2015; 14(9):1023–1026

[10] Dayan SH, Arkins JP, Patel AB, Gal TJ. A double-blind, randomized, placebo-controlled health-outcomes survey of the effect of botulinum toxin type a injections on quality of life and self-esteem. Dermatol Surg. 2010; 36 Suppl 4:2088–2097

[11] Carruthers A, Carruthers J. Prospective, double-blind, randomized, parallel-group, dose-ranging study of botulinum toxin type A in men with glabellar rhytids. Dermatol Surg. 2005; 31(10):1297–1303

2 Tincture of Time: Facial Aging and Anatomical Considerations

Jose Raúl Montes and Jonathan J. Dutton

Summary

Genetic aging and photoaging result in thinning of all layers, effacement of the dermal-epidermal junction, loss of collagen, disorganization of elastin fibers, clumping of melanocytes, and advancing dermal elastosis. This process driven by extrinsic and intrinsic factors occurs equally across genders, male and female, however it has been published that extrinsic factors such as sun exposure and tobacco usage are more associated with male behavior. Therefore, the skin aging changes are expected to be accelerated in the male patient population sooner than in females.

The face and scalp are arranged in six concentric tissue which are thicker and heavier in men, accounting for more gravitational pull with aging and consequential tissue descend, which translates into lowering eyebrows with aging, more pronounced than in females. Furthermore, the forehead is greater in height and width, and the supraorbital rims form a more prominent ridge in men than in women. In men, temples are expected to be flat or slightly convex in contrast to their woman counterpart where temples are flat or slightly concave. The midface region in the male patient is characterized by a nose with a more straight and wider dorsum. In general, the female cheek fuller with a higher point light reflection (or projection) laterally. Men's cheeks are usually flatter and present with a wider bizygomatic distance. On this chapter anatomic male features will be discussed as a guiding compass for surgical and non-surgical cosmetic treatment planning in the male patient.

Keywords: anatomy of aging, male anatomy, male and female anatomic differences, male aesthetic procedures, approachs to facial aging

2.1 Background

The number of aesthetic procedures performed in the United States has significantly increased over the past several decades. Between 1997 and 2016, there was a 99.2% increase in the number of cosmetic surgical procedures performed annually in the United States, and a massive 650.2% increase in nonsurgical procedures.[1] In 2014, Americans spent more than $12 billion on combined surgical and nonsurgical cosmetic procedures, of which eyelid surgery, nose surgery, botulinum toxin, fillers, and chemical peels ranked among the top procedures performed. More than 40% of all cosmetic procedures were performed on individuals between the ages of 35 and 50 years. Almost 70% of adults in the United States are currently considering a cosmetic procedure.[2] While 90% of cosmetic procedures are performed in females, interest among males continues to increase. Between 1997 and 2014, there was a 273% increase in the number of cosmetic procedures performed on men, with botulinum neurotoxin and dermal fillers being the most common. This compares to a 429% increase for females during the same period.

Facial aging is a multifactorial process and results in a broad range of physiologic and morphologic changes affecting every tissue system, including bones, ligaments, muscles, fascia, deep and subcutaneous fat, and skin. The process of aging is the same for everyone, although the age of onset and the rate of aging changes vary considerably between different individuals, genders, ethnic groups, and among various lifestyles. Age-related changes of the facial skeleton underlie alterations in the soft tissues that are suspended from it, and are recognized as key elements in the aging process.[3,4,5,6]

Men age differently than women largely because of differences in genetic and hormonal characteristics, facial anatomy, environmental exposure, and behavior. In a survey of 600 aesthetically oriented men, facial areas of primary concern were facial and forehead wrinkles, baggy eyelids, tear troughs, sagging skin, and hair loss reflecting the importance of the upper face in social interaction.[7] Considering the growing number of men seeking surgical, and especially noninvasive cosmetic, procedures each year, the aesthetic provider must become comfortable with the facial anatomy of men, and the most important aspects of facial aging. Although the procedures performed in men and women are similar, anatomical details may vary, as do aesthetic objectives of men.[8]

2.2 Male Facial Anatomy and Aging Changes

2.2.1 Aging and Gender

Numerous soft-tissue changes gradually evolve during the aging process in the face. Both intrinsic and extrinsic factors contribute to skin aging. Smoking and ultraviolet (UV) radiation are the most important extrinsic risk factors for aging skin and for the formation of coarse wrinkles.[9,10,11,12] Smoking reduces capillary blood flow, decreasing collagen and elastin fibers in the dermis and impairing elasticity. UV exposure leads to accelerated degradation of dermal collagen matrix. In general, men develop more wrinkles earlier in life than women. Although these have sometimes been attributed to higher occupational sun exposure in men, the difference remains significant even after adjusting the wrinkling for occupational sun exposure.[13] Other extrinsic

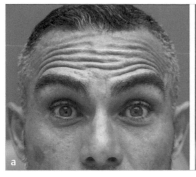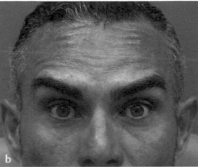

Fig. 2.1 A male patient with deep frontal ridges and wrinkles before and after neuromodulator treatment (45 units total on glabella, lateral orbicularis oculi, and frontalis muscle). **(a)** Before. **(b)** After.

factors include gravity, which acts on facial soft tissues, as well as other environmental insults, such as pollutants (e.g., heavy metals), and pesticides. Personal habits, such as diet and lack of sleep, also contribute to the onset and degree of aging changes.

Age and genetic background are the major intrinsic factors related to facial aging and the formation of fine wrinkles. Men tend to show aging phenomena more than women because of reduced innate antioxidant capacity, and increased levels of oxidative stress.[14] Men are more likely to participate in behavior such as smoking, alcohol use, and UV exposure, which accelerate the aging process.[15] The facial skeleton is larger in men and facial muscles have increased mass, which contribute to contraction-induced static wrinkles over time. Under the influence of these intrinsic and extrinsic factors, all of the facial skin undergoes major changes with age that progress at variable rates for each individual. Genetic aging and photoaging result in thinning of all layers, effacement of the dermal–epidermal junction, loss of collagen, disorganization of elastin fibers, clumping of melanocytes, and advancing dermal elastosis.[16] This results in loss of dermal understructure with the development of ridges and wrinkles, uneven pigmentation, loss of elasticity, and stretching of small blood vessels with areas of patchy redness (▶ Fig. 2.1).

2.2.2 Forehead and Temple

The face and scalp are arranged in six concentric tissue layers that consist of skin, subcutaneous tissue, superficial musculoaponeurotic layer, loose areolar tissue, deep fascia and periosteum, and bone.[17] Except for thickness, the skin and subcutaneous layers are basically the same over the entire face and scalp. The musculoaponeurotic fascial layer is attached above to the skin and subcutaneous layers by fine connective tissue bands called *retinacula cutis* fibers. Over the scalp and forehead, the musculoaponeurotic layer is formed by galea aponeurotica and its two muscular components, the occipitalis muscle posteriorly and frontalis muscle anteriorly. Here, the skin, subcutaneous layer, and galea form a single functional unit that

is mobile over an underlying loose avascular areolar tissue layer.

These six tissue layers are thicker and heavier in men, accounting for more gravitational pull with aging and consequential tissue descend, which translates into lowering eyebrows with aging, more pronounced than in females. In the skull, however, older females have thicker bone thickness as compared to males.

The **eyebrows** are part of the **forehead** and scalp anatomy, and their mobility is part of the complex system of facial expression. They are situated over the superior bony orbital rims, at the junction between the upper eyelid and the forehead. The brows extend from just above the trochlear fossa medially, near the frontozygomatic suture line laterally. The flattened glabellar region is central in the midline and separates the two eyebrows. Above the brows, the forehead is covered by skin that becomes thinner closer to the top of the head and thicker closer to the eyebrows. The eyebrow is separated from the superior orbital rim by a prominent underlying fat pad. The skin in this region contains short, course eyebrow hairs that emerge at an oblique angle. Medially these hairs may be directed slightly upward, but they are usually directed more horizontally or slightly downward and laterally in the central and lateral brow. These variable orientations are important to consider during direct brow elevations with resection of skin immediately above the brow line, because cutting the hair follicles will result in loss of cilia and exposure of the scar line.

The **eyebrow** is capable of a wide range of vertical movement. These movements are accomplished by the interaction of five striated muscles that insert into the dermal tissues along the brow. These are the frontalis, procerus, depressor supercilii, corrugator supercilii, and orbicularis oculi muscles.[18] All are innervated by the seventh cranial, or facial, nerve. The frontalis muscle fibers are oriented vertically on the forehead and form the anterior belly of the occipitofrontalis musculofascial complex. The galea aponeurotica covers and invests the frontalis and occipitalis muscles on either end, and carries a rich supply of blood vessels and nerves. The galea is attached to the overlying skin by a firm dense adipose layer, and is separated from the underlying cranial periosteum by a loose areolar fascial space that allows for mobility of the scalp. At 8 to 10 cm above the superior orbital rim, the galea splits into superficial and deep layers that extend anteriorly and surround the forehead muscles. The deep layer of the galea extends below the frontalis muscle and fuses to periosteum 8 to 10 mm above the superior orbital rim. The superficial layer continues downward over the anterior surface of the frontalis muscle to the orbital rim, where it inserts onto a fusion line, the arcus marginalis, around the margin of the orbital rim. From the arcus marginalis, the anterior galea continues downward into the upper eyelid, where it continues as the anterior layer of the orbital septum.

This explains the contribution of the frontalis muscle, not only on eyebrow position but also on the eyelid height. On patients with low borderline eyelid position or documented eyelid ptosis, avoid neurotoxin forehead injections or be very conservative, because an underlying eyelid droop clinically insignificant will be dramatically revealed.

The frontalis muscle is paired and has no bony attachments. Its proximal fibers originate from the galea aponeurotica at about the level of the coronal suture line and extend toward the supraorbital rim (▶ Fig. 2.2).

Frontalis muscle fibers interdigitate with the corrugator and the orbital portion of the orbicularis muscles.[19] The medial fibers blend with those of the procerus and depressor supercilii muscles. The frontalis muscle does not extend beyond the junction of the middle and lateral thirds of the brow, so that the lateral brow lacks an elevator. Because of this relationship, the lateral brow is under the depressor influence of the lateral portion of the orbicularis muscle.

Owing to the lack of frontalis action, lateral eyebrow or eyebrow tail tends to descend with aging. Neurotoxin injection on the lateral orbicularis is indicated to elevate the lateral eyebrow.

The superficial fascia over the forehead and brows is relatively thin. The skin is closely applied to the superficial layer of the galea over the frontalis muscle by fibrous septa that extend through the galea and superficial fat to the dermis. On its deep surface, the frontalis muscle is separated from the underlying periosteum by a fat layer within the deep fascia of the forehead. This has been referred to as the sub-brow fat pad or the superior retro-orbicularis oculi fat, or ROOF.[20] This fat pad measures approximately 1 cm vertically and is about 5 mm in thickness, and helps cushion the brow during movement over the supraorbital bony rim. This sub-brow fat pad may get deflated with aging and is one of the target zones at the periocular area for injectable implants. The frontalis muscle elevates the brow and, together with the posterior occipitalis belly, tightens the scalp providing mobility of the skin along the temples (▶ Fig. 2.3 and ▶ Video 2.1).

Forehead and brow ptosis is a prominent feature of the aging face.[21,22,23] As brow ptosis progresses, dermatochalasis of the upper eyelids may become more pronounced. When a patient is evaluated for blepharoplasty, it is important to evaluate whether the dermatochalasis is the result of redundant upper eyelid skin, or a manifestation of downwardly displaced forehead skin, or both. Failure to recognize the etiology of this deformity may result in failure to correct the responsible anatomic defect (▶ Fig. 2.4).

In selected cases, neurotoxin injection, specifically at the glabellar brow depressor muscles and the lateral orbicularis, may result in eyebrow elevation that may correct a "pseudo dermatochalasis".

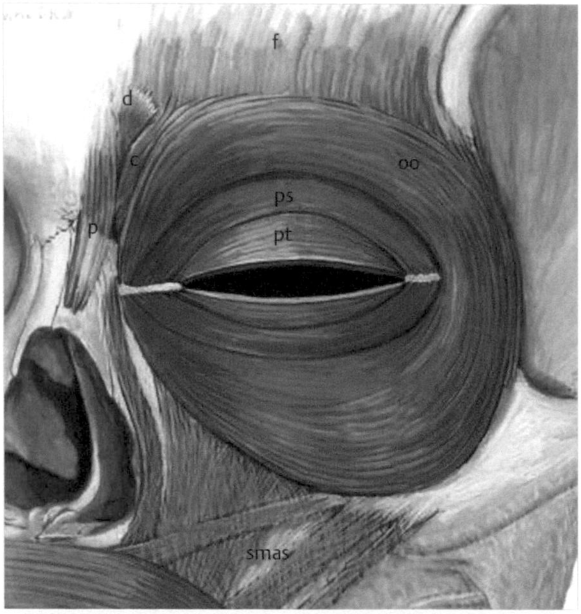

Fig. 2.2 Forehead muscles (c, corrugator; ds, depressor supercilii; f, frontalis; oo, orbicularis oculi; p, procerus; smas, musculoaponeurotic system superficial; ps, preseptal; pt, pretarsal).

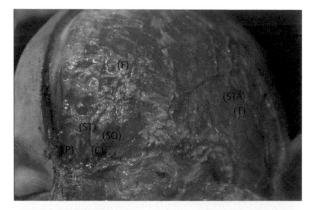

Fig. 2.3 The procerus and corrugator muscles with supraorbital and supratrochlear arteries.

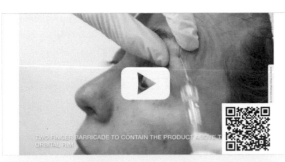

Video 2.1 Roof Injection.

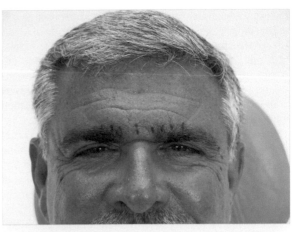

Fig. 2.4 An aging male face with horizontal forehead furrows, and horizontal and vertical glabellar creases.

Three anatomic findings that may help you predict an effective brow elevation with neurotoxin:

- Patients with thin skin on forehead/eyebrow, usually women.
- Patients with preexisting tarsal plate show.
- Patients with strong lateral orbicularis action (crow's feet).

The **procerus** is a small pyramidal muscle closely related to the frontalis muscle complex. It arises by tendinous fibers from periosteum on the lower portion of the nasal bone. The muscle passes vertically upward between the brows and separates into its paired heads, which interdigitate with the medial borders of the frontalis muscle on either side and insert onto the dermis of the skin over the lower central forehead (▶ Fig. 2.2). Contraction of the procerus muscle draws the medial portion of the brow downward and produces transverse wrinkles over the glabella and the nasal bridge. The depressor supercilii muscle was previously believed to be part of the orbicularis muscle, but it is now considered a separate structure.[24] It arises from the frontal process of the maxillary bone as two distinct heads, runs superiorly deep to the lateral edge of the procerus, and inserts into the dermis of the medial brow (▶ Fig. 2.2).

Patients with a strong nasalis muscle contraction or "bunny lines" usually have strong depressor supercilii recruitment as well. On these patients, extend your glabellar neurotoxin pattern of injections to include these muscles.

The **corrugator supercilii** muscle forms a pyramidal band of fibers beneath the medial fibers of the frontalis and orbicularis muscles (▶ Fig. 2.2). It arises from the medial end of the frontal bone at the superomedial orbital rim and divides into two separate heads. The oblique head runs superiorly and slightly laterally and interdigitates through the frontalis and orbicularis muscles to insert into dermis along the medial eyebrow. This head, along with the depressor supercilii, the procerus, and the medial slip of the orbital portion of the orbicularis muscle, acts to depress the medial brow.[25] The larger transverse head of the corrugator muscle passes laterally and slightly superiorly beneath the orbital portion of the orbicularis muscle within the galeal fat pad and inserts

into the deep fascia of the frontalis and orbicularis muscles along the central one-third of the brow. Contraction of the corrugator muscle pulls the brow medially and downward, and produces vertical glabellar folds.

In gross shape, the forehead is greater in height and width, and the supraorbital rims form a more prominent ridge in men than in women.[26] The medial supraorbital ridges in men blend into the central glabella, so that the glabellar region is more prominent than in women.[27] Although the orbit is absolutely larger and more rounded in men, the male orbit is proportionally smaller in relation to the overall size of the skull.[28] The eyebrow is flatter in contour and sits lower along the orbital rim.[29] Men with deep-set eyes and more prominent supraorbital rim may exhibit a slightly lower brow position (▶ Fig. 2.4).[30]

Stronger and bigger muscles at glabella in men required more units of neurotoxin.[31] Low-set eyebrows in men required careful assessment of frontalis muscle action before neuromodulator injection to prevent potential eyebrow droopiness. In the heavy low-set male patient, consider neurotoxin injection at the glabella and the lateral orbicularis; avoid forehead injections (▶ Fig. 2.4).

The **temple** refers to the anatomic area of the temporal fossa. The borders are the superior temporal line superiorly, the frontal process of the zygoma anteriorly, the zygomatic process of the temporal bone and zygoma inferiorly, and the temporal hairline and the ear posteriorly.[32] The temporal fossa contains the temporalis muscle, which originates from the superior temporal fusion line and inserts inferiorly on the coronoid process of the mandible. The surface of the temporalis muscle is covered by a dense fibrous layer, the deep temporal fascia that contains a temporal fat pad inferiorly. Superficial to the deep temporal fascia is a loose areolar layer, the temporoparietal or superficial temporal fascia. The superficial temporal artery runs superiorly, and the temporal branches of the facial nerve course diagonally through this facial layer. These are important structures to be avoided in temporal forehead lift procedures and during temporal zone filler placement since it is recognized as one of the "danger zones."

Forehead, temples, glabella eyelid, nose, mid face, nasolabial fold are facial "danger zones" because they are connected to the very complex orbital circulation. Accidental intra-arterial filler injection may produce a retrograde embolization reaching to the orbital and retinal circulation with catastrophic outcomes such as blindness[33] (▶ Fig. 2.5).

It is well recognized that bone remodeling occurs throughout life, with a gradual additive projection of bone in the forehead by thickening of the frontal bone.[34,35] The upper forehead also shows some regression due to loss of calvarial height and volume with increasing age.[36] Temporal hollowing is a prominent feature of the aging face, often attributed to atrophy of the temporal fat pad. However, more recent studies suggest that redistribution of fat inferiorly rather than atrophy is more likely responsible for the relative superior hollowing in this region.[37]

In men, supraorbital or frontal bossing is common with an increased concavity at central forehead with aging; consider a combination of neurotoxin and filler injections in selected cases to improve the appearance of deep rhytids without lowering the "heavy" brow complex (▶ Fig. 2.6 and ▶ Video 2.2).

The "young" women temples are usually flat; with aging, they may become dramatically concaved. In men, temples are expected to be flat or slightly convex. For filler injection to temple, there are two schools of thought:

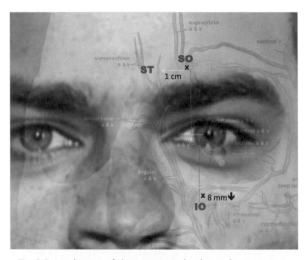

Fig. 2.5 Localization of the main periorbital vascular structures. Note: The best way to locate the main vessels around the eye is to use your patient's pupil as your guiding compass. For instance, to find the foramen (or cleft where the bundle of supraorbital nerves and vessels emerges), use the iris' medial limbus and the orbit's superior margin. The neurovascular structures of the infraorbital foramen are aligned between the iris' medial limbus and the pupil at approximately 8 mm to 1 cm from the lower orbital rim. Remember that the supratrochlear artery is located approximately 1 cm medial to the supraorbital artery. All these structures emerge from deep within these foramina.

superficial/subcutaneous injection or deep supraperiosteal injection. In our opinion, deep injection over bone is safer (▶ Fig. 2.7 and ▶ Video 2.3).

2.2.3 Eyelids and Periorbital Region

In the young adult, the interpalpebral fissure measures 10 to 11 mm in vertical height, but with advancing years the upper eyelid assumes a more ptotic position, resulting in a fissure of only about 8 to 9 mm (▶ Fig. 2.8). The horizontal length of the fissure is 30 to 31 mm by the age of about 15 years. The upper and lower eyelids meet medially and laterally at an angle of approximately 60 degrees. The interpalpebral fissure is usually inclined slightly upward at its lateral end, such that the lateral canthal angle generally is about 2 to 3 mm higher than the medial canthal angle. In the primary position of gaze, the upper eyelid margin usually lies at the superior corneal limbus in children and 1.5 to 2.0 mm below it in the adult. The upper eyelid marginal contour usually reaches its highest point just nasal to the pupil, and the lower eyelid margin rests at the inferior corneal limbus. These anatomic landmarks are similar in both men and women.

Patients with upper eyelids that rest close to their pupils, at less than 3 mm of a light reflex to the pupil, may have an underlying eyelid droop that can be aggravated by neurotoxin treatment to the forehead complex. Likewise, if lower eyelid margin is resting lower to the inferior corneal limbus, with scleral show, neurotoxin injections at the pretarsal orbicularis or the lower eyelid should be avoided, since they will only accentuate an "undesired" lid retraction or descend.

The orbicularis oculi is a periocular striated muscle sheet that lies just below the skin. It is divided anatomically into three arbitrary segments: the orbital, preseptal, and pretarsal portions in the upper and lower eyelids (▶ Fig. 2.9). The orbital portion overlies the bony orbital rims. It arises from insertions on the frontal process of the maxillary bone, the orbital process of the frontal bone, and from the common medial canthal ligament. The fibers pass around the orbital rim to form a continuous circle, and insert medially just below their points of origin. The palpebral portion of the orbicularis muscle overlies the mobile eyelid from the orbital rims to the eyelid margins. Although this portion forms a single anatomic unit in each eyelid, it is customarily further divided topographically into two parts, the preseptal and pretarsal orbicularis.

The preseptal part is positioned over the orbital septum in both upper and lower eyelids, and the pretarsal part overlies the tarsal plates. The postorbicular fascial plane is an avascular loose areolar layer between the orbicularis muscle and the orbital septum–levator aponeurosis fascial complex. This plane is an important surgical reference that allows easy and bloodless dissection and identification of the underlying orbital septum. The orbital septum is a fibrous, multilayered membrane that

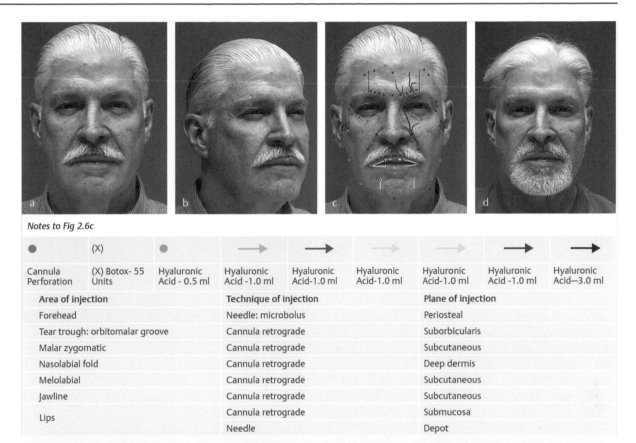

Notes to Fig 2.6c

●	(X)	●	→	→	→	→	→	→	→
Cannula Perforation	(X) Botox- 55 Units	Hyaluronic Acid - 0.5 ml	Hyaluronic Acid -1.0 ml	Hyaluronic Acid-1.0 ml	Hyaluronic Acid-1.0 ml	Hyaluronic Acid-1.0 ml	Hyaluronic Acid-1.0 ml	Hyaluronic Acid -1.0 ml	Hyaluronic Acid—3.0 ml

Area of injection	Technique of injection	Plane of injection
Forehead	Needle: microbolus	Periosteal
Tear trough: orbitomalar groove	Cannula retrograde	Suborbicularis
Malar zygomatic	Cannula retrograde	Subcutaneous
Nasolabial fold	Cannula retrograde	Deep dermis
Melolabial	Cannula retrograde	Subcutaneous
Jawline	Cannula retrograde	Subcutaneous
Lips	Cannula retrograde	Submucosa
	Needle	Depot

Fig. 2.6 A 61-year-old patient with exemplary men's features: low set eyebrows, frontal bossing, prominent chin, and squared jawline. (a) Before (front). (b) Before (right side). (c) Marking for injection. (d) After.

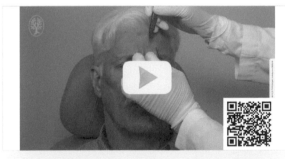

Video 2.2 Mid forehead injection in combination with neurotoxin; lip augmentation with cannula; injection jawline with cannula.

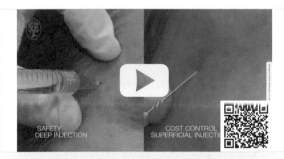

Video 2.3 Temporal fossa injection, deep needle injection technique.

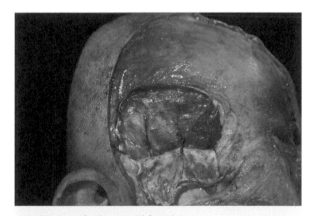

Fig. 2.7 Superficial temporal fascial.

begins anatomically at the arcus marginalis along the orbital rim (▸ Fig. 2.10).

The multilayered structure of the orbital septum is easily noted in most individuals during eyelid surgery and provides a critical landmark that separates the anterior from the posterior eyelid lamellae. Immediately behind the orbital septum are the yellowish preaponeurotic fat pockets. These are anterior extensions of extraconal or peripheral orbital fat (▸ Fig. 2.11). There are two pockets in the upper eyelid, medial and central, and three in the

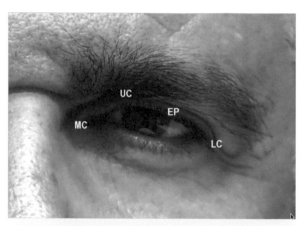

Fig. 2.8 External eyelid and the periorbital region (EP, eyelid platform; LC, lateral canthal angle; MC, medial canthal angle; UC, upper eyelid crease).

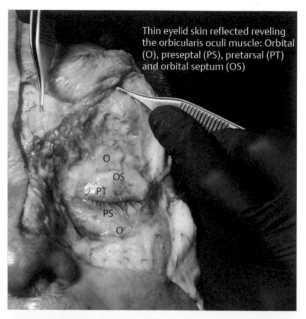

Fig. 2.9 Orbicularis oculi muscle.

lower eyelid, medial, central, and lateral. These fat pockets are surgically important landmarks that help identify a plane immediately anterior to the major eyelid retractors, the levator aponeurosis in the upper eyelid and the capsulopalpebral fascia in the lower eyelid.

With aging, upper eyelid fat pads experience changes. The medial fat pad tends to grow and the central fat pad gets atrophic.[38] These fat pad volume changes make the upper eyelid look deflated or sunken centrally, more prominently in women due to thinner upper eyelid skin. A low-concentration hyaluronic acid filler placement below the orbicularis muscle may correct this involutional change (▶ Video 2.4).

The major eyelid retractor of the upper eyelid is the levator palpebrae superioris muscle. It arises deep in the orbit from the lesser sphenoid wing and passes forward along the superior orbit. At the orbital rim, the fibrous sheath surrounding the muscle thickens to form a horizontal condensation that extends horizontally across the superior orbit attached medially and laterally to the orbital fascia and bones. This is the superior transverse orbital ligament of Whitnall that contributes support for anterior orbital fascial suspensory systems that maintain spatial relationships between a variety of anatomic structures in the superior orbit and the upper eyelid (▶ Fig. 2.11). It appears to function as a hammock sling supporting the levator aponeurosis, where it changes the vector from horizontal to vertical. It may also serve as a check ligament against excessive posterior excursion of the levator muscle.

From Whitnall's ligament, the levator aponeurosis continues downward 14 to 20 mm to its insertions. Contrary to previous teaching, only a small percentage of the terminal fibers of the aponeurosis inserts directly onto the tarsus. Most aponeurotic fibers insert into the pretarsal fascia and onto the interfascicular septa of the pretarsal orbicularis muscle. Some fibers continue through the muscle to fuse with fibers of the subcutaneous fascia. These multilayered

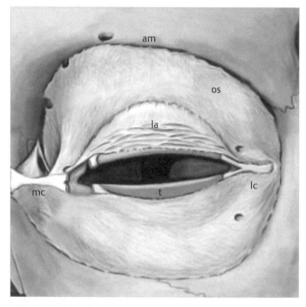

Fig. 2.10 Orbital septum (am, arcus marginalis; la, levator aponeurosis; lc, lateral canthal ligament; mc, medial canthal ligament; t, tarsus; os, orbital septum).

slips maintain a close approximation of the skin, muscle, aponeurosis, and tarsal lamellae in the marginal portion of the eyelids, contributing to the formation of the marginal eyelid platform that is aesthetically important in the Caucasian eyelid. Men tend to have a smaller tarsal plate than women, and this finding is consistent with aging.

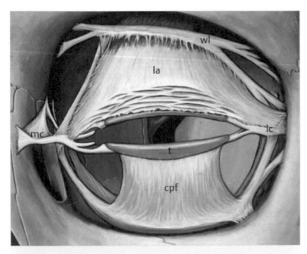

Fig. 2.11 Superior eyelid suspensory apparatus (cpf, capsulo-palpebral fascia; la, levator aponeurosis; lc, lateral canthal ligament; mc, medial canthal ligament; t, tarsal plate; wl, Whitnall's ligament).

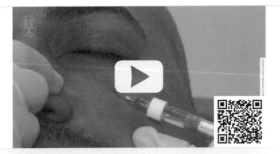

Video 2.4 Tear through orbito malar grove correction with hyaluronic and cannula techniques.

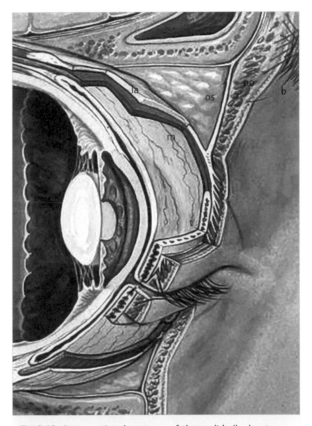

Fig. 2.12 Cross-sectional anatomy of the eyelids (la, levator aponeurosis; mm, Müller sympathetic muscle; oo, orbicularis oculi muscle; os, orbital septum; t, tarsal plate with meibomian glands).

Smooth muscle fibers innervated by the sympathetic nervous system are present in both upper and lower eyelids. In the upper eyelid, the supratarsal muscle of Müller originates from the undersurface of the levator muscle just anterior to Whitnall's ligament. It runs downward, posterior to the levator aponeurosis, to which it is loosely adherent. Müller's muscle inserts onto the anterior edge of the superior tarsal border via a zone of dense connective tissue. In the lower eyelid, smooth muscle fibers are present along the posterior surface of the capsulopalpebral fascia, a short distance distal to Lockwood's ligament. The tarsal plates provide the firm structural integrity of the upper and lower eyelid margins (▶ Fig. 2.12).

Tarsal plates consist of dense fibrous tissue approximately 1.0 to 1.5 mm thick. The central vertical height of the tarsal plate is 12 mm in the upper eyelid, and 3.5 to 5.0 mm in the lower eyelid. Within each tarsus are the sebaceous meibomian glands, approximately 25 in the upper lid and 20 in the lower lid. Medially and laterally, the tarsal plates pass into fibrous bands that form the medial and lateral canthal ligaments. These lie between the orbicularis muscle anteriorly and the conjunctiva posteriorly. The medial canthal ligament divides into a complex pattern of anterior, superior, and posterior crura that surround the lacrimal sac and insert onto crests of the maxillary and lacrimal bones. Laterally, the tarsal plates pass into less well-developed fibrous strands that form the lateral canthal ligament that inserts onto the periosteum just inside the lateral orbital rim.

The lateral canthal position may descend with aging irrespective of gender. In man who are obese and have sleep apnea, the fibrous tissues of the tarsal plates get progressively stretched with a conundrum of signs and symptoms known as floppy eyelid syndrome. These patients require surgical intervention to correct eyelid malposition due to excessive tissue laxity.[39] The lower eyelid becomes lax and droops downward, especially laterally, and can be significantly more severe in older men.[40,41] The orbital septum becomes lax allowing herniation of the anteroinferior orbital fat above the orbitomalar ligament, resulting in bulging lower lids commonly seen in the aging male face. Infraorbital hollowing is a related phenomenon seen along the eyelid–cheek interface, exacerbated by downward descent of the malar fat compartments.

Entropion and ectropion are among the most common acquired lower eyelid malpositions associated with aging. Resorption of the inferolateral bony orbital rim and laxity of the orbicularis retaining ligaments cause drooping of the lateral lower eyelid and downward displacement of the lateral canthal angle.[8]

The male "negative vector patient" who presents with poor anterior maxillary projection may show early signs of lower eyelid malposition (like ectropion) and orbital fat prolapse, creating an abrupt transition between the inferior orbit and midface (▶ Fig. 2.13 and ▶ Video 2.4). The midface concavity of the "negative vector" patient demands convexity; our filler landing platforms for the "negative vector patient" are the bony tear trough and the maxillary face lateral to the infraorbital artery. A buttress will be created by injecting at these two sites.

One of the areas of main concern for the aesthetically oriented male patient is the eye region, specifically the under-eye depression. For the negative vector patient, consider two-pronged approaches: infraorbital injections and concomitant maxillary filler injection (▶ **Video 2.5**).

2.2.4 Midface Anatomy and Aging

The male dorsal nose is wider and straighter compared with females, where it is relatively narrower and laterally concave.[42]

The male dorsal nose is expected to be straight and wider than in females. Be very careful on patients who have had previous nasal surgery since anatomy may be disturbed and injection safety may be more challenging (▶ **Video 2.6**).

The male cheek has more fullness, a broader based malar prominence, and an apex that is more medial and subtly defined.[43] The frontal and zygomatic processes are wider in males, creating a flatter appearance.[44] The skin of the midface is structurally and histologically similar to other areas of the face, but the thickness of the epidermis and dermis is greater than on the eyelids, and similar to that of the forehead.[45] As in other skin areas of the face,

aging changes occur both from intrinsic genetic mechanisms and from environmental exposure, primarily UV light. Smoking may have a deleterious effect by disrupting its microvasculature with loss of collagen and elastin, replacement of ground substance by fibrous tissue, and decrease in the rate of cell renewal. Dry skin results from loss of sebaceous glands, and hyperpigmentation occurs from increased melanin.

In the midface, the superficial musculoaponeurotic system (SMAS) is a part of the subcutaneous fascia of the head and neck. It is continuous superiorly with the galea aponeurotica over the forehead, and laterally with the temporoparietal or superficial temporal fascia over the temporal fossae. Inferiorly, the SMAS is continuous with the platysma of the neck and lower face. The SMAS invests the muscles of facial expression, and separates the subcutaneous fat into superficial and deep layers. Fibrous septa extend from the SMAS, through the superficial fat layer, to the overlying dermis. Motor nerves to the facial muscles lie just inferior to the SMAS.

Midface subcutaneous fat deposits influence the mechanical properties of the overlying skin. Progressive changes in these fat compartments are considered to be major factors contributing to facial aging. Facial fat is broadly divided into superficial and deep layers, above and below the SMAS, and these are further subdivided into distinct fat compartments, separated by fascial ligaments, septa, and muscles.[46] The various fat compartments differ in types of fat depending upon adipose cell size, collagenous composition of their extracellular matrix, and mechanical characteristics.[47] They also vary in physiological properties that differ from fat elsewhere in the body, such as the abdomen, and even differ from one localized compartment to another in the face.[48] These differences result in disparate aging changes in various parts of the face. The result is structural instability and wrinkles in the overlying skin, as well as fat atrophy or redistribution that manifests as general midfacial volume deflation, loss of volume in the temple, periorbital, and chin regions, and relative fat volume increase in the jowls and lateral nasolabial folds. Men show a greater loss of facial volume than females.[49] The downward force of gravity and loss of elasticity from photoaging result in

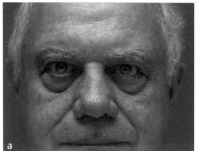 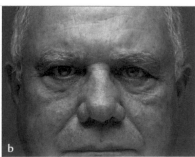

Fig. 2.13 Negative vector patient before and after treatment of injectable biostimulant agent, poly-L-lactic acid (PLLA; Sculptra) at the junction of the maxilla and the infraorbital orbitomalar ligaments. **(a)** Before. **(b)** After poly-L-lactic acid.

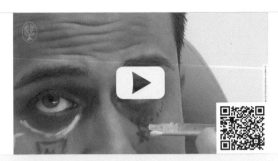

Video 2.5 Negative vector patient.

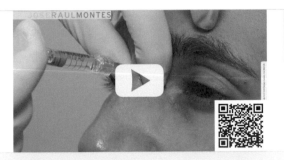

Video 2.6 Dorsal nose injection.

drooping of facial soft tissues, downward redistribution of facial fat compartments, and age-related changes in the overlying skin. Males have greater facial muscle mass and larger facial movements.[50] These result in a higher degree and wider distribution of midfacial wrinkles, and these tend to appear at an earlier age.[51] Men also have less subcutaneous fat, accentuating the appearance of deep wrinkles in aged males.[52]

Craniofacial growth was thought to end in early adulthood except for minor degenerative changes. The concept that the facial skeleton was in a state of continual change was introduced by Humphrey[53] in 1858, and later elaborated upon by Enlow,[54] who developed the idea of growth fields. According to this concept, the frontonasal bones lay down new bone in the upper face and drift forward, whereas the midfacial skeleton resorbs and shows gradual posterior drift.[34,55] This theoretical model postulated that the facial skeleton, as viewed from the right, shows a gradual rotation around the orbit, such that the forehead rotates anteriorly and slightly inferiorly, whereas the midface rotates posteriorly and slightly superiorly.[34,35,56,57,58]

It was also shown that the orbital aperture increased in diameter in the superomedial and inferolateral directions along with a flattening of the glabellar–maxillary angle.[59] These changes in the facial skeleton with aging cause the maxillary, pyriform, and glabellar angles to become more acute, with significant effects on the draping of overhanging soft tissues. This regression of bony projection affects the suspensory understructure of all facial soft tissues, and contributes to some of the common midface aging changes, including volume deflation, sagging, development of prominent folds over retaining ligaments, and loss of dentition.[60]

Bony retrusion and soft-tissue atrophy or redistribution along midface occur in men and women. However, the connection of these involutional changes requires an individual and tailored approach that preserves gender differences. In general, women demand a fuller cheek and higher point of light reflection (▶ Fig. 2.14), whereas men require softening of the under eye depression to midface, or support at the submalar and anteromalar maxillary platforms.

2.2.5 Jawline and Lower Face

The male face is usually square and with more jagged contours, especially on the lower face, and male attractiveness is usually defined by a strong jawline and more anteriorly projected chin complex. "Female attractiveness" lies in the cheekbones and for men, it lies in the chin.[15] Men have a larger mouth with thinner lips, especially the upper lip.[61] As observed in women, men's lips become thinner during the aging process. Despite the aging changes, lip reshaping is not a common procedure requested by men. Examination of old photographs is a powerful tool when evaluating the male or female patient and counseling them about the involutional changes of the perioral area (▶ **Video 2.2**).

A common misconception about cosmetic facial shaping with injectables is that it is only about adding volume. However, the possibility of reduction plays a role especially on the lower face. Contrary to men, in women, masseteric hypertrophy may be an "undesired" feature since this conveys masculinization to the lower face. This can be improved with neurotoxin treatment (▶ Fig. 2.15).

Another area where reduction plays a role is the under-chin bulge or submental fullness. Upon the approval of Kybella, deoxycholic acid for submental fat reduction, by the Food and Drug Administration (FDA), many cosmetic practices experienced an increase in the number of male patients looking for a nonsurgical solution to double chin.

When planning treatment on the lower face in men, the goals are to improve jawline definition, whereas for women it is more about jowl reduction and jawline definition. Facial shaping with injectables requires a comprehensive approach including all facial zones and combination of products. The possibility of reductions plays a role especially on the lower face (▶ Fig. 2.16 and (▶ **Video 2.7**). One

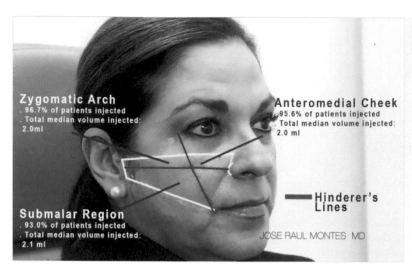

Fig. 2.14 Hinder's line. Point of light reflection is above the lines of intersection.

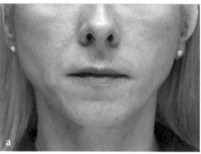 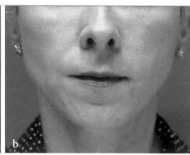

Fig. 2.15 Female masseteric hypertrophy. (a) Before and (b) after neurotoxin treatment.

of the areas of highest concern for men is the under-chin fullness.[62]

2.2.6 Hairline and Male Pattern Hair Loss

Hair loss is a common condition that will impact men and women at some point in their lives. The most common cause of alopecia in men is male pattern hair loss.[63] Studies suggest that by the age of 35 years 66% of American men will experience some degree of appreciable hair loss.[64] Male pattern hair loss is a very common problem that increases with age. Current treatment options are discussed and compared in ▶ Table 2.1. Options include minoxidil, 5-alpha-reductase inhibitors, follicular cells implantation, hair transplantation, platelet-rich plasma, low-level light therapy, and nutritional supplementation (▶ Fig. 2.17). This will be addressed in greater detail in Chapter 5.

2.3 Conclusion

Men's preference in nonsurgical aesthetic procedures is similar to women ranking neurotoxin first and injectable implants second. In terms of surgical procedures, eyelid surgery is among the most sought-after treatments for both men and women. This explains the importance of the periocular zone as a focus for facial rejuvenation.

There are significant anatomical differences between men and women, and clinical implications:

- Men have thicker skin and increased muscle mass and strength. This has an impact on neurotoxin treatments requiring higher doses.
- Involutional changes in the male lower eyelid may require surgical correction and concomitant midface support with injectables to compensate for maxillary retrusion and lack of orbital support. Midface injectable implants in men are more commonly needed at the anteromalar or submalar face of the maxilla, whereas in woman the injections are more commonly placed at the superolateral malar zone to create a "higher point of light reflection."
- On the lower face, for women, it is about lips and the perioral area. For men, it is about jawline definition and chin projection.
- Reduction plays a role in facial shaping with injectables. For women, neurotoxin injections are effective to reduce masseteric hypertrophy, and deoxycholic acid (Kybella)

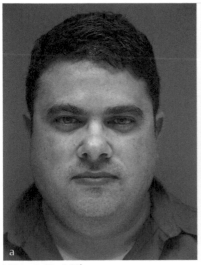 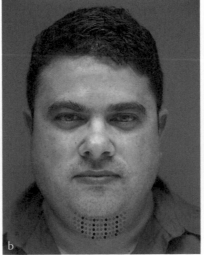 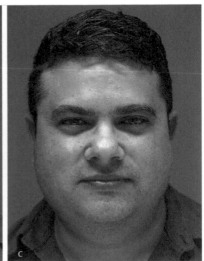

Notes to Fig. 2.16b

● ● ● Deoxycholic acid injection: 6.0 mL

Area of injection	Technique of injection	Plane of injection
Double chin	Needle	Subdermal preplatysma

Fig. 2.16 A patient with severe submental fat. Treated with three vials (6 mL total) of deoxycholic acid (Kybella) on first session. **(a)** Before. **(b)** Marks Injection. **(c)** After.

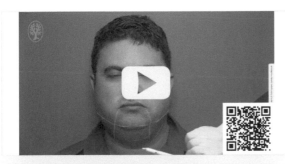

Video 2.7 Submental fat injection with Kybella.

is effective for double chin or submental fat reduction in both men and women.

- We tend to say that "Men are from Mars and Women are from Venus." With the advent of less invasive cosmetic procedures, the distance between these two planets is getting smaller every day.

2.4 Pearls

- On patients with low borderline eyelid position or documented eyelid ptosis, avoid neurotoxin forehead injections or be very conservative.
- On patients with a strong nasalis muscle contraction or "bunny lines" extend your glabellar neurotoxin pattern of injections to the depressor supercilii because usually have strong recruitment as well.
- Stronger and bigger muscles at glabella in men required more units of neurotoxin. Low-set eyebrows in men required careful assessment of frontalis muscle action before neuromodulator injection to prevent potential eyebrow droopiness.
- For the negative vector patient, consider two-pronged approaches: infraorbital injections and concomitant maxillary filler injection.
- When planning treatment on the lower face in men, the goals are to improve jawline definition.

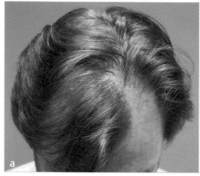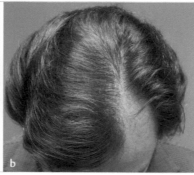

Fig. 2.17 Typical male pattern hair loss treated with oral nutraceutical supplement. **(a)** Before. **(b)** After 3 months of Nutrafol.

Table 2.1 Current treatments for male pattern hair loss

Treatment		Mechanisms	Findings	Pros	Cons
Minoxidil		Acts by shortening telogen phase and increasing hair diameter[64]	40% of male patients experience hair regrowth with 5% minoxidil[65]	Effectiveness is proven in men and women[66,67]	Process is difficult to incorporate into a daily hair care routine[68]
5-alpha-reductase inhibitors	Finasteride	Prevents conversion of testosterone to its active form 5-dihydrotestosterone[69]	1% finasteride gel has the most dermal absorption and it will be a good replacement of oral therapy[60]	Topical finasteride can be considered for hair density maintenance[70]	Erectile dysfunction is the most common side effect, followed by ejaculatory dysfunction and loss of libido[70] Patients are required to use for 1 y to see results[71]
	Dutasteride	Was proved to reduce serum dihydrotestosterone[72]	Dutasteride seems to provide a better efficacy compared with finasteride in treating androgenetic alopecia[73]	Is more potent than finasteride[70,71]	Was associated with higher prevalence of sexual complaints[74]
Follicular cell implantation (FCI)		New follicles are induced by the cultured dermal papilla cells in conjunction with existing epidermis in the scalp[75]	70% of the patients had 11.8% average increase in hair density[64]	Would be permanent and is not to be limited by the quantity of donor hair[75]	Graft rejection by the host[75]
Hair transplantation	Follicular transfer unit (FTU)	A strip of individual follicular unit is removed from a large section of scalp tissue by surgery[76]	A significant positive effect on men with regard to attractiveness and age perception has been observed by evaluators after undergoing the treatment[77]	Higher number of obtained grafts and less transected follicles[64]	Time-consuming, leaves a line scar, and can cause dysesthesia at the donor site[64,78]
	Follicular unit extraction (FUE)	Is a technique that uses punches of 0.8–1 mm in diameter to extract the follicular units[77]	The main advantages of robotic FUE compared with the standard ellipse are its minimally invasive nature and the lack of a linear scar. The average transection rate with the robot to date is 6.6% (range: 0.4–32.1%)[78]	Linear scar is avoided	Was limited by the clinical skill of the operator removing the grafts[79]

(Continued)

Table 2.1 (*Continued*) Current treatments for male pattern hair loss

Treatment	Mechanisms	Findings	Pros	Cons
LLLT (low-level laser therapy)	Increases adenosine triphosphate (ATP) production, causing cell proliferation, oxygenation of tissues, and increasing growth factors by acting on mitochondria[80]	37% of treatment group had increase in hair growth compared to the placebo group[81]	Might be an effective, safe, well-tolerated treatment, specifically for patients unwilling to undergo more invasive options[82,83]	Optimum parameters such as wavelength, coherence, and dosimetric remain to be determined[84]
Platelet-rich plasma (PRP) and microneedling	Autologous preparation of platelets in concentrated plasma. Contains numerous growth factors that are presumably released into the tissue where PRP is introduced[85]	28% of the patients reported an excellent improvement and 64% reported a moderate improvement[86]	Better penetration of a topical drug such as minoxidil[86]	Most of the evidence is anecdotal
Nutraceutical supplement	Capsules with multimodal approach composed of standardized phytoactives with clinically proven anti-inflammatory properties, stress adapters, antioxidants, and dihydrotestoster-one (DHT)[87]	81% reported improvement in overall hair growth. Also, enhances subjects' quality of life (QOL) and self-perceived hair parameters[87]	Multitarget the numerous triggers that compromise hair health at the follicle level: microinflammation, stress, hormonal imbalances, and oxidative damage[88]	A minimum of 3 mo of use is required

References

[1] American Society of Aesthetic Plastic Surgery. Statistics. Available at: http://www.surgery.org/media/statistics. Accessed December 28, 2018

[2] American Society for Dermatologic Surgery. ASDS Consumer Survey. 2018. Available at: https://www.asds.net/consumer-survey/. Accessed December 28, 2018

[3] Enlow DH. A morphogenetic analysis of facial growth. Am J Orthod. 1966; 52(4):283–299

[4] Pessa JE, Chen Y. Curve analysis of the aging orbital aperture. Plast Reconstr Surg. 2002; 109(2):751–755, discussion 756–760

[5] Kahn DM, Shaw RB, Jr. Aging of the bony orbit: a three-dimensional computed tomographic study. Aesthet Surg J. 2008; 28(3):258–264

[6] Kim SJ, Kim SJ, Park JS, Byun SW, Bae JH. Analysis of age-related changes in Asian facial skeletons using 3D vector mathematics on picture archiving and communication system computed tomography. Yonsei Med J. 2015; 56(5):1395–1400

[7] Jagdeo J, Keaney T, Narurkar V, Kolodziejczyk J, Gallagher CJ. Facial treatment preferences among aesthetically oriented men. Dermatol Surg. 2016; 42(10):1155–1163

[8] Farhadian JA, Bloom BS, Brauer JA. Male aesthetics: a review of facial anatomy and pertinent clinical implications. J Drugs Dermatol. 2015; 14(9):1029–1034

[9] Vierkötter A, Schikowski T, Ranft U, et al. Airborne particle exposure and extrinsic skin aging. J Invest Dermatol. 2010; 130(12):2719–2726

[10] Daniell HW. Smoker's wrinkles. A study in the epidemiology of "crow's feet.". Ann Intern Med. 1971; 75(6):873–880

[11] Green AC, Hughes MC, McBride P, Fourtanier A. Factors associated with premature skin aging (photoaging) before the age of 55: a population-based study. Dermatology. 2011; 222(1):74–80

[12] Gunn DA, Dick JL, van Heemst D, et al. Lifestyle and youthful looks. Br J Dermatol. 2015; 172(5):1338–1345

[13] Hamer MA, Pardo LM, Jacobs LC, et al. Lifestyle and physiological factors associated with facial wrinkling in men and women. J Invest Dermatol. 2017; 137:1692e–1699

[14] Keaney TC. Aging in the male face. Intrinsic and extrinsic factors. Dermatol Surg. 2016; 42(7):797–803

[15] Keaney TC. "Man-some": a review of male facial aging and beauty. J Drugs Dermatol. 2017; 16(6):91–93

[16] Kimball AB, Alora-Palli MB, Tamura M, et al. Age-induced and photo-induced changes in gene expression profiles in facial skin of Caucasian females across 6 decades of age. J Am Acad Dermatol. 2018; 78 (1):29–39.e7

[17] Mendelson BC, Jacobson SR. Surgical anatomy of the midcheek: facial layers, spaces, and the midcheek segments. Clin Plast Surg. 2008; 35 (3):395–404, discussion 393

[18] Dutton JJ. Atlas of Surgical Orbital Anatomy. 2nd ed. Philadelphia, PA: Elsevier, Saunders; 2011:130–131

[19] Knize DM. An anatomically based study of the mechanism of eyebrow ptosis. Plast Reconstr Surg. 1996; 97(7):1321–1333

[20] Most SP, Mobley SR, Larrabee WF, Jr. Anatomy of the eyelids. Facial Plast Surg Clin North Am. 2005; 13(4):487–492, v

[21] Dutton JJ. Atlas of clinical and Surgical Orbital Anatomy. 2nd ed. Philadelphia, PA: Elsevier, Saunders; 2011:131

[22] Lavker RM. Structural alterations in exposed and unexposed aged skin. J Invest Dermatol. 1979; 73:59–66

[23] Lavker RM, Zheng PS, Dong G. Aged skin. J Invest Dermatol. 1987; 88 s uppl:44s–51s

[24] Cook BE, Jr, Lucarelli MJ, Lemke BN. Depressor supercilii muscle: anatomy, histology, and cosmetic implications. Ophthal Plast Reconstr Surg. 2001; 17(6):2001–404–411

[25] Knize DM. Muscles that act on glabellar skin: a closer look. Plast Reconstr Surg. 2000; 105(1):350–361

[26] Dempf R, Eckert AW. Contouring the forehead and rhinoplasty in the feminization of the face in male-to-female transsexuals. J Craniomaxillofac Surg. 2010; 38(6):416–422

[27] Ferembach D, Schwindezky I, Stoukal M. Recommendation for age and sex diagnoses of skeletons. J Hum Evol. 1980; 9:517–549

[28] Pretorius E, Steyn M, Scholtz Y. Investigation into the usability of geometric morphometric analysis in assessment of sexual dimorphism. Am J Phys Anthropol. 2006; 129(1):64–70

[29] Spiegel JH. Facial determinants of female gender and feminizing forehead cranioplasty. Laryngoscope. 2011; 121(2):250–261

[30] Russell MD, Brown T, Garn SM, et al. The supraorbital torus. Curr Anthropol. 1985; 26:337–360

[31] Flynn TC. Botox in men. Dermatol Ther. 2007; 20(6):407–413

[32] Rihani J. Aesthetics and rejuvenation of the temple. Facial Plast Surg. 2018; 34(2):159–163

[33] Scheuer JF, III, Sieber DA, Pezeshk RA, Campbell CF, Gassman AA, Rohrich RJ. Anatomy of the facial danger zones: maximizing safety during soft-tissue filler injections. Plast Reconstr Surg. 2017; 139(1): 50e–58e

[34] Shaw RB, Jr, Kahn DM. Aging of the midface bony elements: a three-dimensional computed tomographic study. Plast Reconstr Surg. 2007; 119(2):675–681, discussion 682–683

[35] Richard MJ, Morris C, Deen BF, Gray L, Woodward JA. Analysis of the anatomic changes of the aging facial skeleton using computer-assisted tomography. Ophthal Plast Reconstr Surg. 2009; 25(5):382–386

[36] Frank K, Gotkin RH, Pavicic T. Age and gender differences of the frontal bone: a computed tomographic (CT)-based study. Aesthet Surg J. 2019; 39(7):699–710

[37] Foissac R, Camuzard O, Piereschi S, et al. High-resolution magnetic resonance imaging of aging upper face fat compartments. Plast Reconstr Surg. 2017; 139(4):829–837

[38] Oh SR, Chokthaweesak W, Annunziata CC, Priel A, Korn BS, Kikkawa DO. Analysis of eyelid fat pad changes with aging. Ophthal Plast Reconstr Surg. 2011; 27(5):348–351

[39] Abenavoli FM, Lofoco G, DeGaetano C. A technique to correct floppy eyelid syndrome. Ophthal Plast Reconstr Surg. 2008; 24(6): 497–498

[40] van den Bosch WA, Leenders I, Mulder P. Topographic anatomy of the eyelids, and the effects of sex and age. Br J Ophthalmol. 1999; 83: 347–352

[41] Sadcik NS. Volumetric structural rejuvenation for the male face. Dermatol Clin. 2018; 36:43–48

[42] Swift A. The mathematics of facial beauty. In: Jones D, ed. Injectable Fillers: Principles and Practice. Hoboken, NJ: Blackwell Pub.; 2010:140

[43] Koudelová J, Brůžek J, Cagáňová V, Krajíček V, Velemínská J. Development of facial sexual dimorphism in children aged between 12 and 15 years: a three-dimensional longitudinal study. Orthod Craniofac Res. 2015; 18(3):175–184

[44] Chopra K, Calva D, Sosin M, et al. A comprehensive examination of topographic thickness of skin in the human face. Aesthet Surg J. 2015; 35(8):1007–1013

[45] Saban Y, Polselli R, Bertossi D, East C, Gerbault O. Facial layers and facial fat compartments: focus on midcheek area. Facial Plast Surg. 2017; 33(5):470–482

[46] Kruglikov I, Trujillo O, Kristen Q, et al. The facial adipose tissue: a revision. Facial Plast Surg. 2016; 32(6):671–682

[47] Wollina U, Wetzker R, Abdel-Naser MB, Kruglikov IL. Role of adipose tissue in facial aging. Clin Interv Aging. 2017; 12:2069–2076

[48] Rossi AM. Men's aesthetic dermatology. Semin Cutan Med Surg. 2014; 33(4):188–197

[49] Janssen I, Heymsfield SB, Wang ZM, Ross R. Skeletal muscle mass and distribution in 468 men and women aged 18–88 yr. J Appl Physiol (1985). 2000; 89(1):81–88

[50] Tsukahara K, Hotta M, Osanai O, Kawada H, Kitahara T, Takema Y. Gender-dependent differences in degree of facial wrinkles. Skin Res Technol. 2013; 19(1):e65–e71

[51] Sjöström L, Smith U, Krotkiewski M, Björntorp P. Cellularity in different regions of adipose tissue in young men and women. Metabolism. 1972; 21(12):1143–1153

[52] Humphrey GM. A Treatise on the Human Skeleton. Cambridge, England: MacMillan; 1858

[53] Enlow DH. The Human Face: An Account of the Postnatal Growth and Development of the Craniofacial Skeleton. New York, NY: Harper and Row; 1968

[54] Pessa JE. An algorithm of facial aging: verification of Lambros's theory by three-dimensional stereolithography, with reference to the pathogenesis of midfacial aging, scleral show, and the lateral suborbital trough deformity. Plast Reconstr Surg. 2000; 106(2):479–488, discussion 489–490

[55] Pessa JE, Zadoo VP, Mutimer KL, et al. Relative maxillary retrusion as a natural consequence of aging: combining skeletal and soft-tissue changes into an integrated model of midfacial aging. Plast Reconstr Surg. 1998; 102(1):205–212

[56] Paskhover B, Durand D, Kamen E, Gordon NA. Patterns of change in facial skeletal aging. JAMA Facial Plast Surg. 2017; 19:413–417

[57] Mendelson B, Wong CH. Changes in the facial skeleton with aging: implications and clinical applications in facial rejuvenation. Aesthetic Plast Surg. 2012; 36:753–760

[58] Mendelson B, Wong CH. Changes in the facial skeleton with aging: implications and clinical applications in facial rejuvenation. Aesthetic Plast Surg. 2012; 36(4):753–760

[59] de Maio M. Ethnic and gender considerations in the use of facial injectables: male patients. Plast Reconstr Surg. 2015; 136(5) Suppl: 40S–43S

[60] Chatham DR. Special considerations for the male patient: things I wish I knew when I started practice. Facial Plast Surg. 2005; 21(4): 232–239

[61] Santos LD, Shapiro J. Update on male pattern hair loss. J Drugs Dermatol. 2014; 13(11):1308–1310

[62] McAndrews P. American Hair Loss Association: Men's Hair Loss/Introduction. 2010. Available at: https://www.americanhairloss.org/men_hair_loss/introduction.html

[63] Santos LD, Shapiro J. Update on male pattern hair loss. J Drugs Dermatol. 2014; 13(11):1308–1310

[64] Fabbrocini G, Cantelli M, Masarà A, Annunziata MC, Marasca C, Cacciapuoti S. Female pattern hair loss: a clinical, pathophysiologic, and therapeutic review. Int J Womens Dermatol. 2018; 4(4):203–211

[65] Blume-Peytavi U, Hillmann K, Dietz E, Canfield D, Garcia Bartels N. A randomized, single-blind trial of 5% minoxidil foam once daily versus 2% minoxidil solution twice daily in the treatment of androgenetic alopecia in women. J Am Acad Dermatol. 2011; 65(6):1126–1134.e2

[66] Gupta AK, Foley KA. 5% Minoxidil: treatment for female pattern hair loss. Skin Therapy Lett. 2014; 19(6):5–7

[67] Farris PK, Rogers N, McMichael A, Kogan S. A novel multi-targeting approach to treating hair loss, using standardized nutraceuticals. J Drugs Dermatol. 2017; 16(11):s141–s148

[68] Mella JM, Perret MC, Manzotti M, Catalano HN, Guyatt G. Efficacy and safety of finasteride therapy for androgenetic alopecia: a systematic review. Arch Dermatol. 2010; 146(10):1141–1150

[69] Hajheydari Z, Akbari J, Saeedi M, Shokoohi L. Comparing the therapeutic effects of finasteride gel and tablet in treatment of the androgenetic alopecia. Indian J Dermatol Venereol Leprol. 2009; 75(1):47–51

[70] Price VH, Menefee E, Sanchez M, Kaufman KD. Changes in hair weight in men with androgenetic alopecia after treatment with finasteride (1 mg daily): three- and 4-year results. J Am Acad Dermatol. 2006; 55(1):71–74

[71] Clark RV, Hermann DJ, Cunningham GR, Wilson TH, Morrill BB, Hobbs S. Marked suppression of dihydrotestosterone in men with benign prostatic hyperplasia by dutasteride, a dual 5alpha-reductase inhibitor. J Clin Endocrinol Metab. 2004; 89(5):2179–2184

[72] Zhou Z, Song S, Gao Z, Wu J, Ma J, Cui Y. The efficacy and safety of dutasteride compared with finasteride in treating men with androgenetic alopecia: a systematic review and meta-analysis. Clin Interv Aging. 2019; 14:399–406

[73] Traish AM, Mulgaonkar A, Giordano N. The dark side of 5α-reductase inhibitors' therapy: sexual dysfunction, high Gleason grade prostate cancer and depression. Korean J Urol. 2014; 55(6):367–379

[74] Teumer J, Cooley J. Follicular cell implantation: an emerging cell therapy for hair loss. Semin Plast Surg. 2005; 19(02):193–200

[75] Bicknell LM, Kash N, Kavouspour C, Rashid RM. Follicular unit extraction hair transplant harvest: a review of current recommendations and future considerations. Dermatol Online J. 2014; 20(3):doj_21754

[76] Bater KL, Ishii M, Joseph A, Su P, Nellis J, Ishii LE. Perception of hair transplant for androgenetic alopecia. JAMA Facial Plast Surg. 2016; 18(6):413–418

[77] Rashid RM, Morgan Bicknell LT. Follicular unit extraction hair transplant automation: options in overcoming challenges of the latest technology in hair restoration with the goal of avoiding the line scar. Dermatol Online J. 2012; 18(9):12

[78] Jiménez-Acosta F, Ponce-Rodríguez I. Follicular unit extraction for hair transplantation: an update. Actas Dermosifiliogr. 2017; 108(6):532–537

[79] Avram MR, Watkins SA. Robotic follicular unit extraction in hair transplantation. Dermatol Surg. 2014; 40(12):1319–1327

[80] Keaney T. Emerging therapies for androgenetic alopecia. J Drugs Dermatol. 2015; 14(9):1036–1040

[81] Leavitt M, Charles G, Heyman E, Michaels D. HairMax LaserComb laser phototherapy device in the treatment of male androgenetic alopecia: a randomized, double-blind, sham device-controlled, multicentre trial. Clin Drug Investig. 2009; 29(5):283–292

[82] Lanzafame RJ, Blanche RR, Chiacchierini RP, Kazmirek ER, Sklar JA. The growth of human scalp hair in females using visible red light laser and LED sources. Lasers Surg Med. 2014; 46(8):601–607

[83] Jimenez JJ, Wikramanayake TC, Bergfeld W, et al. Efficacy and safety of a low-level laser device in the treatment of male and female pattern hair loss: a multicenter, randomized, sham device-controlled, double-blind study. Am J Clin Dermatol. 2014; 15(2):115–127

[84] Afifi L, Maranda EL, Zarei M, et al. Low-level laser therapy as a treatment for androgenetic alopecia. Lasers Surg Med. 2017; 49(1):27–39

[85] Avci P, Gupta GK, Clark J, Wikonkal N, Hamblin MR. Low-level laser (light) therapy (LLLT) for treatment of hair loss. Lasers Surg Med. 2014; 46(2):144–151

[86] Rose PT. Hair restoration surgery: challenges and solutions. Clin Cosmet Investig Dermatol. 2015; 8:361–370

[87] Shah KB, Shah AN, Solanki RB, Raval RC. A comparative study of microneedling with platelet-rich plasma plus topical minoxidil (5%) and topical minoxidil (5%) alone in androgenetic alopecia. Int J Trichology. 2017; 9(1):14–18

[88] Ablon G, Kogan S. A six-month, randomized, double-blind, placebo-controlled study evaluating the safety and efficacy of a nutraceutical supplement for promoting hair growth in women with self-perceived thinning hair. J Drugs Dermatol. 2018; 17(5):558–565

[89] Sadick NS, Callender VD, Kircik LH, Kogan S. New insight into the pathophysiology of hair loss trigger a paradigm shift in the treatment approach. J Drugs Dermatol. 2017; 16(11):s135–s140

3 Taking a Hard Look: Soft Tissue Augmentation

Shino Bay Aguilera, Cameron Chesnut, Michael B. Lipp, and Luis Soro

Summary

As the number of male patients seeking cosmetic enhancements continues to rise, the need to understand the differences and similarities between both genders to tailor techniques most suitable for the male aesthetic patient is crucial for optimal results. In order to avoid feminizing a male face, it is important to appreciate the areas on the face that represent sexual dimorphism. Along with increased awareness of these key facial characteristics, injectors must understand rheological properties of injectable fillers to both preserve and create masculinity of the face, yielding strong and defined borders which are generally perceived as more attractive in men. In this chapter, we cover these principles to better help providers achieve successful outcomes with their male patients.

Keywords: dimorphism, symmetry, chiseled, masculine

3.1 Background

According to the American Society of Plastic Surgeons' 2017 National Plastic Surgery Statistics, 14.1 million cosmetic procedures were performed, with men making up 1.1 million cases.[1] This represents 8% of the market, which has grown significantly (76%) since 2000.[1] Soft-tissue fillers are one of the top five nonsurgical, minimally invasive, cosmetic procedures performed on men. In a study of over 52,000 men and women, women outnumbered men by a 9:1 ratio of cosmetic procedures performed. Interestingly, women only outnumbered men by a 2:1 ratio in their interest in cosmetic procedures,[2] suggesting that there is an unmet need for the male aesthetic patient. Despite the rising demand of aesthetic procedures for men, there is limited literature available to guide clinicians in understanding treatment preferences of the male aesthetic patient as well as treatment approaches.

In a survey of treatment-naive men interested in cosmetic procedures, men were most motivated to consider injectable procedures "to look good for my age" and "to look more youthful."[3] The most concerning facial areas most likely to be prioritized for treatment were the tear troughs and crow's feet, highlighting that the periorbital areas are most likely the primary focus of aesthetically oriented men. The least concerning facial areas and least likely to be prioritized for treatment included lip volume and perioral lines. Respectively, this may be due to concerns of feminization and because men are less susceptible to the development of perioral wrinkles due to the inherent larger numbers of skin appendages and thicker skin.[4,5,6] The top reasons men would not consider an injectable cosmetic procedure were, in the following order: thinking they did not need it yet, concerns of side effects/safety, concerns about injecting a foreign material into their body, cost, maintenance of procedures, and concerns about not looking natural.[3]

The survey suggested that many of the barriers to trying aesthetic treatments such as dermal fillers are rooted from a low level of awareness and lack of education about the procedures. As a cosmetic physician, it is crucial to educate the male cosmetic patient, understand their interests and needs, and approach treatments with attention to the unique facial dimorphisms between genders.

Volumetric changes are a key component of male facial aging and the aforementioned areas of concern, and there are numerous options available to revolumize the male face. Poly-L-lactic acid (PLLA) is a biostimulatory nonhyaluronic acid filler that produces a natural look by stimulating collagen production and in the authors' opinion helps maintain and imitate the architecture of the bone when properly placed.[7] PLLA has both rejuvenative and prejuvenative properties, which are ideal for male aesthetic patients concerned with looking "overdone or feminized" or feeling they "do not need it yet."

To achieve a masculine look, one that is more chiseled, angulated, and squared, the cosmetic physician must choose the appropriate filler products. An understanding of rheological properties of fillers is essential to understanding each fillers personality.[8] One of the most highly referenced and used measurement of fillers is G prime (G'). G' is most often used to describe the fillers' hardness and ability to cause tissue projection. High-G' fillers such as calcium hydroxylapatite (CaHA) or hyaluronic acid (HA) when properly placed can correct and enhance masculine features. An exception would be fillers placed in the tear trough or lip region, which require a low-G' HA filler. Fat transfer presents an autologous option for revolumization that can offer similar variation in characteristics based on harvest and preparation, allowing specific structural properties for use in specific areas. Soft-tissue augmentation with volume is a balance between anatomy and aesthetic goals. With an understanding of facial dimorphism between genders along with age-related changes, the proper placement and volume can be used to achieving a masculine and natural look.

3.2 Facial Dimorphisms

The dimorphic features that characteristically differentiate a man's face from a woman's face are a result of the hormonal influences that occur during puberty.[9] In an adult male, differences can be seen in the skin, subcutaneous tissue, and bone structure. The epidermis and dermis in men are overall thicker compared to women and are largely due to increased collagen density in men.[6] This is likely influenced by androgens since skin collagen density is increased in females with primary cutaneous virilism compared to normal female controls.[10] However, men have less facial subcutaneous fat.[9]

As a generality, excluding ethnic variations, a man's face is more square shaped compared to the heart-shaped or inverted triangular shape of a woman. When evaluating a male patient, the temple width should ideally line up with the lateral zygoma, which should also line up with the projection of the mandible. Balancing these three areas will help achieve a squared look, which is considered an ideal masculine feature by experts.[9]

3.3 The Aging Face

Keeping in mind masculine features, changes in bone structure also occur in the aging face, and failure to address these foundational changes may limit the benefits of rejuvenated procedures. Men tend to age more linearly compared to women who undergo greater age-related changes after menopause.[11] Bone mineral density studies of the skulls of men and women have shown that both men and women experience a decrease in bone densities, particularly the maxilla and mandible, between young (20–40 years) and middle-aged (41–60 years) individuals.[12] Bone resorption also occurs in the orbital apertures, pyriform aperture, maxilla, zygomas, and mandible, and is described in more detail below (► Fig. 3.1).

The orbital aperture increases with age. This is largely due to resorption that tends to occur in the inferolateral and superomedial quadrant of the orbit.[13] The midface, formed by the maxilla and the zygoma, undergoes retrusion.[14,15,16] Much like the orbital aperture, the pyriform aperture also increases. Resorption occurs in the inferior and lateral walls. Posterior resorption is greatest in the lower pyriform aperture, which is the major supporting structure of the lateral crura and external nasal valves.[17] The anterior nasal spine, which supports the columella, also undergoes resorption. These changes manifest as a clinical lengthening of the nose, tip drooping, and a columella and lateral crura displacing posteriorly.[18] Supporting this area with supraperiosteal injections in the pyriform fossa with a high-G′ filler can help soften and lift the perinasal and nasolabial folds. PLLA can be used in this area to build collagen and provide supplemental support to the soft tissues acting as a proxy where bone resorption has occurred.[7] In dentate men and women, the maxilla and mandible experience resorption changes, despite it traditionally being thought to occur only in nondentulous individuals.[19] An accelerating factor may be seen in patients with bruxism, an unconscious clenching and grinding of the teeth.[20] The ramus height, mandibular body height, and mandibular body length decrease with age in both genders, whereas the mandibular angle increases

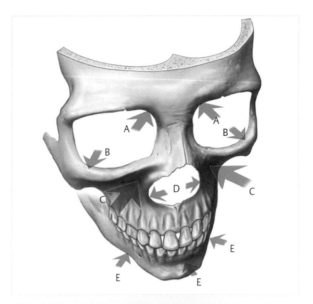

Fig. 3.1 Bone resorption of the human skull with aging. The *arrows* indicate areas were resorption tends to occur with aging. (A) Superomedial orbital rim. (B) Inferomedial, orbital rim. (C) Maxilla. (D) Pyriform aperture. (E) Mandible.

with age.[21] The increase in mandibular angle is likely due to the combination of decreasing lengths in the ramus body height and mandibular body length. CaHA along the inferior borders of the mandible can help mask these changes by maintaining mandibular proportions.

3.3.1 Upper Third

A major contributing factor to the appearance of aging in the upper one-third of the face is the frontal concavity. Brow ptosis and eventual furrowing of the brows is a result of diminished soft-tissue volume on the forehead, creating projected expressions of anger, sadness, and tiredness. Gender and genetics play a role in the presentation of variations of frontal concavity.[22,23,24]

The upper third of the face of the bony structures of a woman's forehead and glabella is more curvilinear and less pronounced. The supraorbital rim of a woman is less noticeable than that of a man. A man has a more oblique forehead, a glabella that is more prominent, and a supraorbital rim that is more pronounced. The pronounced supraorbital rim establishes the position of the male eyebrow, which sits flat along the orbital rim compared to women who have a more arched brow. As a result, women tend to dominate in the upper one-third of the face with higher arched brows and a more open appearance of the eyes.[25] Conversely, men dominate in the lower one-third of the face due to pronounced jaw lines, yet also present with lower set eyebrows, bossing brow bones, and less soft-tissue volume in the upper one-third of the face. Due to these combined factors, a pronounced frontal concavity is naturally more prevalent in men. Premature aging in the upper one-third of the face may also be due to genetic differences. Asian and Mestizo ethnicities specifically have deficiency in soft-tissue volume contributing to very flat or even concave frontal projection. Therefore, presence of frontal concavity appears earlier in certain populations, usually by the fourth decade.

Male brow position rests on the superior orbital rim, and the shape is flat with less of a lateral peak than the female brow. This lower, flatter position at baseline puts the male brow in a position to become notably ptotic with age. As brow lifting techniques for men are often limited and less than desirable due to hairline recession, the progressive use of volume to control brow position and shape becomes especially important via frontoplasty. Volumization can affect and raise the medial two-thirds of the brow via the frontalis muscular connection, whereas augmentation of lateral brow fat pad, retro-orbicularis oculi fat compartment can elevate the third of the brow lateral to the conjoint tendon.

Neurotoxins, although excellent for reducing rhytids, when used in a frontalis muscle that is already volume depleted, can lead to an exaggerated aging appearance and worsening of brow and lid ptosis.[26] To circumvent this potential undesirable outcome, we hereby describe a technique utilizing a low-viscosity, low-G' HA filler to volumize frontal concavity.

Anatomy

Understanding the anatomical boundaries and danger zones in the frontal region is of utmost importance when injecting to avoid any complications. Most important is a clear knowledge of nerves and the vascular supply of the area. The main arterial danger zones to be aware of when using this technique include the supratrochlear, supraorbital arteries, and branches of the superficial temporal artery.

The frontal branch of the superficial temporal artery courses superiorly and medially to anastomose with the supratrochlear and supraorbital arteries, which are branches of the ophthalmic artery. Bilaterally, these supply the majority of the frontal region. The glabella is predominantly supplied by small arterial branches from the supratrochlear and supraorbital arteries with limited collateral circulation.[7] The veins in the frontal region accompany the arteries and drain to the angular vein and the internal jugular vein. The supratrochlear and supraorbital nerves branch off of the trigeminal nerve and provide sensory innervation to the region (▶ Fig. 3.2).

The anatomical plane of all structures should be taken into consideration before the injection of filler to decrease complications such as vascular compromise. Vascular occlusion can occur by external compression of the blood supply by adjacent filler injection, direct intra-arterial injection of product, and by vascular injury during injection.[26,27,28] Symptoms of vascular compromise

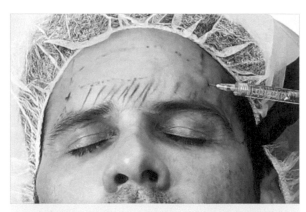

Fig. 3.2 Injecting in the subgaleal space proves to be safe and effective when doing frontoplasty with injectable fillers.

are blanching of the skin, a progressive dusky color change of the skin, and eventual ulceration with eschar formation. In the glabellar region specifically, vascular occlusion may lead to blindness. Finally, in addition to vessel injury, nerve damage can occur, and may present as discomfort during the injection, headache, neuralgia, and/or paresthesia.

If adverse events are suspected, treatment protocols should be utilized.[27,28] Risk of these events can be minimized by careful selection of the injection site, aspiration prior to injection, injecting in the subgaleal space, and continually monitoring for signs and symptoms of vessel occlusion.

Frontoplasty Technique

Always keeping in mind important vascular landmarks (▶ Fig. 3.3a), find the temporal crest as a landmark and demarcate this area. Depending on how wide and deep the frontal concavity of the individual is, mark two to four entry points on each side of the temporal crest (▶ Fig. 3.3b). Prior to injections, the face is cleansed (e.g., hypochlorous acid or chlorhexidine) to promote an aseptic and sterile technique. A 21-gauge needle can be used to create the openings and a 25- or 22-gauge, 2-inch cannula can be used to fill the frontal concavity in the subgaleal plane by lifting the frontalis muscle between the thumb and the forefinger and sliding the cannula into the subgaleal space (▶ Fig. 3.3c). HA can be deposited in a linear retrograde fashion. Using small-gauge cannulas (i.e., 25- or 22-guage cannulas), knowing where the tip of the cannula is at all times, moving at least 1 to 2 mm retrograde before beginning to deposit small aliquots of the product, knowing the trajectory of the important arteries, and making sure to always inject perpendicular to them can help prevent canalization of the artery and will help reduce the risk of intravascular occlusion. The end point of each injection occurs when visualization of the deficit is no longer appreciated (▶ Fig. 3.3d). Of note, it is important

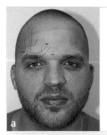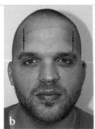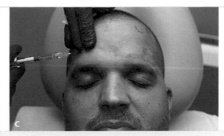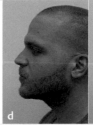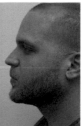

Fig. 3.3 **(a)** Important vascular landmarks to be considered when preparing to treat frontal concavity. **(b)** Entry points marked here with an *X* may vary according to the size and location of the frontal concavity defect. A small bolus of lidocaine 1% with epinephrine is injected until blanching is noted at each marked entry site. **(c)** Prior to injections, the face is cleansed with a chlorhexidine sponge or hypochlorous acid and the pencil markings are removed to promote an aseptic or sterile technique. The entry points are injected with lidocaine 1% with epinephrine for anesthesia. A 21-gauge needle is used to create the openings and a 25-gauge, 2-inch cannula is used to fill the frontal concavity in the subgaleal plane. **(d)** Patient treated with a total of 1.8 mL of hyaluronic acid to alleviate moderate frontal concavity.

to encourage patient feedback while injecting to assess for nerve impingement or compromise. Most patients show a great improvement with small volumes such as 1- to 2-mm syringe of product. When using HA, it is important to choose a product with the right consistency that allows for easy flow (i.e., low viscosity) through the subgaleal space, but with enough lift capacity (i.e., low G′) to volumize the forehead. When utilizing fat transfer for this region, one author (C.C.) prefers to use a moderately structural, less homogenized, or emulsified microfat graft with the objective of a smooth, durable correction, as the overlying frontalis muscle and skin overlie a deeper plane with which to structurally graft and provide such contour correction.

The lateral brow fat pad can be addressed through a similar cannula entry site and injection plane; blending with any temporal augmentation can also be performed. When using autologous fat, the forgiving depth in the temporal fossa allows the use of a more coarse, structural millifat graft with the objective of projecting the overlying dense mass of soft tissue. The larger, generally 19-gauge, cannula size utilized with such millifat grafts allows the injector to feel penetration of the deep temporal fascia for deep graft placement to yield such soft-tissue projection.

In summary, injection of a cohesive, low-viscosity, low-G′, HA filler, or structural fat graft via the use of a safer subgaleal cannula injection technique allows for the effective rejuvenation of frontal concavity. A filler placed appropriately in the mid-forehead brings a more youthful and fresh appearance to the face and patients indicate a high level of satisfaction with the treatment outcome. Most treated patients observe a durability of this diluted HA filler technique of about 2 to 3 years.

3.3.2 Midface (Middle Third)

In the middle third of the face, women's cheeks are rounder and fuller with an apex more anterolateral. This is due to a combination of more subcutaneous fat in the cheeks[29,30,31] along with a more curvilinear zygoma.[32] Men have an apex that is more anteromedial and subtle with a broader based malar prominence.[33] This is largely due to zygomatic processes that are wider and zygomatic arches that are larger in men.[11] Men also have less superficial subcutaneous fat in the midface/cheeks.[30,31,34] Injecting fillers in the cheeks of men should be done with a high-G′ filler balancing a 1:1 ratio between the medial and lateral cheek.[11] In comparison, the medial-to-lateral cheek thickness ratio is 1.5:1 in women.[35] A cosmetic physician injecting a filler in this region should be aware of these differences to not cause feminization when injecting in the cheeks.

Revolumizing the midface and augmenting the zygomatic arch is safe and effective. This technique addresses flattening and sagging of the midface, which naturally occurs due to aging, and in many cases also enhances overall facial attractiveness. Studies have shown that a larger bizygomatic width-to-facial height ratio as measured from the upper lip to the upper eyelid or brow is perceived as being more attractive.[25]

Anatomy

Several anatomical structures must be considered in the appropriate use of all filler injections. When using a product that is harder to dissolve such as CaHA, this is imperative. With surgical procedures, it is of paramount importance to be mindful of the danger of transection of nerves and vessels. With filler injections, the same awareness applies. Focus should be intently on the underlying vasculature, since occlusion from injection of a product into a vessel lumen or external compression is the most fundamental complication to avoid. Vascular occlusion is fortunately rare, and the potential is further minimized when injecting a product in the periosteal region as described with this technique.[36]

Due to the variable nature of facial anatomy, while working around primary named arteries and nerves, extra caution is warranted. In the midface region, these include the infraorbital artery arising from the infraorbital foramen, the transverse facial artery that traverses just inferior to the lower border of the zygomatic arch, and the torturous facial artery with its anastomosing angular artery (► Fig. 3.4). The primary nerve to pay attention to in this region is the infraorbital nerve, which also emerges from the palpable infraorbital foramen. Injury to this nerve can result in intractable neuralgia for a prolonged period, and therefore extreme caution is to be applied when injecting around the foramen.

Midface with Calcium Hydroxyapatite

Prior to injecting CaHA in areas of danger, consider transferring the product to a 1-mL BD syringe, which allows for easier aspiration and assurance that the needle tip is not placed intravascularly.[36] Utilizing a retrograde injection technique and avoiding large boluses can also help minimize inadvertent occlusion.

Using Hinderer's lines, the apex of the cheek is slightly more anteromedial in a male compared to a woman. A combination of needle and cannula techniques can be useful in this area to create a masculine look that is well defined and chiseled. Using a cannula and entering from behind the zygomatic eminence, small aliquots of continuous product should be injected in a retrograde fashion parallel along the supraperiosteal plane across the zygoma, keeping in mind that the zygoma should thin

laterally. This accentuates and defines the malar cheek while using the zygoma as a platform to directly lift the midface. Using a needle, small aliquots of CaHA can be placed perpendicular to bone at the apex to provide additional lift (► Fig. 3.5a–g).

Midface with Hyaluronic Acid

HA is the most commonly utilized of all injectable fillers for facial rejuvenation. It has a low level of adverse reactions due to its biocompatibility with human tissue and the benefit of reversibility with hyaluronidase enzyme.[37] For the male patient, when selecting an injectable HA filler, it is important to use the highest G' option to lift the midface or achieve adequate contour and angularity that defines a male face. Restylane Lyft HA is one reasonable option for use in male patients due to its stiffness or higher G'.

The following technique, described here by the authors to elevate and contour the midface of the male patient, uses four injections focused on retaining the ligaments of the face to lift and simultaneously contour the midface of a male patient with respect to sexual dysmorphism.[38]

First, the apex of the cheek is identified either by glance or using Hinderer's lines as previously described. The first injection can then be made approximately 1 cm posterior to the apex where 0.1 mL of HA is placed supraperiosteally (► Fig. 3.6a). Next, a larger bolus of 0.2 mL is made directly into the apex (► Fig. 3.6b). These injection points alone help lift and anchor the midface. A 0.1-mL bolus is then

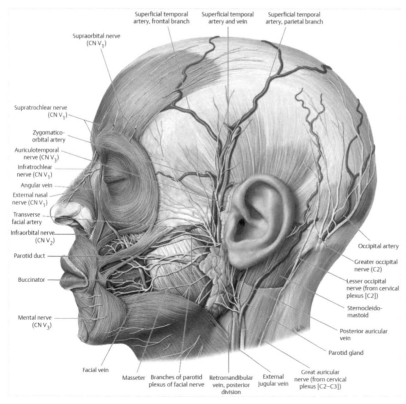

Fig. 3.4 Superficial arteries and veins of face and scalp. (Reproduced with permission from Schünke M et al., ed. Thieme Atlas of Anatomy, Volume 3: Head, Neck, and Neuroanatomy. 3rd Edition. New York: Thieme; 2020.)

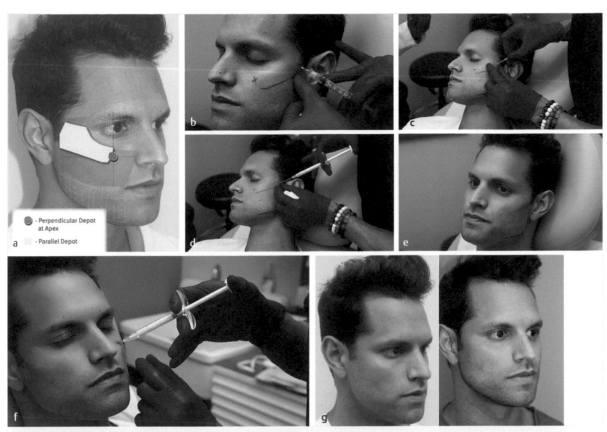

Fig. 3.5 Midface with calcium hydroxyapatite. **(a)** Schematic drawing of product injection at the midface. The *blue circle* represents the apex where a depot injection at a 90-degree angle is placed supraperiosteally. The *yellow region* represents the path along which product should be placed in a retrograde fashion with a 25-gauge cannula supraperiosteally. **(b)** Numbing the area with 1% lidocaine with epinephrine. **(c)** Create a point of entrance with a 21-gauge needle. **(d)** Introduce the cannula at a 30-degree angle. Once in the supraperiosteal plane, decrease the angle to 10 degrees and keep the syringe parallel to the zygoma. The tip of the cannula should be 1 to 2 mm behind the zygomatic eminence. **(e)** Inject while moving retrograde and laterally toward the hairline, placing 0.1 mL of product continuously with a final total of 0.5 mL having been placed along the zygoma. **(f)** Place 0.2 mL of product perpendicular to the zygoma at the apex with provided needle. **(g)** The patient was treated with Radiesse + in the midface, jawline, and chin.

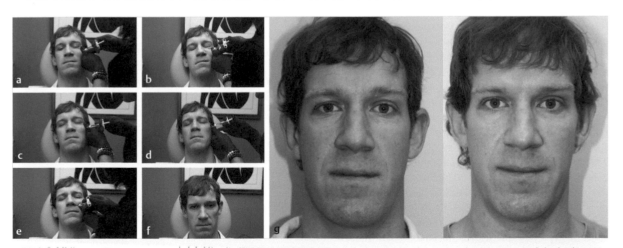

Fig. 3.6 Midface with hyaluronic acid. **(a)** After finding the apex, we move 1 cm posterior to the apex and inject 0.1 mL of the hyaluronic acid (HA) perpendicular to the periosteum (supraperiosteal). **(b)** Inject 0.2 mL of the product right at the apex, which is our position no. 2 (injection is perpendicular supraperiosteal). Position nos. 1 and 2 lift and anchor the face. **(c)** After injecting the apex, inject 0.1 mL of product in front of the zygomatic ligament (McGregor's patch). **(d)** After injecting McGregor's patch, we continue to follow the zygoma with small aliquots of 0.05 mL until reaching the hairline (usually spacing injections about 0.5 cm apart). **(e)** 0.2 mL was injected supraperiosteally on the canine fossa to alleviate a deep nasolabial fold. **(f)** Split face showing the treated and untreated side. Showing a much more define, strong, and masculine zygoma and zygomatic arch. **(g)** Before and after HA injections to the midface demonstrating a more refreshed masculine, youthful look.

injected approximately 5 mm lateral to the initial injection point (McGregor's patch) to further lift the midface (▶ Fig. 3.6c). Finally, a series of injections at 5-mm intervals with small aliquots of 0.05 mL are made until reaching the hairline (▶ Fig. 3.6d). If needed and product remains, the canine fossa or the submalar area can also be injected using a serial puncture approach or a fanning retrograde technique with a needle or cannula (▶ Fig. 3.6e).

One pearl to consider is that when treating male patients in this area, it is important to avoid overcorrecting the medial cheek so as to avoid creating a rounder "ogee curve" often sought by female patients. More emphasis should then be placed on enhancing the lateral zygoma.

Infraorbital Hollows

Perhaps one of the earliest signs of visible aging of the face for men and women is changes to the periocular region. Lipoatrophy of the deep fat compartments in the infraorbital space in particular leads to a sunken, hollow look resulting from more of the underlying orbicularis oculi muscle being visible and less light reflectance in the area. To combat this, use of a low-G' HA filler and ideally one with a lower HA concentration to prevent delayed swelling reactions can be very beneficial to patients concerned with changes in this zone.

With fat transfer in the infraorbital region, a graft with smaller cellular structure, such as a stromal vascular fraction-based graft with a microfat or nanofat preparation (Tulip Medical, San Diego, California, United States), allows grafting to multiple planes within the more delicate tissues around the orbicularis oculi and thin overlying skin, which allows each aging tissue type to be addressed independently. The stem cell component of this particular type of graft also shows benefit to surrounding tissue quality via paracrine effects, which are especially useful in this area of relatively thin tissue that is especially prone to photodamage and structural breakdown from repeated movement. A more structural millifat graft can simultaneously be placed in the deep fat compartment to address deep atrophy and descent. Placing specific types of fat grafts in multiple planes ensures excellent graft survival and outcomes by addressing specific areas of volumetric change.

When treating with HA, total volume used should be conservative, typically not exceeding more than 0.5 mL per side or 1 mL of product total. The product should be placed deeply along the orbital rim to ensure the filler stays beneath the orbicularis oculi muscle. Unless used in exceedingly small quantities, placement of HA that is too superficial can lead to delayed swelling and an undesirable puffy appearance to the area and Tyndall's effect.

The technique for treating male patients in this area is essentially no different than that for treating female patients. Each individual will have variable volume deficiencies that should be assessed and localized prior to injecting. Filler injections of the infraorbital hollows are ideally done using a 25- to 27-gauge cannula to minimize trauma and potential for bruising. One technique found to be successful is creating two entry ports per side with a 23- to 25-gauge needle, one inferior to the tear trough and just lateral to the midpupillary line and another point that is inferior to the lateral infraorbital hollow. Insertion of the cannula through these two points allows easy access to target treatment zones. It is important to ensure proper depth. The injector should ideally not be able to see the tip of the cannula through the dermis. Once the tip of the cannula is in the site of intended revolumization, a retrograde fanning approach using no more than 0.1 to 0.2 mL to each zone provides natural volume correction. It is often preferred to undercorrect this area, as product hydration over time can lead to swelling and puffiness.

3.3.3 Lower Face

Jawline and Chin

A squared, well-defined jawline is a widely accepted sexually dimorphic feature associated with male attractiveness. Patients with jowls, poor delineation of the lateral jawline from the neck or those simply looking to enhance lower face volume and definition can greatly benefit from this procedure. Use of a stiffer, high-G' filler such as CaHA or structural millifat injected supraperiosteally via a cannula can offer cosmetically pleasing outcomes.

In the lower third of the face, men have larger mandibles and a chin and jawline with clear-cut angles resulting in a more square-shaped contour of the face. The chin has well-developed tubercles and the mandibular ramus has prominent angulation.[39,40] Men also have large masseter muscles, which give more projection and definition to the jawline. These features are perceived as highly masculine. Women have smaller and more subtle angles of the mandible. In a study where subjects were asked the prototypical gender of a female face superimposing masculine features, the jaw was perceived as the most significant change in gender. This was followed by eyebrows/eyes and then the chin.[41] In the authors' opinion, a high-G' filler, ideally CaHA, can be placed supraperiosteally along the jawline to provide projection and build a strong jawline.

Jawline and Chin with Calcium Hydroxyapatite

The ramus height, mandibular body height, and mandibular body length decrease with age, whereas the mandibular angle increases with age.[21] The increase in mandibular angle is likely due to the combination of decreasing lengths in the ramus body height and mandibular body length. CaHA injected along the inferior borders of the mandible can help mask these changes by maintaining more youthful mandibular proportions. For jawline contouring, CaHA can be injected with a needle along the inferior and posterior borders creating a smaller mandibular angle. Injections placed laterally will broaden the jaw, creating masculine features, and are more often avoided when treating women. To address the prejowl sulcus, small aliquots can be injected supraperiosteally with a needle along the border avoiding injection into the apex of the jowl, as this can worsen the appearance of the jowl. Great care must be taken to avoid injecting the facial artery past the anterior border of the masseter insertion point. The antegonial notch along the midportion of the mandibular body can often be palpated as a landmark indicating the artery's location as it crosses the mandible and continues tortuously along the nasal labial fold splitting into the inferior and superior labial arteries and angular artery. In the antegonial region, a cannula technique is recommended placing small aliquots subcutaneously in a retrograde linear fashion to bridge the prejowl sulcus and masseteric regions of the jawline.

When addressing the jawline, the chin must also be evaluated and addressed as it is continuum with the jawline. Ideally, the gnathion should be positioned within 1 to 2 mm of the lower lip vermillion border when evaluated from a lateral position in the Frankfort horizontal plane. Treating the chin and adding projection lengthens the mandible helping reduce the appearance of marionette lines and jowls. Injections in the pogonion will increase projection, whereas injections in the menton will increase vertical height. Injections in the gnathion will increase both projection and vertical height of the chin. For a masculine effect, injections can be placed more laterally to square the chin. It is important to avoid the infraorbital foramen, which lies approximately 1.5 cm superior to the mandibular border in line with the first and second premolars, as this is a danger zone for intravascular injection and nerve injury.

Fat transfer for jawline and chin augmentation aligns well with addressing those sexual dimorphic features and performs especially well due to the musculature and supporting vasculature's ability to support a tissue graft in the specific areas of need along the mentalis and masseter. Chin augmentation is performed in and around the highly vascular mentalis muscle, blended into the prejowl sulcus and added to the posterior rami of the mandible both superficial and deep to the masseter. All of these areas can be accessed via one cannula entry site midway along the mandibular body. The superficial musculoaponeurotic system (SMAS)/platysma integrates and inserts to function as a lip depressor in the region just superior to the inferior border of the mandible; thus, it serves as excellent support during fat transfer to the jawline.

Lip Rejuvenation

Just like females, males can experience subtle volume loss to their lips over time. When treating male patients with this concern, it is of paramount importance to retain a naturally appearing lip and avoid artificial overinflation. Simple volume replacement, not enhancement, should be the goal. The authors find that avoidance of enhancing or defining the vermilion border, sometimes a telltale sign of lip augmentation, is also best avoided. Utilizing a soft, low-G′ filler yields the best outcomes in this region. In particular, some of the authors (S.B.A., L.S.) have found the HA product Versa by Revanesse to be an excellent choice for a cosmetically pleasing result and a high patient satisfaction. Injecting approximately 0.2 mL of the product evenly throughout each of the four quadrants of the vermilion body is usually sufficient for a subtle and natural-looking result. Given that bruising can be a bigger concern for male patients in this region, the authors also recommend injecting filler with a cannula technique to allow for less trauma to the lip and less swelling postprocedure.

3.3.4 Pan Facial Revolumization with Poly-L-Lactic Acid

Poly-L-lactic acid (PLLA) is unique in its ability to stimulate the host's own type 1 collagen, thus volumizing tissue in a gradual, progressive, and predictable manner.[42] It is now well understood that facial aging is a result of architectural changes in several layers of tissue contributing to changes in the topography, shape, ratios, and proportions of a youthful face. As we age, fibroblast production of collagen decelerates after the age of 25 years and eventually stops. In addition, around the fourth decade, fat malposition becomes apparent. Fat loss, particularly in the deep fat compartments, creates descent and deflation of the midface, resulting in a gaunt and tired appearance.[43] The loss of superficial fat compartments further contributes to contour deformities. After the fifth decade and beyond, craniofacial skeletal changes decrease the structural scaffolding of the face, diminishing support of the facial retention ligaments resulting in a concertina effect and sagging of the face (▶ Fig. 3.7).[14]

To alleviate the changes of the deep medial fat compartments and the periosteum of the maxilla, two insertion points are used using a fanning retrograde injection technique (▶ Fig. 3.8a, b).

The anteromedial cheek is best recreated by crosshatching these two points of entrance. It is important to avoid placing the tip of the needle near the infraorbital foramen, pulling back slowly on the plunger for 6 to 10 seconds prior to injecting to confirm the needle is not in a vessel.

The zygoma and zygomatic arch change with the passing of time. This causes a loss of support from the periosteum

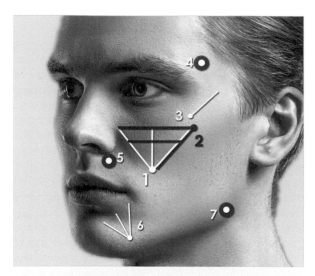

Fig. 3.7 Precise sculpt technique with poly-L-lactic acid.

and the zygomatic ligament resulting in an anteroinferior descent of the midface and the acquisition of elderly-looking features. Restoring this area with PLLA has proven to be beneficial with repeated anterograde injections parallel to bone allowing the product to track along the zygoma moving laterally toward the hairline (▶ Fig. 3.8c).

The temporal fossa is one of the most overlooked areas in the upper third of the face and contributes to a significantly aged appearance if not addressed during the rejuvenation process with PLLA. When injecting into this area, it is best to ask patients to open their mouth wide, in order to relax the temporalis muscle and the fascia. This reduces postinjection discomfort while chewing and also allows the needle to penetrate both the temporalis fascia and muscle with not much pain. The needle is introduced perpendicular to the skin over the temporal fossa using caution to avoid any visible vessels. It is important to pull back on the plunger and wait 6 to 10 seconds prior to injecting to confirm the needle is not in a vessel.

A pronounced nasolabial fold can cause one to look tired and older and continues to be one of the first anatomical changes that a patient may see with advanced age. The contributing factors can be multifactorial, but the most common causes are the descent of the overlying midfacial structures caused by retrograde bone remodeling in the upper maxilla and bone loss in the canine fossa and pyriform aperture. It is postulated that when the retention ligaments in the face loosen from a lack of support from the deeper tissues, this contributes to grooves and folds on the face (▶ Fig. 3.8e, f). Injections of PLLA directed deep toward the alar groove as well as to the deep medial fat compartments (described earlier) with a 6- to 10-second aspiration safety checks can help build support to the retention ligaments through its collagen-producing properties.

The melomental folds are often caused by lack of support from the periosteum, deep fat compartments, and the mandibular septum. Using PLLA supraperiosteal can help imitate these deeper tissues and at the same time provide support to the ligaments in this area (▶ Fig. 3.8g).

To treat this area, the mentalis muscle and soft tissue are pinched and lifted up with the injector's nondominant hand just medial to the prejowl sulcus. The needle should be introduced making sure that the tip of the needle is not inside a muscle. Again, it is important to pull back on the plunger for 6 to 10 seconds prior to injecting to confirm the needle is not in a vessel.

The ramus of the jaw can be the major contributor of jowl formation with advanced age, but often not thought of as such when trying to improve the formation of a jowl. Other contributing factors of a jowl formation are lateral fat depletion, mandibular fat accumulation, and relaxation of the mandibular septum. As we age, the ramus of the jaw remodels and loses skeletal height causing the soft tissue to slide forward. If this bony structure is recreated with the help of PLLA, one can appreciate marked improvement or resolution of a jowl depending on the gravity of the other contributing factors forming the jowl (▶ Fig. 3.8h). To treat this area with PLLA, the needle is introduced perpendicular to the skin over the most posterior portion of the ramus of the jaw bone. A 6- to 10-second aspiration safety check is recommended to confirm the needle is not in a vessel before a supraperiosteal bolus is delivered.

The variable dilution ratios, reconstitution times, injection techniques, and risk of nodule formation with PLLA can be intimidating to new injectors. The risk of nodule and papule formation in early clinical studies was 17.2%; however, in these Food and Drug Administration (FDA) studies, the reconstitution volumes were 5 mL using crosshatching injection techniques into deep dermis. Today, most experienced injectors of PLLA use greater reconstitution volumes and inject deeper onto bone or into the deep fat pads.

Patients should be instructed to massage at home using the "rule of 5s" (5 minutes, 5 times per day for 5 days). The scheduled follow-up should be in 8 to 12 weeks. Depending on the degree of volume loss, a second and even third treatment may be necessary for optimal results. Results can be maintained with yearly "touch-ups."

3.4 Complications

Injectable filler techniques are all considered blind procedures; therefore, a good understanding of facial anatomy is imperative to prevent the possibility of common adverse reactions and severe complications when injecting fillers. In addition, one must factor in that there are always variations to normal anatomy and other steps must be taken to reduce the incidence of such adverse

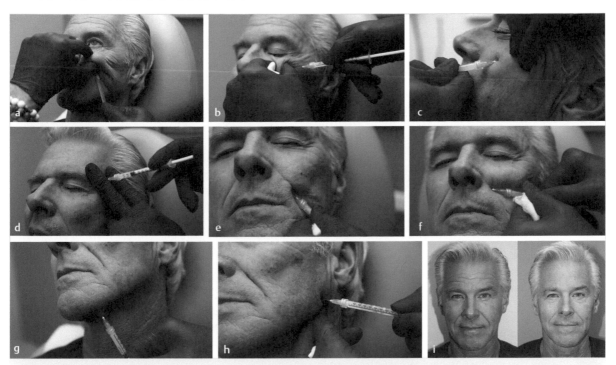

Fig. 3.8 Pan facial revolumization with poly-L-lactic acid. **(a)** Syringe no. 1: fanning retrograde. The needle is introduced approximately 2 cm inferior to the zygoma with the tip of the needle directed toward the medial canthus. Slowly inject approximately 0.2 to 0.3 mL in a retrograde fashion. Partially withdraw the needle, redirect 15 to 20 degrees laterally, and repeat the process. A total of three linear retrograde injections are performed with the last injection angled toward the lateral canthus. **(b)** Syringe no. 2: parallel retrograde/crosshatched. Slowly inject approximately 0.2 to 0.3 mL periosteally along the anteromedial cheek in a retrograde fashion. Partially withdraw the needle, redirect inferior and parallel to the first injection, and repeat the process, injecting in a retrograde fashion. Partially withdraw the needle, redirect approximately 45 degrees inferiorly, and inject the remaining 0.1 to 0.2 mL. These injections should crosshatch with those of syringe no. 1. **(c)** Syringe no. 3: anterograde push. The needle is inserted at a 30- to 45-degree angle directed laterally. Once in the subcutis, the needle angle is reduced to 5 to 10 degrees. Slowly inject in an anterograde fashion approximately 0.2 to 0.3 mL periosteally along the zygoma while holding the needle stationary. **(d)** Syringe no. 4: temporal fossa bolus. The needle is introduced perpendicular to the skin over the temporal fossa using caution to avoid any visible vessels. Advance the needle to the temporal periosteum. Pull back on the plunger prior to injecting to confirm the needle is not in a vessel. Slowly inject a periosteal bolus. The entire syringe may be used if clinically necessary. **(e)** Syringe no. 5: retrograde injection (part 1). The needle is introduced to the skin of cheek just medial to the midpoint of the nasolabial fold with the tip of the needle directed toward the alar groove. Slowly inject approximately 0.2 to 0.3 mL in a retrograde fashion parallel to the nasolabial fold. **(f)** Syringe no. 5: anterograde push (part 2). Reintroduce the needle just medial to the superior pole of the nasolabial fold injecting an anterograde push of approximately 0.2 to 0.3 mL at the pyriform aperture. **(g)** Syringe no. 6: fanning retrograde. The needle is introduced to the skin anterior and parallel to the mental tubercle with the needle directed superiorly. Advance the needle and pull back on the plunger prior to injecting to confirm the needle is not in a vessel. Slowly inject approximately 0.2 to 0.3 mL in a retrograde fashion. **(h)** Syringe no. 7: bolus at the ramus. The needle is introduced perpendicular to the skin over the most posterior portion of the ramus of the jaw bone using caution to avoid any visible vessels. Advance the needle toward the periosteum. Slowly inject a periosteal bolus. The entire syringe may be used if clinically necessary. **(i)** Before and 8 weeks after the postprocedure. The patient was treated with poly-L-lactic acid on the temple, midface, chin, and jawline. This technique is supraperiosteal with a 6-mL dilution.

reactions. The anatomical plane of all structures should be considered before injection of any fillers to decrease complications such as vascular compromise. Vascular occlusion can occur due to external compression of the blood supply by adjacent filler injection, but is more commonly associated with direct intra-arterial injection of product. Symptoms of vascular compromise are blanching of the skin, a progressive reticulated dusky or purpuric color change, and eventual ulceration with eschar formation. In the glabellar region or during frontoplasty, vascular occlusion may lead to blindness. Nerve

damage can also occur, and may present as discomfort during the injection, headache, neuralgia, and/or paresthesia postinjection.

Prior to injection of any fillers, ensure that the skin is thoroughly cleansed and devoid of any makeup or moisturizers. It is important to avoid injecting skin that has visible inflammatory lesions such as acne, rosacea, or herpes simplex. To optimize safety when injecting HA, it is important to always pull back on the plunger and count for 6 to 10 seconds before injecting to reduce the risk of an intravascular injury. However, having a negative blood flash does not guarantee that the needle is not inside a blood vessel. Utilizing a retrograde injection technique when injecting intradermal and avoiding large boluses, greater than 0.3 mL, will further reduce risk potential.

When using CaHA as an injectable filler, consider using a cannula when injecting intradermally or transferring the product to a 1-mL syringe with a rubber plunger to create suction for easier aspiration due to the fact that the provided syringe does not allow aspiration of the product.

During the frontoplasty technique, extreme precautionary measures must be taken into consideration to prevent nerve injury or vascular occlusions. Side effects are diminished by careful selection of the injection site, aspiration prior to injection if using a needle, injecting in the subgaleal space with 25- or 22-gauge cannula, and monitoring closely for signs and symptoms of vessel occlusion. The authors suggest never following the trajectory of the arteries, but rather staying perpendicular to their course.

PLLA, like any other filler, can be harmful and capable of serious adverse reactions if injected intravascularly. Therefore, the same safety measures must be applied when utilizing this product. In addition, injecting deeply along the periosteum can help reduce visible iatrogenic nodule formation.

Injecting intravascularly is one of the greatest fears of all aesthetic injectors. It is important to take all possible precautionary measures to prevent it from occurring. In the event that it does occur, prompt recognition of a potential intravascular injection is critical. Some common signs and symptoms can help alert the injector to initiate a reversal protocol immediately. The first indication is immediate blanching of the skin. The patient expressing disproportionate pain to injection is another suggestive symptom; however, due to the addition of lidocaine in most injectable fillers, not every patient may experience this. Several hours postinjection, a maroon reticulated patch appears, which tends to move superiorly from the injection site, consistent with the trajectory of the artery. A day or two later, there can be a development of pustule formation, which can be mistaken for herpes zoster or impetigo by inexperienced injectors. Subsequent darkening of the tissue indicates impending necrosis. There are several protocols in place on suspicion of an intravascular injection, but first line of defense is using hyaluronidase (500–1,500 units), avoidance of cold compresses in favor of warm compresses to increase blood flow, aspirin daily, and red LED (light-emitting diode) light treatment to increase microcirculation. Hyperbaric oxygen treatments should be considered if these steps do not lead to sign of reversal of impending necrosis. The authors also strongly recommend learning how to perform retrobulbar injections of hyaluronidase, or being able to refer the patient to a physician proficient in retrobulbar injections of hyaluronidase to prevent the risk of a vision loss from an intravascular injury.

3.5 Conclusion

More and more men are seeking out minimally invasive aesthetic procedures. In order to meet this rising demand, aesthetic practitioners must be well versed in the important anatomical differences between males and females as well as the respective differences in standards of beauty. Given that male beauty is generally associated with more angularity to the face as opposed to softer curves and contours associated with females, males can often benefit from selection of stiffer, higher G′ fillers and more structural fat grafting when injecting the mid- and lower face. Proper volume placement in the midface is of utmost importance to avoid a feminized appearance. Injecting higher quantities of filler along the mandible can help achieve a stronger, more defined jawline in keeping with a desirable male aesthetic. Use of a soft, low-G′ filler will often give the best outcome for subtle revolumization of the male lip when indicated. For long-term maintenance of the bony architecture of the face and for general skin conditioning, PLLA injections are another great tool in the armamentarium to counter the effects of aging. As with female patients, particular care should be taken to avoid outcomes that may look overdone or unnatural. A thorough understanding of underlying facial anatomy, as well as the signs and symptoms of intravascular injection, will help ensure the safety of these procedures in all patients.[44]

3.6 Pearls

- A square-shaped face is an ideal masculine feature. The temple width should line up with the lateral zygoma and projection of the mandible.
- Men's facial bone structure tends to age more linearly compared to women who undergo greater age-related changes after menopause.
- Male beauty is associated with angularity compared to softer curves and contours associated with females. As such, males often benefit from correction with stiffer high-G′ fillers and structural fat grafts.
- Upper face rejuvenation:
  - Brow position rests lower in males and can become notably ptotic with age. Frontoplasty can help correct brow positioning and shape with the progressive addition of cohesive, low-viscosity, low-G′ HA fillers or structural fat grafts.
  - A clear knowledge of anatomical boundaries and danger zones (i.e., nerves and vessels) is of paramount importance to avoid complications.

- ○ Subgaleal injections using a cannula are a safe technique and effective treatment for rejuvenation of the frontal cavity.
- Midface rejuvenation:
  - ○ A larger bizygomatic width-to-facial height ratio as measured from the upper lip to the upper eyelid or brow is perceived as being more attractive.
  - ○ Supraperiosteal injections to the midface with a high-G′ filler maximize lift and can be used to achieve a more chiseled look.
- Infraorbital hollows:
  - ○ A low-G′, low-concentration HA filler is ideal for infraorbital hallows.
  - ○ Fat transfer to the infraorbital region requires a graft with smaller cellular structure.
- Lower face rejuvenation:
  - ○ A square, well-defined jawline is a widely accepted sexually dimorphic feature associated with male attractiveness. The use of a stiff, high-G′ filler or structural fat graft placed supraperiosteally can achieve cosmetically pleasing outcomes.

References

[1] American Society of Plastic Surgeons. 2017 Plastic Surgery Statistics: Cosmetic Surgery Gender Distribution—Male. Available at: https://www.plasticsurgery.org/news/plastic-surgery-statistics. Accessed May 12, 2019

[2] Frederick DA, Lever J, Peplau LA. Interest in cosmetic surgery and body image: views of men and women across the lifespan. Plast Reconstr Surg. 2007; 120(5):1407–1415

[3] Jagdeo J, Keaney T, Narurkar V, Kolodziejczyk J, Gallagher CJ. Facial treatment preferences among aesthetically oriented men. Dermatol Surg. 2016; 42(10):1155–1163

[4] Paes EC, Teepen HJ, Koop WA, Kon M. Perioral wrinkles: histologic differences between men and women. Aesthet Surg J. 2009; 29(6):467–472

[5] Lindsey S, Rosen A, Shagalov D, Weiss E. Sex differences in perioral rhytides-does facial hair play a role? Dermatol Surg. 2019; 45(2):320–323

[6] Shuster S, Black MM, McVitie E. The influence of age and sex on skin thickness, skin collagen and density. Br J Dermatol. 1975; 93(6):639–643

[7] Aguilera SB, Branch S, Soro L. Optimizing injections of poly-L-lactic acid: the 6-step technique. J Drugs Dermatol. 2016; 15(12):1550–1556

[8] Pierre S, Liew S, Bernardin A. Basics of dermal filler rheology. Dermatol Surg. 2015; 41 Suppl 1:S120–S126

[9] Rossi AM, Fitzgerald R, Humphrey S. Facial soft tissue augmentation in males: an anatomical and practical approach. Dermatol Surg. 2017; 43 Suppl 2:S131–S139

[10] Burton JL, Johnson C, Libman L, Shuster S. Skin virilism in women with hrsutism. J Endocrinol. 1972; 53(3):349–354

[11] Keaney TC, Anolik R, Braz A, et al. The male aesthetic patient: facial anatomy, concepts of attractiveness, and treatment patterns. J Drugs Dermatol. 2018; 17(1):19–28

[12] Shaw RB, Jr, Katzel EB, Koltz PF, Kahn DM, Puzas EJ, Langstein HN. Facial bone density: effects of aging and impact on facial rejuvenation. Aesthet Surg J. 2012; 32(8):937–942

[13] Kahn DM, Shaw RB, Jr. Aging of the bony orbit: a three-dimensional computed tomographic study. Aesthet Surg J. 2008; 28(3):258–264

[14] Pessa JE. An algorithm of facial aging: verification of Lambros's theory by three-dimensional stereolithography, with reference to the pathogenesis of midfacial aging, scleral show, and the lateral suborbital trough deformity. Plast Reconstr Surg. 2000; 106(2):479–488, discussion 489–490

[15] Shaw RB, Jr, Kahn DM. Aging of the midface bony elements: a three-dimensional computed tomographic study. Plast Reconstr Surg. 2007; 119(2):675–681, discussion 682–683

[16] Mendelson BC, Hartley W, Scott M, McNab A, Granzow JW. Age-related changes of the orbit and midcheek and the implications for facial rejuvenation. Aesthetic Plast Surg. 2007; 31(5):419–423

[17] Pessa JE, Peterson ML, Thompson JW, Cohran CS, Garza JR. Pyriform augmentation as an ancillary procedure in facial rejuvenation surgery. Plast Reconstr Surg. 1999; 103(2):683–686

[18] Rohrich RJ, Hollier LH, Jr, Janis JE, Kim J. Rhinoplasty with advancing age. Plast Reconstr Surg. 2004; 114(7):1936–1944

[19] Mendelson B, Wong CH. Changes in the facial skeleton with aging: implications and clinical applications in facial rejuvenation. Aesthetic Plast Surg. 2012; 36(4):753–760

[20] Aguilera SB, Brown L, Perico VA. Aesthetic treatment of bruxism. J Clin Aesthet Dermatol. 2017; 10(5):49–55

[21] Shaw RB, Jr, Katzel EB, Koltz PF, Kahn DM, Girotto JA, Langstein HN. Aging of the mandible and its aesthetic implications. Plast Reconstr Surg. 2010; 125(1):332–342

[22] Henderson JL, Larrabee WF, Jr. Analysis of the upper face and selection of rejuvenation techniques. Otolaryngol Clin North Am. 2007; 40(2):255–265

[23] Lambros V. Observations on periorbital and midface aging. Plast Reconstr Surg. 2007; 120(5):1367–1376, discussion 1377

[24] Charles Finn J, Cox SE, Earl ML. Social implications of hyperfunctional facial lines. Dermatol Surg. 2003; 29(5):450–455

[25] Valentine KA, Li NP, Penke L, Perrett DI. Judging a man by the width of his face: the role of facial ratios and dominance in mate choice at speed-dating events. Psychol Sci. 2014; 25(3):806–811

[26] Emer J, Waldorf H. Injectable neurotoxins and fillers: there is no free lunch. Clin Dermatol. 2011; 29(6):678–690

[27] Glaich AS, Cohen JL, Goldberg LH. Injection necrosis of the glabella: protocol for prevention and treatment after use of dermal fillers. Dermatol Surg. 2006; 32(2):276–281

[28] Van Loghem J, Humzah D, Kerscher M. Cannula versus sharp needle for placement of soft tissue fillers: an observational cadaver study. Aesthet Surg J. 2017; 38(1):73–88

[29] Wysong A, Joseph T, Kim D, Tang JY, Gladstone HB. Quantifying soft tissue loss in facial aging: a study in women using magnetic resonance imaging. Dermatol Surg. 2013; 39(12):1895–1902

[30] Codinha P. Facial soft tissue thicknesses for the Portuguese adult population. Forensic Sci Int. 2009; 184(1–3):80.e1–80.e7

[31] Cha KS. Soft-tissue thickness of South Korean adults with normal facial profiles. Korean J Orthod. 2013; 43(4):178–185

[32] Toledo Avelar LE, Cardoso MA, Santos Bordoni L, de Miranda Avelar L, de Miranda Avelar JV. Aging and sexual differences of the human skull. Plast Reconstr Surg Glob Open. 2017; 5(4):e1297

[33] Farhadian JA, Bloom BS, Brauer JA. Male aesthetics: a review of facial anatomy and pertinent clinical implications. J Drugs Dermatol. 2015; 14(9):1029–1034

[34] Wysong A, Kim D, Joseph T, MacFarlane DF, Tang JY, Gladstone HB. Quantifying soft tissue loss in the aging male face using magnetic resonance imaging. Dermatol Surg. 2014; 40(7):786–793

[35] Keaney TC. Aging in the male face: intrinsic and extrinsic factors. Dermatol Surg. 2016; 42(7):797–803

[36] Aguilera SB, Tivoli YA, Seastrom SJ. How to make calcium hydroxylapatite injections safer. J Drugs Dermatol. 2014; 13(9):1015

[37] Snozzi P, van Loghem JAJ. Complication management following rejuvenation procedures with hyaluronic acid fillers-an algorithm-based approach. Plast Reconstr Surg Glob Open. 2018; 6(12):e2061

[38] Furnas DW. The retaining ligaments of the cheek. Plast Reconstr Surg. 1989; 83(1):11–16

[39] Thayer ZM, Dobson SD. Sexual dimorphism in chin shape: implications for adaptive hypotheses. Am J Phys Anthropol. 2010; 143(3):417–425

[40] Loth SR, Henneberg M. Mandibular ramus flexure: a new morphologic indicator of sexual dimorphism in the human skeleton. Am J Phys Anthropol. 1996; 99(3):473–485

[41] Brown E, Perrett DI. What gives a face its gender? Perception. 1993; 22(7):829–840

[42] Sculptra® Aesthetic. Instructions for Use. Fort Worth, TX: Galderma Laboratories, L.P.; 2016

[43] Fitzgerald R, Vleggaar D. Facial volume restoration of the aging face with poly-l-lactic acid. Dermatol Ther (Heidelb). 2011; 24(1): 2–27

[44] Chesnut C. Restoration of visual loss with retrobulbar hyaluronidase injection after hyaluronic acid filler. Dermatol Surg. 2018; 44(3): 435–437

4 High Brow Approach to Neuromodulators

Edith A. Hanna, Matthew K. Sandre, and Vince Bertucci

Summary

Although women represent the majority of patients seen in many aesthetic practices, the number of male patients is increasing. This heightened demand has been attributed to a multitude of factors including interest in enhancing one's appearance, ageism, competition in the workplace, increasing acceptance of cosmetic procedures, as well as ever-growing societal and social media pressures. Botulinum toxin A (BTX-A) treatments constitute the most popular minimally invasive cosmetic procedure by far. Whereas the general principles of BTX-A treatment for men and women are similar, it is important to acknowledge unique male characteristics that impact assessment and treatment paradigms. Attending to the distinctive needs of the male patient is paramount in order to achieve optimal clinical outcomes and enhance the overall patient experience.

Keywords: botulinum toxin, botulinum neurotoxin A, botulinum toxin serotype A, neurotoxins, neuromodulators, BTX-A, male, men

4.1 Background

The introduction of botulinum toxin A (BTX-A) to the armamentarium of cosmetic practitioners has revolutionized the field of facial rejuvenation, initiating a seismic shift in patient preferences in favor of minimally invasive procedures. In the past 15 years, BTX-A injections have become increasingly popular as a noninvasive cosmetic procedure with a 759% increase.[1] Whereas women much more commonly undergo BTX-A treatments, the number of men availing BTX-A injections has increased by 337% since 2000.[2] Men are becoming increasingly attentive to their appearance, and societal norms are evolving to create a more accepting environment for men to express their concerns and seek appropriate treatments. According to the American Society for Aesthetic Plastic Surgery, 1,638,940 women and 162,093 men underwent BTX-A treatment in 2018. Men constituted 9% of BTX-A treatments and this number continues to increase.[3] According to the American Society of Plastic Surgeons, botulinum toxin treatments were by far the most popular minimally invasive procedure in males in 2018 with a 41% share, an almost threefold margin over laser hair removal, the second-most popular.[4]

4.1.1 Motivation

From 2000 to 2018, the use of BTX-A among men increased by 381% according to the Plastic Surgery Statistics Report conducted annually by the American Society of Plastic Surgeons.[4] Even though BTX-A reduces unwanted wrinkles and rejuvenates the skin, vanity is not the only motivator behind decisions to undergo such treatment. This increase in the rate of BTX-A injections among men may be attributed to multiple factors. First and foremost, from an evolutionary perspective, an improved appearance is always desirable.[5] BTX-A treats wrinkles, thus softening facial lines, improving skin quality, and enhancing the overall appearance of the face.[6] Second, given that ageism exists in some workplaces, an aged appearance could potentially interfere with promotions, career opportunities, and personal growth.[7] As a result, men have shown more interest in receiving BTX-A injections to improve their appearance and become more competitive with their younger-looking colleagues. Third, there are shifting expectations around aging. As life expectancies rise, so are expectations for graceful aging. According to a project led by Dr Scherbov, from the International Institute for Applied Systems Analysis in Austria, given that life expectancy is increasing, people are now being viewed as "old" when they hit 65.[8] Men who are in their 60 s do not feel their age and thus avail themselves of noninvasive procedures such as BTX-A injections to maintain a youthful appearance that better matches how they feel. Finally, social media has become an integral part of society that has generated enormous pressures to look youthful. According to a report conducted by Nuffield Council on Bioethics, pressure from social media is linked to a significant rise in cosmetic procedures such as BTX-A injections.[9]

4.1.2 Demographics

Data on the demographics of men undergoing BTX-A injections are limited. According to the 2018 Plastic Surgery Statistics Report,[4] 1% of men undergoing BTX-A treatment fell into the age range between 20 and 29 years, followed by 18% of those who were in the age range between 30 and 39 years, 57% were in the age range between 40 and 45 years, whereas 23% were aged 55 and over.

In a recent systematic review by Roman and Zampella on 19 randomized controlled trials (RCTs) on BTX-A injections for facial rhytids and 22 RCTs on hyaluronic acid injectable fillers for soft-tissue augmentation, men represented 11.8% of all patients and 13.9% patients receiving BTX-A.[10] Caucasian patients represented 67.1% of the total patients, whereas Asian, Hispanic, and black patients represented 16.8, 6.5, and 5.4% of study participants, respectively.

4.2 Anatomy

4.2.1 Assessment of the Face

When assessing the male face (▶ Fig. 4.1), care must be taken to review not only the musculature that is to be

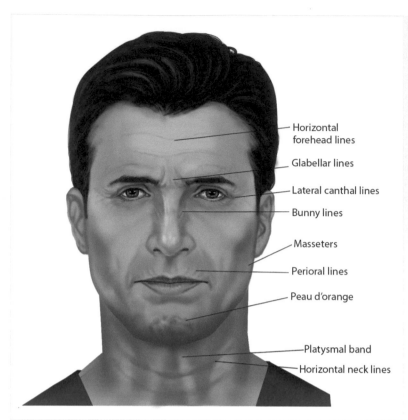

Fig. 4.1 Facial areas amenable to neuro-modulator treatment.

Horizontal forehead lines

Glabellar lines

Lateral canthal lines

Bunny lines

Masseters

Perioral lines

Peau d'orange

Platysmal band

Horizontal neck lines

targeted with neurotoxin (► Fig. 4.2) but also the skeletal shape, vasculature, and the hairline. This ensures that the physician takes into account sexual dimorphism, which is the intraspecies phenotypic difference between sexes.[11]

Bone

There are a number of differences between the male and female skull (► Fig. 4.3). Men are characteristically seen to have larger skulls than females. In reality, this reflects the observation that female skulls are roughly 80% the size of male skulls.[12,13] Starting at the more anterior aspects of the skull, men appear to have a higher, wider, flatter, and greater sloped forehead compared to females.[11,14]

Looking at the periorbital area of the male skull, the supraorbital ridge is more prominent in males, giving greater glabellar anterior projection and acting as the common landmark for male brow position.[11,12,15,16] In contrast, the female supraorbital ridge is less prominent, with the brow positioned just superior to the ridge.[17] The shape of the male brow is often flat, whereas the female brow usually peaks or arches in its lateral third portion.[17,18] Additionally, the male orbits themselves frequently have a larger height and a less oval shape.[19]

The more notable skeletal differences on the lower portion of the face between sexes are in the cheeks and chin.[12,20,21] Male cheeks or zygomas are frequently flatter but more angulated than females.[20] Finally, the male chin is seen as wider and larger than females, with male chins also having more anterior projection.[21]

Musculature

Males have approximately 1.5 times more muscle mass overall than females, yet studies are lacking that confirm if this increase also specifically applies to facial muscle mass.[22] After adjusting for facial size, men also appear to have greater facial muscle movement during lip pursing, cheek puffing, and eye-opening animations.[23] A 2009 study showed that males have greater upward motion in both of the study's analyzed facial movements—posed smile and lip pucker.[24] With regard to rhytid formation, a 2013 Japanese study of 173 males and females aged 21 to 75 years found that men have greater forehead rhytid formation across all age groups.[25] Furthermore, the study found that males had statistically significant higher rhytid scores in additional facial areas within specific age categories: 21- to 28-year-old males had higher glabellar, nasal root, and cheek rhytid scores; 35- to 41-year-old males had higher nasal root rhytid scores; and finally 47- to 59-year-old males had higher periocular rhytid scores.[25]

Males do not have more rhytids in all facial areas. For example, aging females typically have deeper rhytids than males in the perioral area.[25,26] This may be due to

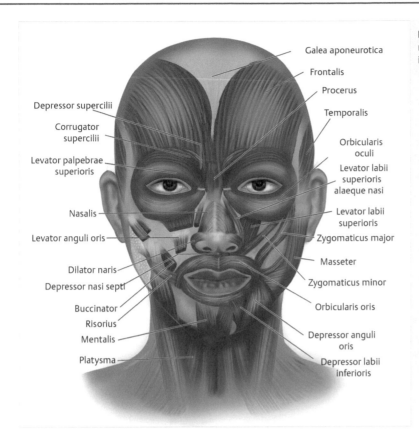

Fig. 4.2 Facial muscles relevant to botulinum toxin treatment. Note the close muscle interrelationships.

Galea aponeurotica

Frontalis

Procerus

Temporalis

Depressor supercilii

Corrugator supercilii

Levator palpebrae superioris

Orbicularis oculi

Levator labii superioris alaeque nasi

Levator labii superioris

Nasalis

Levator anguli oris

Zygomaticus major

Masseter

Dilator naris

Depressor nasi septi

Zygomaticus minor

Buccinator

Orbicularis oris

Risorius

Mentalis

Depressor anguli oris

Platysma

Depressor labii inferioris

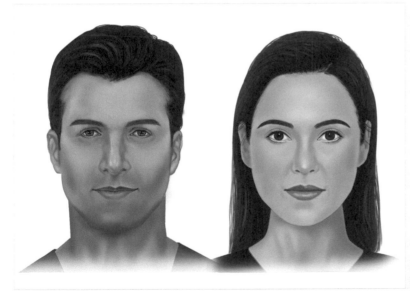

Fig. 4.3 Youthful male and female faces. Detailed knowledge of gender differences is important in optimizing male aesthetic treatment outcomes.

smaller size of the perioral pilosebaceous unit in females compared to males.[26] Thicker adipose layers are seen in female faces, which could also explain why females often have fewer or more shallow rhytids than in their male counterparts.[11,27] Of note, it has also been shown that male skin, including facial skin, can be 10 to 20% thicker than in women, which may impact injection technique.[28]

Certain facial rhytid patterns are more commonly seen in men secondary to larger facial muscle bulk and recruitment of nearby muscles.[12] For example, the "U" glabellar wrinkle pattern is seen more often in men as a result of their larger procerus muscle.[29] Men also more commonly have a downward fan lateral canthal wrinkle pattern, whereas women are seen to have central, full, or downward fan patterns.[30] The higher prevalence of the downward fan pattern in males may be secondary to greater recruitment of the zygomaticus major muscle.[12]

Some authors also suggest that the corrugator supercilii are broader in men and their distal fibers extend more laterally than in females.[31] The same author emphasizes that the frontalis is more sheetlike in men, whereas in women, it is thought of as two separate muscle bellies with absent or reduced central muscle mass.[31] Both of the aforementioned differences should be considered when planning injection patterns in male patients.

Vasculature

There appears to be an increase in vasculature in the male face when compared to the female face.[32,33] It has been hypothesized that this finding is secondary to the increased blood supply needed for the coarse terminal facial hairs in men.[11] Furthermore, an increase in the number of dermal capillaries often corresponds to greater diameter of the patient's hair follicles.[34] This increase in local vasculature is thought to increase a male's bruising risk with facial neurotoxin injection.[11] However, given that the increase in vasculature is thought to be located in areas of coarse facial hair, Keaney and Alster postulate that injecting the frontalis would not carry a similar increased risk of bruising.[11]

Hairline

A regression of the anterior, especially the anterolateral, aspects of the hairline can often occur in male androgenic alopecia.[12,35] As a result of this regression, the male forehead can appear larger.[12] The authors suggest that care should be taken to assess the most superolateral aspects of male forehead rhytids, especially if the patient has androgenetic alopecia, as failure to treat this area could draw unnecessary attention to a receding hairline.

4.3 Approach

Male patients have varying degrees of knowledge about BTX-A treatments, making it important to take the time to fully explain the process, and set realistic expectations to optimize patient satisfaction.[12] Male patients are also more likely to seek out cosmetic procedures that require less downtime and fewer visits.[12,36] The authors suggest booking a follow-up visit for all newly treated patients 2 to 3 weeks after treatment in order to optimize outcomes, build trust, and improve retention rates. Data suggest that male patients are less likely to return on their own even if they deem the outcome less than desirable.[12,37]

Minimal data exist that specifically address male neurotoxin dosing with most of it focusing on the glabella. Given increased muscle mass and strength, men generally tend to require higher doses than women.[38] As with all medical procedures, neurotoxin treatments must be individualized

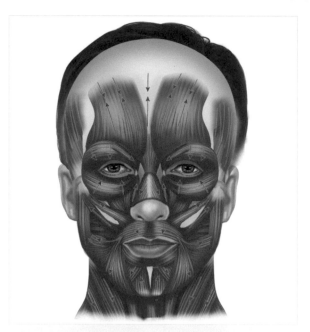

Fig. 4.4 Facial muscle vectors. Understanding precise muscle activity allows one to customize treatments and optimize outcomes.

based on unique male characteristics in order to achieve optimal clinical outcomes and enhance the overall patient experience.

The approach to BTX-A treatment involves proper assessment of muscle bulk and activity with corresponding vectors of movement (▶ Fig. 4.4), as these determine dose required and treatment pattern, respectively.[70] For the purposes of this chapter, dosing will be stated in onabotulinumtoxinA equivalents unless otherwise noted and the focus will primarily be on treatment of the upper face (▶ Table 4.1). It is important to note that dosing between BTX-A formulations is not interchangeable and units cannot be converted on a 1:1 basis.

4.3.1 Forehead and Brow

Brow height, shape, and position are key determinants of nonverbal cues perceived by others and overall facial appearance. Brow ptosis occurs naturally over time, making careful inspection of brow height critical when assessing the upper face.[12,39] Although the product monograph recommends injecting at least 2 cm superior to the eyebrow to reduce the risk of neurotoxin-induced ptosis, the authors suggest considering individual anatomy and muscle depth so as to avoid lowering the brow by inadvertently targeting the frontalis muscle.[35,40] Males typically have more noticeable forehead rhytids as they may contract the frontalis more frequently in order to raise the brow and maximize visual fields.[31] Many males have a tall forehead, meaning that one row of injections may not be

Table 4.1 Upper face botulinum toxin applications

Upper face botulinum toxin applications[a]			
Indication	Muscle(s) targeted	Injection site and dose	Tips
Forehead rhytids	Frontalis	1–2 units per site; most commonly 3–5 sites but up to 14 sites based on forehead height, brow position, and tendency to peaked brows	Assess for upper eyelid dermatochalasia and low-set eyebrows Stay ≥2 cm above brow Consider additional superior injection sites for tall foreheads
Glabellar rhytids	Procerus, corrugator supercilii, depressor supercilii	20–50 units divided among 1–2 procerus injection sites and 2–6 corrugator supercilii sites	Inject medial corrugators deeply and lateral corrugators superficially
Lateral canthal lines	Orbicularis oculi	1–4 units per site to 3–4 injection sites	Assess LCL pattern. Stay ≥1 cm outside orbital rim and superior to maxillary prominence. Consider lower dose for inferior injection sites to avoid "shelflike" cheek appearance when smiling
Lateral brow lift	Orbicularis oculi	1 unit superficially per site to 1–3 sites into the tail of the eyebrow	Works best when brows move lower with tight eye closure
Prominent infraorbital muscular ridge ("jelly roll")	Orbicularis oculi	0.5–2 units superficially 2–3 mm below ciliary margin into each of 1–2 injection sites	Perform "snap test" to assess lower eyelid elasticity to avoid ectropion and infraorbital festoons

Abbreviation: LCL, lateral canthal line.
[a]Onabotulinumtoxin A units.

adequate to achieve the desired degree of wrinkle reduction. Thus, in some cases, two rows of four to eight injection points may be needed to fully treat upper and lower frontalis rhytids.[12,39,41] One author suggests approaching this in two visits, treating the upper forehead lines at the first visit, and then subsequently treating any residual lower forehead lines at a second appointment.[31] It is also important to assess the most superolateral aspects of the forehead in male patients with a receding hairline to determine whether or not additional neurotoxin injections in this area would help reduce wrinkles in the area of temporal recession.[20,37,39,41] The authors recommend starting with conservative forehead dosing given that the frontalis is highly responsive to treatment. Additionally, because the frontalis muscle is the only brow elevator, it should not be injected without also treating the glabella. Failure to do so will result in unopposed brow depressor activity and could theoretically contribute to medial brow ptosis, especially in older male patients.

The line of convergence (C-line) is a more recently introduced concept[42] that describes a horizontal line located at approximately 60% of the total forehead height measured from the orbital rim. Below this line, the frontalis muscle lifts the eyebrows, while above the C-line, it

depresses the hairline. It is important to consider this during forehead injection planning.

Given that most men prefer flatter brow shape, it is important to consider lower lateral frontalis activity when treating the forehead. In men with prominent activity in this area, failure to treat may lead to overly peaked lateral brows, resulting in a more feminine brow appearance.[12,31,37,39,41] To avoid this, or to rectify it if it occurs, 2 units of onaBTX-A/incoBTX-A or 6 units of aboBTX-A may be injected into the lower lateral frontalis above the lateral brow or where the brow is peaking.[12,31,41] Caution is advised in individuals with upper eyelid dermatochalasis.

In less common instances where a browlift is desired in men, two approaches are suggested by one author. Treatment of only the medial aspect of the glabella, the procerus muscle, can result in elevation of the medial brow,[31] whereas neurotoxin injection into the most lateral aspect of the eyebrow targeting a portion of the orbicularis oculi muscle will elevate the lateral brow.[31] Both techniques can be combined if complete brow elevation is desired.[31] A 2016 paper by Scherer recommends a different approach for a browlift in men, which aims to raise the entire brow without a change in shape.[39] This author utilizes four injection points along the length of the superior aspect of the eyebrow itself to relax the corrugator and the upper orbital portion of the orbicularis muscle.[39] Moving medial to lateral, the injection points include the head of the eyebrow, followed by an intermediate point, then a third injection in the relative brow curvature point, and finally into the brow tail.[39] That author suggests 2.5 to 5 units per injection point, except for the medial head of the brow where 5 units are recommended.[39]

A large consensus developed recommendations in 2017 for incoBTX-A injections into male and female foreheads.[38] They divided the forehead into 12 zones (3 vertical by 4 horizontal) with the lowest four zones positioned 1.5 to 2 cm superior to the eyebrow to lower the risk of brow ptosis.[38] Separate protocols were developed for males and females, each being subdivided into normal kinetic, hyperkinetic, and hypertonic.[38] Other considerations impacting their recommended doses included forehead size, presence of palpebral weakness, hairline, and tendency to develop a Mephisto sign ("Spocking" or peaked brow).[38] The dose per injection point did not exceed 1 unit in hypertonic males or females. Slightly higher varying doses of 1 to 2 units per injection point are recommended in hyperkinetic males and females.[38] Similarly, the suggested doses for normal kinetic males and females per injection point are 1 to 2 units.[38] However, one exception is a recommendation of 3 units into each of the two central forehead zones if the normal kinetic male has palpebral weakness.[38]

4.3.2 Glabella

The glabellar complex consists of left and right corrugator supercilii muscles and the central procerus muscle that pull the brows inferomedially with contraction. When treating the glabellar area, patients should be examined both at rest and at maximal frown. The authors find it helpful to rate glabellar frown severity as mild, moderate, or severe based on the depth and width of the wrinkles. This, combined with muscle bulk, helps guide BTX-A dosing, with higher dosing required in cases of more severe dynamic wrinkles and larger muscle bulk. It is imperative to keep in mind that deep static glabellar lines, colloquially referred to as "the 11 s," are not commonly eliminated with neurotoxin treatment alone and that complementary soft-tissue filler treatment may be required to improve the contour and smoothen the "hill and valley" glabellar appearance that is sometimes evident. Interestingly, the authors find that repeated, consistent BTX-A treatments do sometimes eventually significantly improve static wrinkles.

The muscles of the glabellar complex interdigitate and are intimately related. Because of this, knowledge of anatomy and muscle depth is critical in order to maximize efficacy and minimize complications that may arise by inadvertently treating adjacent muscles. Asking the patient

to frown allows the belly of the procerus and corrugators to be visualized and grasped between the thumb and the index finger, facilitating injection accuracy. Whereas Food and Drug Administration (FDA) product monographs for all approved BTX-A products suggest staying at least 1 cm above the bony supraorbital rim when injecting the corrugators, the authors recommend individual evaluation in order to allow treatments to be tailored to the individual's unique anatomy. Note that injecting the glabellar area could potentially stimulate the trigeminal nerve and thus trigger a sneezing sensation or response.

The first injection is centrally placed perpendicularly into the procerus over the area of greatest muscle bulk. If the procerus muscle is long and demonstrates significant activity, two separate midline injection sites rather than the standard single injection may be advantageous.[43] Once again, injection depth must be tailored to procerus muscle depth with more inferior injections being deeper than more superior ones. Given that more men appear to have a "U" glabellar pattern, injecting both the superior and inferior portions of the procerus muscle may be advisable.[29]

When injecting the corrugators, it is important to consider the origin and insertion of the muscle. Because the corrugator originates on bone medially and then becomes more superficial laterally, interdigitating with the frontalis muscle, it is best to inject deeply medially and more superficially laterally. Failure to inject superficially laterally may result in brow ptosis due to inadvertent weakening of the frontalis muscle. The number of injections will be determined by factors such as the extent of the corrugator muscle and the desire to avoid brow ptosis in individuals with low-set brows, as detailed later.

Glabellar BTX-A injection patterns are best determined based on the five described muscle contraction patterns, namely, the "U," "V," "omega," "converging arrows," and "inverted omega" dynamic wrinkle patterns.[44] In Koreans, the patterns described include "U," "11," "X," "π (pi)," and "I."[29]

Care should be taken to assess brow position, shape, and symmetry when treating the glabellar complex. All of this must be done in conjunction with assessment of the forehead as the frontalis muscle greatly influences brow position, serving as the only brow elevator. If the brows are asymmetric, it is important to point this out to the patient prior to treatment. In deciding how to proceed in such cases, analysis of the medial, central, and lateral portions of the brow should be considered. When the medial portion of the brow is low, this may sometimes be corrected by injecting the belly of the medial corrugator muscle deeply over the inferomedial portion of the brow, thus reducing the downward pull of the medial head of the corrugator muscle, thus allowing for more superolateral positioning of the medial brow. On the other hand, if the lateral portion of the brow is low, this may be due to contraction of the descending lateral orbicularis oculi muscle fibers that pull the tail of the brow inferomedially in a purse-string fashion. Ascertaining the contribution of lateral orbicularis oculi activity to lateral brow position may be done by asking the patient to tightly close the eyes and observing changes in brow position. When the lateral brow moves inferomedially, this implies that the orbicularis oculi muscle plays a significant role in lowering the lateral brow and, thus, a series of one to three low-dose BTX-A injections into the tail of the brow can minimize the downward pull and lead to lateral brow lift. Conversely, if there is no downward movement of the lateral brow when tightly closing the eyes, such injections are unlikely to help lift the lateral brow.

Reshaping the brow area may also be accomplished by strategic placement of BTX-A in the frontalis muscle. Injections in the lower portion of frontalis will lessen the ability to raise the brow, thus resulting in lower brow position, whereas injections higher up on the forehead typically have the opposite effect, elevating the brows. Utilizing a "**V**"- or "**M**"-shaped forehead injection pattern will typically create a more arched brow, whereas forehead injections carried out in a straight horizontal line typically yield a straighter brow.

Brow position and eyelids must be assessed carefully prior to treating the glabellar complex. Individuals who manifest upper eyelid dermatochalasis or who have naturally low-set brows may be at higher risk of brow ptosis with treatment of the glabella. Injection of the lateral corrugators may weaken the lower frontalis fibers, causing the brows to drop and eyelids to become heavier. Thus, in these cases, it is critical to reduce the number of lateral injection sites and/or dose of BTX-A. Alternatively, lateral corrugator treatment may be omitted altogether as an added precautionary measure. Unfortunately, this will lead to residual lateral corrugator activity, leading to medial movement of the skin and thus contributing to incomplete effacement of glabellar furrows. Patients that desire a more "frozen" look over the glabella must be advised that this may come at the expense of heavier brows and eyelids, potentially producing a more tired appearance.

One of the first neurotoxin dose response studies in men was published by Carruthers and Carruthers in 2005.[45] The study evaluated 20-, 40-, 60-, and 80-unit doses of BTX-A distributed among seven glabellar complex sites in 80 men.[45] The 40-, 60-, and 80-unit doses were consistently more effective with longer duration, higher peak response rate, and greater improvement from baseline compared to the 20-unit dose in a dose-dependent manner. Importantly, the incidence of adverse events was not increased with higher doses.[45] The authors concluded that the FDA- and Health Canada–approved glabellar dose of 20 units of BTX-A is too low in male patients and they recommended starting at 40 units.

A randomized, placebo-controlled study of 50 units of aboBTX-A for glabellar lines found that women had a substantially better response as measured by none or mild wrinkles at day 30 than men (93 vs. 67%).[46] The authors similarly concluded that 50 units of aboBTX-A is too low of a starting dose for the male glabellar complex.[46]

A second randomized, placebo-controlled trial of aboBTX-A injection into the glabellar complex was conducted with dosing adjustments based on gender and glabellar muscle mass.[47] Male patients enrolled in the study received 60 to 80 units of aboBTX-A, whereas female dosing ranged from 50 to 60 units. Overall, despite higher dosing, males were still less likely to respond than females; however, the response rate was higher than that reported by other studies using 50 units of aboBTX-A.[47]

A 2009 study suggested a 7-point injection approach for treating the glabella where all injections are located between the midpupillary vertical lines and focus on targeting the lateral corrugator insertion point.[48] Failure to treat the lateral corrugators can result in an irregular contraction pattern.[12,31,48]

Finally, when treating the glabellar complex, it is important to realize that splaying of the eyebrows may occur as a result of reduced inferomedial muscle movement, leading to change in facial appearance.[48]

4.3.3 Lateral Canthus

Lateral periorbital rhytids are a product of orbicularis oculi muscle contraction and, to a lesser extent, contraction of the zygomaticus major muscle. It is imperative to ascertain the relative contribution of each muscle in order to formulate an appropriate injection pattern. Similar to other areas, the deeper the dynamic lateral canthal lines (LCLs), the higher the dose generally needed. Additionally, the more extensive the area of involvement, the greater the number of injection sites required.

Diagnostically, the relative contribution from orbicularis oculi and zygomaticus muscles may be determined by having the patient make expressions that utilize different muscle groups. A big smile that includes cheek movement is caused by a combination of orbicularis oculi and zygomaticus major activity. In contrast, "squinting" as if in a sandstorm without cheek movement is mostly caused by orbicularis oculi movement. Thus, wrinkles in patients who have LCLs with a big smile but not with squinting are predominantly due to zygomaticus major muscle activity and, thus, they will have a suboptimal response to orbicularis oculi treatment. Conversely, if wrinkles are also present with squinting, it is expected that orbicularis oculi treatment will give significant improvement. Communicating this to the patient prior to treatment is paramount in achieving patient satisfaction.

The standard on-label injection pattern for LCLs consists of 4 units into each of three sites per side for a total of six injection points, and a total of 24 units of BTX-A or equivalent per point.[40] The first lateral canthal injection should be placed at least 1 cm temporal to the lateral canthus in order to avoid diffusion to extraocular muscles and the palpebral portion of the orbicularis oculi which can result in strabismus and lid ptosis.

When treating the LCLs, injections should be superficial given that the orbicularis oculi muscle is thin. However, given that males have thicker skin, the depth of injection and dosing may need to be modified accordingly.[28]

In men who have more lateral extension of LCLs, an additional row of injections lateral to the first row may be considered.[31] However, a consensus panel was divided on this approach.[49] Those against it suggested addressing volume loss to treat elongated LCLs, whereas others encouraged the use of a second row of neurotoxin when significant sun damage and cosmetic surgeries, such as facelifts, were the suspected etiology.[49]

As noted earlier, men more frequently exhibit the downward fan LCL pattern. Even in these cases, three injection points are encouraged while paying attention not to venture medial to a vertical line drawn through the lateral canthus or lower than the maxillary prominence.[30] Exercising caution when injecting the lower LCLs will help avoid inadvertent weakening of the zygomaticus major muscle, inability to raise the corner of the mouth when smiling, and a resultant asymmetric or "crooked" smile.

The authors note that naturalness of the smile is frequently overlooked when considering LCL treatment. In individuals with large cheeks, treatment of this area can lead to a shelflike appearance at the LCL–cheek junction consisting of anterior overprojection of the cheeks with a sudden stop at this junction and above which there is no projection, thus creating a linear demarcation between the two zones.[50] To better understand this, reviewing the anatomy of this area is instructional. The zygomaticus major muscle originates from the lateral aspect of the zygomatic bone in the superior cheek region and runs inferomedially inserting at the angle of the mouth. It contributes to lifting of both the middle and superior cheek regions. The authors surmise that the shelflike appearance is caused by weakening of the superior portion of the zygomaticus major muscle with reduced ability to lift the uppermost part of the cheek. The upper noncontractile area appears flatter, in contrast to the contractile portion below which creates volume due to muscle activity, and which combined with the inability to lift the cheek beyond this point means that cheek volume can only move anteriorly. The resultant effect is a shelflike appearance with a line of demarcation separating the overly projected cheek inferior to the line and flattening above it.

These nuances must be addressed during the consultation process to ensure that realistic expectations are set.

4.3.4 Masseters

BTX-A use outside the upper face is less common in males.[12,31] Important considerations when formulating a treatment plan include assessment of facial proportion and shape, especially the lower face, and the presence or absence of jowls. The patient should be examined both at rest and while clenching the teeth. If the facial shape is such that there is excess bulging at and above the mandibular angle and if the muscle is palpable with contraction, treatment may be indicated if a less square shape is desired. However, the presence of jowls or skin laxity may be a relative contraindication as treatment in these cases may lead to worsening of the jowls.

Generally speaking, because men typically prefer a square lower facial contour, treatment of the masseters to reduce muscle bulk is less commonly employed than in women, who often prefer a rounder contour. Having said that, masseter treatment has also been utilized to balance masseter asymmetry[41] and in the treatment of bruxism.[51,52] As with other areas, the larger the muscle mass, the higher the dose of BTX-A required. Injecting 1 cm lateral to the anterior border of the masseter muscle will help prevent inadvertent weakening of the risorius muscle and resultant smile asymmetry. Focusing injections on the lower half of the muscle is considered safest.[53]

A 20 to 50% higher dose than that used in females has been suggested.[12] A consensus group recommended from one to five injection points per side consisting of 5 to 15 units of BTX-A or equivalent per injection point.[49] Three to four injection sites per side is most common in our practice and we recommend titrating the dose so as to achieve the desired degree of muscle bulk reduction and facial contour. Typical total dosing is 15 to 40 units of BTX-A per side.

4.3.5 Other Facial Uses

A myriad of other BTX-A indications have been reported over the years. In the region of the lower eyelid, reduction of the lower eyelid "jelly roll" appearance by treating the hypertrophic orbicularis oculi muscle may be accomplished by injecting 2 to 4 units of BTX-A or equivalent approximately 3 mm below the ciliary margin in the midpupillary line.[54,55] Additionally, it is possible to widen the aperture of the eye and create a more rounded appearance by injecting 0.5 to 1 unit intracutaneously per side in the midpupillary line. This results in lowering of the inferior ciliary margin and creation of "almond-shaped" eyes.[49] We advise against treating the infraorbital region in cases of lower eyelid skin laxity and when there is delayed recoil when tugging on the lower eyelid skin and releasing it so as to avoid excessive scleral show and festooning.

In cases of LCLs that extend inferiorly to form fine, hyperdynamic "accordion" cheek lines, superficial injection of very low doses of dilute BTX-A has been used to improve the depth and extent of the lines.[56] The number of units used varies widely with the area to be covered, but the underlying principle is to inject very low doses over a large surface area in a large volume of reconstitution so as to avoid weakening the zygomaticus muscles.

Usages in the midface include treatment of bunny lines, nasal flare, and nasal tip droop (▶ Table 4.2). Bunny lines are treated by targeting the nasalis muscle and levator labii superioris alaeque nasi (LLSAN). The authors typically utilize one to two injection sites per proximal nasal sidewall and one in the proximal dorsal nose midline with total dosing between 6 and 15 BTX-A units. Nasal flare is treated by targeting the dilator naris muscle, the alar portion of the nasalis muscle, as well as the medial portion of LLSAN. One to 2 units of BTX-A in each mid-nasal ala are

typically used. For individuals with nasal tip droop that is accentuated when enunciating "Peter" or "Bob," nasal tip elevation may be achieved by targeting the depressor septi nasi muscle with 2 to 6 units of BTX-A just above the nasocolumellar junction.

Other neurotoxin indications in the lower face and neck include perioral rhytids, gummy smile, downturned corners of the mouth, mental crease, *peau d'orange* chin, and platysmal bands (▶ Table 4.3).

For dynamic perioral rhytids, the orbicularis oris may be targeted with low doses of BTX-A. Caution is advised so as to avoid adverse events such as lip weakness and

Table 4.2 Midface face botulinum toxin applications

Midface face botulinum toxin applications[a]			
Indication	Muscle(s) targeted	Injection site and dose	Tips
Nasal "bunny" lines	Nasalis	2–5 units into each nasal sidewall muscle belly and into the midline of the nasal dorsum	Stay above the nasofacial groove to avoid inadvertent injection of the levator labii superioris and the lip ptosis
Nasal flare	Dilator naris	1–5 units into each lateral nasal ala	Inject the most active area. Most commonly 1–2 units per ala
Nasal tip droop	Depressor septi nasi	2–3 units just above the base of the columella	Do not inject into the cutaneous upper lip

[a]Onabotulinumtoxin A units.

Table 4.3 Lower face and neck botulinum toxin applications

Lower face and neck botulinum toxin applications[a]			
Usage	Muscle Targeted	Injection site and Dose	Tips
Perioral rhytids	Orbicularis oris	1–2 units per lip quadrant	Avoid in singers and wind-instrument musicians. Avoid lip corners and midline. Exercise caution in individuals with soft-tissue atrophy
Gummy smile	Levator labii superioris alaeque nasi	1–2 units per site (1–3 sites per side) based on gummy smile pattern	Carefully assess gummy smile pattern to determine injection sites
Downturned corners of the mouth ("mouth frown")	Depressor anguli oris	2–5 units into each DAO just above the angle of the mandible and 1 cm lateral to melomental fold	Stay lateral and low to avoid the depressor labii inferioris (DLI) muscle
Peau d'orange chin	Mentalis	1–3 units into each of 1–4 injection points	Avoid injecting too far laterally to avoid DLI
Platysmal bands	Platysma	2–4 units per injection site with 2–4 sites per muscle band, spaced 1–1.5 cm apart	Multiple approaches are possible. Beware of excess muscle weakening. Most effective when there is good baseline cervical skin elasticity

Abbreviation: DAO, depressor anguli oris.

[a]Onabotulinumtoxin A units.

mouth incontinence. These associated adverse events resolved in 21 days in 87% of 60 participants in a randomized clinical trial.[57] By injecting at two to four sites in each of the upper and lower lip perioral region with a total of 1 to 8 units of BTX-A, the lines may be softened. Of note, injecting closer to the vermillion border will result in more lip eversion.

Excessive gingival display, also referred to as gummy smile, is caused by overactivity of one or more muscles including the LLSAN, zygomaticus minor, zygomaticus major, and levator labii superioris. Determining whether the gummy smile is anterior, posterior, or both will dictate the injection site pattern. Typically, one to two injection sites per side with total dosing of 1 to 4 units per side are utilized. However, in some cases, up to three sites and 8 units per side may be required.[49,58,59]

Depressor anguli oris (DAO) activity, which may contribute to downturned corners of the mouth, may be demonstrated by asking the patient to show their bottom teeth or by pronouncing the letter "e" in an exaggerated manner. A total of 2 to 5 units of BTX-A injected at one or two sites per side may be used if there is prominent downward pull of the oral commissures. Injections are typically placed close to the mandible at the origin of the DAO. By staying lateral to the melomental fold, the risk of inadvertent weakening of the depressor labii inferioris (DLI) will be diminished. A split-face clinical trial of 20 patients revealed no difference between 10 units of aboBTX-A and 4 units onaBTX-A in treating the DAO muscle.[60]

Individuals with mentalis muscle overactivity often display dimpling of the chin, also referred to as *peau d'orange*, as well as chin shortening. A total of 2 to 8 units of BTX-A may be injected into the mentalis muscle using one to four injection points to address these issues. This treatment will also help reduce the mental crease. Staying medial to the lateral border of the mentalis will help prevent weakening of the DLI muscle and avoid resultant lower lip asymmetry. This often-overlooked area is especially important in men as it can serve to enhance the chin, thus restoring masculine features.

Dilute, low-dose BTX-A, termed "Microbotox" by one author, has been used to target the superficial muscle fibers that insert into the undersurface of skin that are responsible for fine lines and wrinkles.[61] Low doses of BTX-A reconstituted with large volumes of normal saline have been used with the goal being to avoid weakening of deeper muscles and thereby prevent unwanted facial muscle weakness and asymmetry. Multiple systematic injections at 0.8- to 1-cm intervals with reconstitution ranging from 5 to 10 mL of normal saline per 100 units of BTX-A have been advocated.[62,63,64,65]

Last but not least, the platysma, a superficial muscle of paramount importance in the aging of the lower face and neck, can be modulated with BTX-A. The platysma originates in the superficial fascia of the pectoralis muscle, ascends over the clavicle and mandible, and inserts into the mandible and lateral oral commissures. Importantly, the platysmal fibers are continuous with the superficial musculoaponeurotic system (SMAS) of the face and the lower facial muscles such as the orbicularis oris, DAO, DLI, risorius, and mentalis, thus serving as a lower face depressor.[66] Treatment of the upper platysma with BTX-A therefore impacts the lower face dynamic and contour. De Almeida et al retrospectively analyzed the lower face of 161 patients who had received two injections into the mentalis muscle and two horizontal lines of superficial BTX-A injections above and below the mandible, with a total dose of 14 to 18 units per side.[67] This resulted in a reduction in horizontal lines that appear below the mandible and the chin, reduced horizontal lines in the lower face below the oral commissures, and reduced vertical rhytids lateral to the corners of the mouth.[68]

4.3.6 Scrotal Wrinkling

A less frequently recognized and utilized use of BTX-A in male patients has been for scrotal wrinkling, which has been colloquially termed "Scrotox" by some. Literature on this application is very scant and dose recommendations are anecdotal. It has been hypothesized that treatment of the dartos muscle of the scrotum can result in a smoother scrotal surface.[69]

4.4 Approved Indications and Dosing

It is important to note that FDA-approved injection patterns and dosing for BTX-A are not gender specific. Recommendations contained herein are based on available literature and the senior author's clinical experience.

There are currently four FDA-approved botulinum toxins that are used for the treatment of glabellar, forehead, and LCLs (▶ Table 4.4), and other toxins are presently in development in the United States and Canada, including daxiBTX-A, letiBTX-A, and botulinum toxin E (▶ Fig. 4.5). Additionally, liquid formulations that do not require reconstitution (e.g., MT10109 L by Allergan; QM-1114 by Galderma) are being developed.[71,72] Liquid formulations offer convenience by eliminating the need for reconstitution while minimizing the risk of contamination and errors in reconstitution. One drawback of liquid formulations is that the volume of reconstitution cannot be reduced from that chosen by the manufacturer, meaning that smaller volume injections with less spread of neuromodulator will not be possible.

Table 4.4 FDA-approved indications and dosing for botulinum toxins

Botulinum toxin	Site		
	Glabella	Forehead	Lateral canthus
OnabotulinumtoxinA	20 units divided equally among five injection sites (two sites per corrugator and one in the procerus muscle)	20 units equally divided among five injection sites	12 units per side equally divided among three injection sites
AbobotulinumtoxinA	50 units among five injection sites	N/A	N/A
IncobotulinumtoxinA	20 units among five injection sites	N/A	N/A
PrabotulinumtoxinA	20 units among five injection sites	N/A	N/A

Abbreviation: FDA, Food and Drug Administration.

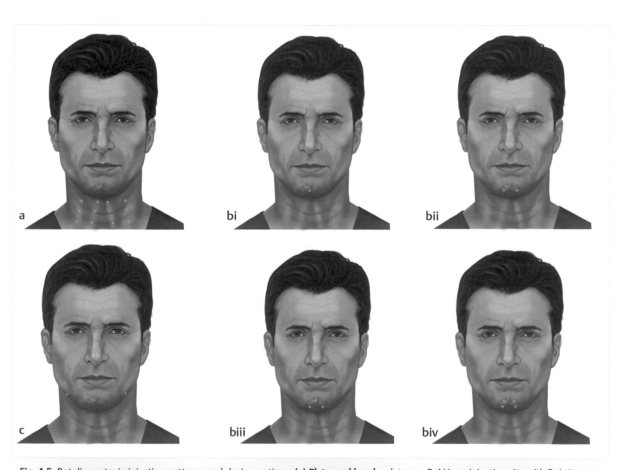

Fig. 4.5 Botulinum toxin injection patterns and dosing options: **(a) Platysmal bands**, *platysma*, 2-4 U per injection site with 2-4 sites per side; (bi-iv) **'peau d'orange' chin**, *mentalis*, 1-3 U into each of 1-4 injection points. The authors choose 3 injection points in many cases; **(c) downturned corners of mouth**, *depressor anguli oris*, 2-5 U into each DAO just above the angle of the mandible and 1 cm lateral to the melomental fold.

(Continued)

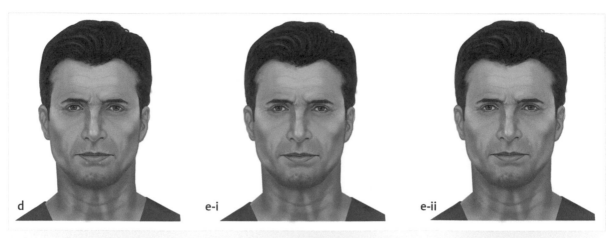

Fig. 4.5 (*Continued*) **(d) Perioral rhytids**, 1-2 U per lip quadrant; **(ei-ii) gummy smile**, *levator labii superioris alaeque nasi, zygomaticus major, zygomaticus* minor, 1-2 U per site (1-3 sites per side) based on gummy smile pattern. **Posterior gummy smile injection sites:** • Inject in nasolabial fold at point of maximal lateral contraction during smile. • 2 cm lateral to the point noted above at level of tragus. **Anterior gummy smile injection sites:** • 1 cm lateral and just inferior to nasal ala.

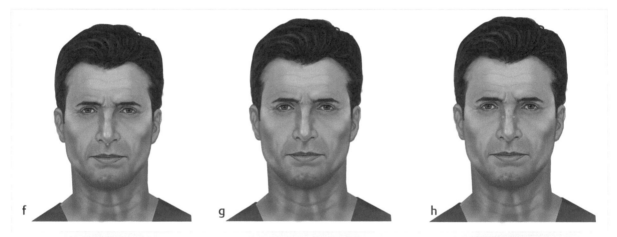

Fig. 4.5 (*Continued*) **(f) Nasal tip droop**, *depressor septi nasi*, 2-3 U just above base of columella; **(g) nasal flare**, *dilator naris*, 1-5 U into each lateral nasal ala, most commonly 1-2 units; **(h) nasal 'bunny' lines**, *nasalis*, 2-5 U into each nasal sidewall muscle belly and into midline of nasal dorsum at area of maximal muscle activity.

(Continued)

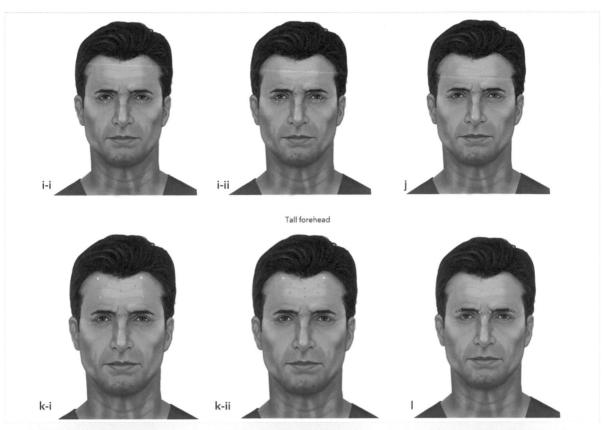

Fig. 4.5 (*Continued*) **(i-i and i-ii) Prominent infraorbital muscular ridge ('jelly roll')**, *orbicular oculi*, 0.5-2 U superficially 2-3 mm below ciliary margin into each of 1-2 injection sites; **(j) lateral canthal lines**, *obicularis oculi*, 1-4 U per site to 3-4 superficial injection sites; **(ki-ii) forehead rhytids**, *frontalis*, 1-2 U per site. Most commonly 3-5 sites but up to 14 sites based on forehead height, brow position, tendency to peaked brows (●) and receding hairline ( ). Pattern is adjusted on a per-patient basis; **(l) lateral brow lift** (●), *orbicularis oculi*, 1 U superficially into each of 1-3 sites over the tail of the eyebrow. **Medial brow lift** ( ), *procerus*, as per glabellar rhytid dosing.

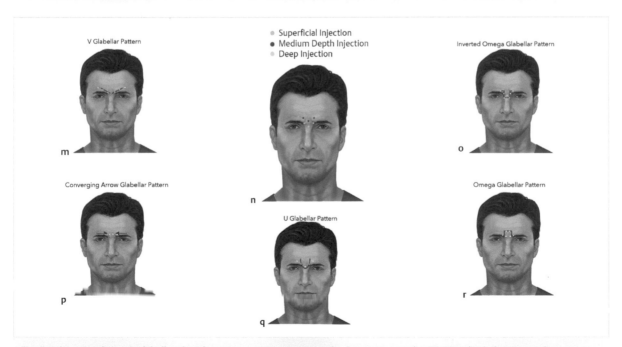

Fig. 4.5 (*Continued*) **(m-r) Glabellar rhytids**, *procerus, corrugator supercilii, depressor supercilia*, 20-50 U divided among 1-2 *procerus* injection sites and 2-6 or more *corrugator* and *depressor supercilii* sites. The solid red lines (—) and arrows (→) reflect the glabellar contraction patterns; the white dots ( ) represent potential injection sites.

4.5 Pearls

- Given the increased popularity of botulinum toxin A (BTX-A) treatments amongst male patients, it is imperative to understand the unique male characteristics that influence assessment and treatment paradigms.
- A number of differences in bone, vasculature, musculature, and hairline imply a distinctive approach when treating the male patient with BTX-A in order to achieve optimal clinical outcomes.

References

[1] American Society of Plastic Surgeons. 2015 Plastic Surgery Statistics Report. Available at: http://www.plasticsurgery.org/Documents/news-resources/statistics/2015-statistics/cosmetic-procedure-trends-2015.pdf. Accessed February 15, 2016

[2] American Society of Plastic Surgeons. 2014 Plastic Surgery Statistics Report. Available at: https://www.plasticsurgery.org/documents/News/Statistics/2014/plastic-surgery-statistics-full-report-2014.pdf

[3] The American Society for Aesthetic Plastic Surgery. Cosmetic (Aesthetic) Surgery National Data Bank STATISTICS. 2018. Available at: https://www.surgery.org/sites/default/files/ASAPS-Stats2018.pdf

[4] American Society of Plastic Surgeons. 2018 Plastic Surgery Statistics Report. Available at: https://www.plasticsurgery.org/documents/News/Statistics/2018/plastic-surgery-statistics-full-report-2018.pdf

[5] Swift A, Remington K. BeautiPHIcation™: a global approach to facial beauty. Clin Plast Surg. 2011; 38(3):347–377, v

[6] Jandhyala R. Impact of botulinum toxin a on the quality of life of subjects following treatment of facial lines. J Clin Aesthet Dermatol. 2013; 6(9):41–45

[7] Hosoda M, Stone-Romero EF, Coats G. The effects of physical attractiveness on job-related outcomes: a meta-analysis of experimental studies. Person Psychol. 2003; 56(2):431–462

[8] Sanderson WC, Scherbov S. Faster increases in human life expectancy could lead to slower population aging. PLoS One. 2015; 10(4): e0121922

[9] Nuffield Council on Bioethics. Cosmetic Procedures: Ethical Issues. 2017. Available at: https://www.nuffieldbioethics.org/wp-content/uploads/Cosmetic-procedures-full-report.pdf

[10] Roman J, Zampella JG. Demographics of men and minorities in cosmetic clinical trials of botulinum toxin and hyaluronic acid fillers. Dermatol Surg. 2020; 46(9):1164–1168

[11] Keaney TC, Alster TS. Botulinum toxin in men: review of relevant anatomy and clinical trial data. Dermatol Surg. 2013; 39(10):1434–1443

[12] Green JB, Keaney TC. Aesthetic treatment with botulinum toxin: approaches specific to men. Dermatol Surg. 2017; 43 Suppl 2:S153–S156

[13] Krogman WM. Craniofacial growth and development: an appraisal. J Am Dent Assoc. 1973; 87(5):1037–1043

[14] Whitaker LA, Morales L, Jr, Farkas LG. Aesthetic surgery of the supraorbital ridge and forehead structures. Plast Reconstr Surg. 1986; 78 (1):23–32

[15] Garvin HM, Ruff CB. Sexual dimorphism in skeletal browridge and chin morphologies determined using a new quantitative method. Am J Phys Anthropol. 2012; 147(4):661–670

[16] Russell MD. The supraorbital torus a most remarkable peculiarity. Curr Anthropol. 1985; 26(3):337–360

[17] Gunter JP, Antrobus SD. Aesthetic analysis of the eyebrows. Plast Reconstr Surg. 1997; 99(7):1808–1816

[18] Goldstein SM, Katowitz JA. The male eyebrow: a topographic anatomic analysis. Ophthal Plast Reconstr Surg. 2005; 21(4):285–291

[19] Pretorius E, Steyn M, Scholtz Y. Investigation into the usability of geometric morphometric analysis in assessment of sexual dimorphism. Am J Phys Anthropol. 2006; 129(1):64–70

[20] Keaney T. Male aesthetics. Skin Therapy Lett. 2015; 20(2):5–7

[21] Thayer ZM, Dobson SD. Sexual dimorphism in chin shape: implications for adaptive hypotheses. Am J Phys Anthropol. 2010; 143 (3):417–425

[22] Janssen I, Heymsfield SB, Wang ZM, Ross R. Skeletal muscle mass and distribution in 468 men and women aged 18–88 yr. J Appl Physiol (1985). 2000; 89(1):81–88

[23] Weeden JC, Trotman CA, Faraway JJ. Three dimensional analysis of facial movement in normal adults: influence of sex and facial shape. Angle Orthod. 2001; 71(2):132–140

[24] Houstis O, Kiliaridis S. Gender and age differences in facial expressions. Eur J Orthod. 2009; 31(5):459–466

[25] Tsukahara K, Hotta M, Osanai O, Kawada H, Kitahara T, Takema Y. Gender-dependent differences in degree of facial wrinkles. Skin Res Technol. 2013; 19(1):e65–e71

[26] Paes EC, Teepen HJ, Koop WA, Kon M. Perioral wrinkles: histologic differences between men and women. Aesthet Surg J. 2009; 29(6): 467–472

[27] Sjöström L, Smith U, Krotkiewski M, Björntorp P. Cellularity in different regions of adipose tissue in young men and women. Metabolism. 1972; 21(12):1143–1153

[28] Bailey SH, Oni G, Brown SA, et al. The use of non-invasive instruments in characterizing human facial and abdominal skin. Lasers Surg Med. 2012; 44(2):131–142

[29] Kim HS, Kim C, Cho H, Hwang JY, Kim YS. A study on glabellar wrinkle patterns in Koreans. J Eur Acad Dermatol Venereol. 2014; 28(10): 1332–1339

[30] Kane MA, Cox SE, Jones D, Lei X, Gallagher CJ. Heterogeneity of crow's feet line patterns in clinical trial subjects. Dermatol Surg. 2015; 41 (4):447–456

[31] Flynn TC. Botox in men. Dermatol Ther. 2007; 20(6):407–413

[32] Mayrovitz HN, Regan MB. Gender differences in facial skin blood perfusion during basal and heated conditions determined by laser Doppler flowmetry. Microvasc Res. 1993; 45(2):211–218

[33] Moretti G, Ellis RA, Mescon H. Vascular patterns in the skin of the face. J Invest Dermatol. 1959; 33:103–112

[34] Montagna W, Ellis RA. Histology and cytochemistry of human skin. XIII. The blood supply of the hair follicle. J Natl Cancer Inst. 1957; 19 (3):451–463

[35] Bolognia J, Schaffer JV, Cerroni L. Alopecias. In: Dermatology: 2-Volume Set. 4th ed. Philadelphia, PA: Elsevier; 2018:1162–1185

[36] Ross EV. Nonablative laser rejuvenation in men. Dermatol Ther. 2007; 20(6):414–429

[37] Rossi AM. Men's aesthetic dermatology. Semin Cutan Med Surg. 2014; 33(4):188–197

[38] Anido J, Arenas D, Arruabarrena C, et al. Tailored botulinum toxin type A injections in aesthetic medicine: consensus panel recommendations for treating the forehead based on individual facial anatomy and muscle tone. Clin Cosmet Investig Dermatol. 2017; 10:413–421

[39] Scherer MA. Specific aspects of a combined approach to male face correction: botulinum toxin A and volumetric fillers. J Cosmet Dermatol. 2016; 15(4):566–574

[40] Allergan Pharmaceuticals Ireland. Full prescribing information: Botox cosmetic (onabotulinumtoxin A) for injection, for intramuscular use. 2020. Available at: https://media.allergan.com/actavis/actavis/media/allergan-pdf-documents/product-prescribing/20190626-BOTOX-Cosmetic-Insert-72715US10-Med-Guide-v2-0MG1145.pdf

[41] Haiun M, Cardon-Fréville L, Picard F, Meningaud JP, Hersant B. Particularités des injections de toxine botulique pour le traitement esthétique du visage chez l'homme. Une mise au point de la littérature. Ann Chir Plast Esthet. 2019; 64(3):259–265

[42] Cotofana S, Freytag DL, Frank K, et al. The bidirectional movement of the frontalis muscle: introducing the line of convergence and its potential clinical relevance. Plast Reconstr Surg. 2020; 145(5):1155–1162

[43] Beer JI, Sieber DA, Scheuer JF, III, Greco TM. Three-dimensional facial anatomy: structure and function as it relates to injectable neuromodulators and soft tissue fillers. Plast Reconstr Surg Glob Open. 2016; 4(12) Suppl Anatomy and Safety in Cosmetic Medicine: Cosmetic Bootcamp:e1175

[44] De Almeida ART, da Marques ERMC, Kadunc BV. Glabellar wrinkles: a pilot study of contraction patterns. Surg Cosmet Dermatol.. 2010; 2 (1):23–28

[45] Carruthers A, Carruthers J. Prospective, double-blind, randomized, parallel-group, dose-ranging study of botulinum toxin type A in men with glabellar rhytids. Dermatol Surg. 2005; 31(10):1297–1303

[46] Brandt F, Swanson N, Baumann L, Huber B. Randomized, placebo-controlled study of a new botulinum toxin type a for treatment of glabellar lines: efficacy and safety. Dermatol Surg. 2009; 35(12): 1893–1901

[47] Kane MAC, Brandt F, Rohrich RJ, Narins RS, Monheit GD, Huber MB, Reloxin Investigational Group. Evaluation of variable-dose treatment with a new U.S. botulinum toxin type A (Dysport) for correction of moderate to severe glabellar lines: results from a phase III, randomized, double-blind, placebo-controlled study. Plast Reconstr Surg. 2009; 124(5):1619–1629

[48] Gassia V. La toxine botulique dans le traitement des rides du tiers supérieur de la face. Ann Dermatol Venereol. 2009; 136 Suppl 6: S299–S305

[49] Sundaram H, Signorini M, Liew S, et al. Global Aesthetics Consensus Group. Global aesthetics consensus: botulinum toxin type A: evidence-based review, emerging concepts, and consensus recommendations for aesthetic use, including updates on complications. Plast Reconstr Surg. 2016; 137(3):518e–529e

[50] Bertucci V, Almohideb M, Pon K. Approaches to facial wrinkles and contouring. In: Kantor J, ed. Dermatologic Surgery. New York, NY: McGraw-Hill Education; 2018; 1244–1270

[51] Lee SJ, McCall WD, Jr, Kim YK, Chung SC, Chung JW. Effect of botulinum toxin injection on nocturnal bruxism: a randomized controlled trial. Am J Phys Med Rehabil. 2010; 89(1):16–23

[52] Long H, Liao Z, Wang Y, Liao L, Lai W. Efficacy of botulinum toxins on bruxism: an evidence-based review. Int Dent J. 2012; 62(1):1–5

[53] Liew S, Dart A. Nonsurgical reshaping of the lower face. Aesthet Surg J. 2008; 28(3):251–257

[54] Carruthers J, Carruthers A. BOTOX use in the mid and lower face and neck. Semin Cutan Med Surg. 2001; 20(2):85–92

[55] Flynn TC, Carruthers JA, Carruthers JA. Botulinum-A toxin treatment of the lower eyelid improves infraorbital rhytides and widens the eye. Dermatol Surg. 2001; 27(8):703–708

[56] Mole B. Accordion wrinkle treatment through the targeted use of botulinum toxin injections. Aesthetic Plast Surg. 2014; 38(2):419–428

[57] Cohen JL, Dayan SH, Cox SE, Yalamanchili R, Tardie G. OnabotulinumtoxinA dose-ranging study for hyperdynamic perioral lines. Dermatol Surg. 2012; 38(9):1497–1505

[58] Mazzuco R, Hexsel D. Gummy smile and botulinum toxin: a new approach based on the gingival exposure area. J Am Acad Dermatol. 2010; 63(6):1042–1051

[59] Duruel O, Ataman-Duruel ET, Tözüm TF, Berker E. Ideal dose and injection site for gummy smile treatment with botulinum toxin-A: a systematic review and introduction of a case study. Int J Periodontics Restorative Dent. 2019; 39(4):e167–e173

[60] Fabi SG, Massaki AN, Guiha I, Goldman MP. Randomized split-face study to assess the efficacy and safety of abobotulinumtoxinA versus onabotulinumtoxinA in the treatment of melomental folds (depressor anguli oris). Dermatol Surg. 2015; 41(11):1323–1325

[61] Wu WTL. Microbotox of the lower face and neck: evolution of a personal technique and its clinical effects. Plast Reconstr Surg. 2015; 136 (5) Suppl:92S–100S

[62] Chang SP, Tsai HH, Chen WY, Lee WR, Chen PL, Tsai TH. The wrinkles soothing effect on the middle and lower face by intradermal injection of botulinum toxin type A. Int J Dermatol. 2008; 47(12): 1287–1294

[63] Kim MJ, Kim JH, Cheon HI, et al. Assessment of skin physiology change and safety after intradermal injections with botulinum toxin: a randomized, double-blind, placebo-controlled, split-face pilot study in rosacea patients with facial erythema. Dermatol Surg. 2019; 45(9): 1155–1162

[64] Sapra P, Demay S, Sapra S, Khanna J, Mraud K, Bonadonna J. A single-blind, split-face, randomized, pilot study comparing the effects of intradermal and intramuscular injectionof two commercially available botulinum toxin a formulas to reduce signs of facial aging. 2017; 10 (2):34–44

[65] Kapoor R, Shome D, Jain V, Dikshit R. Facial rejuvenation after intradermal botulinum toxin: is it really the botulinum toxin or is it the pricks? Dermatol Surg. 2010; 36 Suppl 4:2098–2105

[66] Hoefflin SM. Anatomy of the platysma and lip depressor muscles. A simplified mnemonic approach. Dermatol Surg. 1998; 24(11):1225–1231

[67] de Almeida ART, Romiti A, Carruthers JDA. The facial platysma and its underappreciated role in lower face dynamics and contour. Dermatol Surg. 2017; 43(8):1042–1049

[68] Bertucci V. Commentary on the facial platysma and its under-appreciated role in lower face dynamics and contour. Dermatol Surg. 2017; 43(8):1050–1052

[69] Cohen PR. Scrotal rejuvenation. Cureus. 2018; 10(3):e2316

[70] Hanna E, Pon K. Updates on botulinum neurotoxins in dermatology. Am J Clin Dermatol. 2020; 21(2):157–162

[71] Kim JE, Song EJ, Choi GS, Lew BL, Sim WY, Kang H. The efficacy and safety of liquid-type botulinum toxin type A for the management of moderate to severe glabellar frown lines. Plast Reconstr Surg. 2015; 135(3):732–741

[72] Monheit GD, Nestor MS, Cohen J, Goldman MP. Evaluation of QM-1114, a novel ready-to-use liquid botulinum toxin, in aesthetic treatment of glabellar lines. 24th World Congress of Dermatology; June 10–15, 2019, Milan, Italy. Available at: https://www.wcd2019milan-dl.org/abstract-book/documents/late-breaking-abstracts/03-aesthetic-cosmetic-dermatology/evaluation-of-qm1114-a-novel-490.pdf

5 Following the Pattern: Hair Restoration

Nicole Rogers and Marisa Belaidi

Summary

Hair loss can affect men of all ages, and presents in a variety of patterns. Fortunately, most men respond well to treatment with either medical or surgical treatment. Preferably, patients undergoing a hair transplant procedure will combine it with medical therapy to prevent ongoing loss and potentially enhance the results of their surgery.

Keywords: androgenetic alopecia, male pattern hair loss, minoxidil, finasteride, low-level light therapy, platelet-rich plasma, hair transplant surgery, hair restoration

5.1 Background

The successful treatment of hair loss can improve a man's confidence, relationships, and overall quality of life. It can also increase a man's desire to improve other aspects of his life. He may start dating again, lose weight, or find a better job, all of which contribute to an improved sense of self-worth. When it comes to hair restoration, it is important for men to understand that they have several options spanning from noninvasive medical treatments to more involved procedures: they may choose to start slowly with medical therapy, first trying to achieve maximum growth after 1 to 5 years, or move quickly toward hair transplantation alone or, preferably, in combination with medicine. Cosmetic options like camouflage products or scalp micropigmentation (SMP) can help give them "instant" results in the short term.

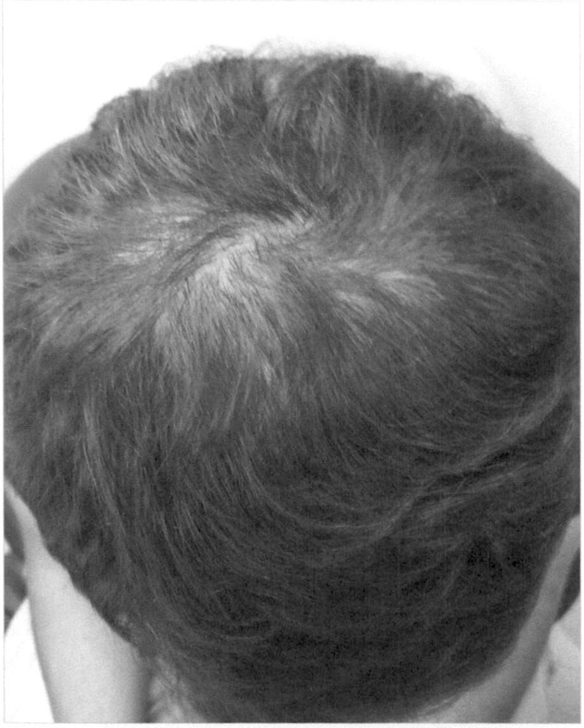

5.2 Diagnosis

Male pattern hair loss presents in a wide array of clinical settings. Onset may begin as early as the teenage years, as shown in ▶ Fig. 5.1, which depicts a young man who was just 16 years when he started to develop thinning in the vertex. Some men may start to notice hair loss as they are heading off to college, presenting as early thinning or recession in the frontal hairline (▶ Fig. 5.2). Others may not necessarily "see" hair thinning; instead, they may just complain of more hair on their pillow or in their hands when they shower.

It is important for clinicians to try to be both compassionate and aggressive in offering treatment to these young men. Do not exclude male pattern hair loss from the differential diagnosis simply due to the patient's young age. With every patient, ask carefully about a family history of hair loss. Be sure to include female relatives in the discussion. Patients may be quick to deny any family history of hair loss, but often forget about the opposite gendered parent or other genetically related individuals.

![Fig. 5.1 Vertex thinning in a 16-year-old adolescent boy.]

Fig. 5.1 Vertex thinning in a 16-year-old adolescent boy.

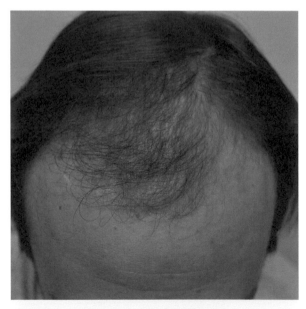

Fig. 5.2 Frontal thinning in a 19-year-old man.

For men, the Hamilton-Norwood system is used to grade the degree of hair loss. It accounts for the different patterns of hair loss, which can start with isolated thinning in the vertex, recession of the frontal bitemporal hairline, or in a diffuse unpatterned alopecia (DUPA) that mimics female pattern hair loss (▶ Fig. 5.3).

Dermoscopy can be an excellent guide in diagnosing male pattern hair loss. The presence of miniaturized hairs along the frontal aspect of a receding hairline or in a thinning vertex can help confirm the diagnosis, especially if the patient also has a family history of hair loss. It is helpful to explain to patients that this miniaturization process is inherited, as thick terminal hairs are replaced by miniaturized versions of themselves over time (▶ Fig. 5.4). Not only are the new hairs coming in finer and thinner, but they are also growing for a shorter period of time. The anagen, or growth, phase can shorten from 5 to 7 years to 3 to 4 years to 1 to 2 years, and as a result of these shorter cycling times, the hairs will appear to fall out more quickly.

5.3 Mimickers of Male Pattern Hair Loss

Occasionally, patients may present with diffuse shedding. This can be the result of telogen effluvium, a temporary shedding often due to a major physiologic or psychologic stressor, or a lab abnormality. Obtaining labwork is recommended for these patients, especially if they have no known family history of hair loss. The most common laboratory abnormalities associated with new-onset hair shedding are observed with thyroid, zinc, iron, and vitamin D.[1] Patients taking Accutane or high-dose vitamin A supplementation may present with temporary hair shedding. Diffuse alopecia areata can also present with diffuse shedding, as in the gentleman depicted in ▶ Fig. 5.5 who quickly experienced hair regrowth with oral prednisone and topical steroid shampoo.

Patients may complain of scalp symptoms like itching, burning, or tenderness in the context of hair loss. This should expand the clinician's differential beyond pattern hair loss. In these cases, obtain a complete history of when the symptoms began and what therapies they have tried (over-the-counter or prescription) and which helped. Such symptoms may point the clinician toward other mimickers of male pattern hair loss, such as frontal fibrosing alopecia (FFA) or lichen planopilaris (LPP), two types of cicatricial alopecia. The patient in ▶ Fig. 5.6 presented with long-standing, asymmetrical frontal hairline recession and also had loss of eyebrows and sideburns to support a diagnosis of FFA. These inflammatory causes of hair loss must first be addressed using topical steroids, oral doxycycline, and/or hydroxychloroquine.

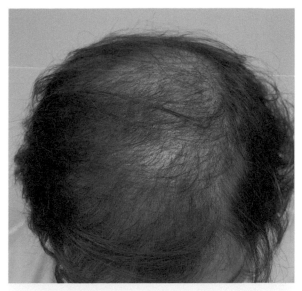

Fig. 5.3 Diffuse unpatterned alopecia (DUPA) in a 30-year-old man.

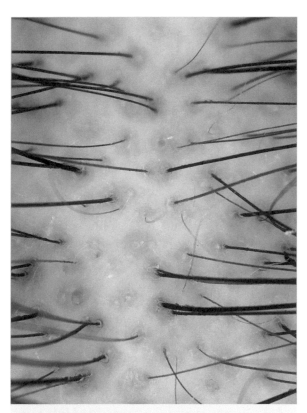

Fig. 5.4 Miniaturized hairs as seen on dermoscopy.

Hair transplantation may be possible on a case-to-case basis, but only after the disease process has been stabilized.

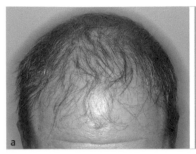 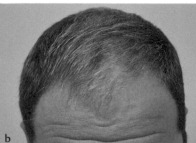

Fig. 5.5 (a) A male patient with diffuse alopecia areata, before treatment. **(b)** A male patient with complete regrowth of alopecia areata, after treatment.

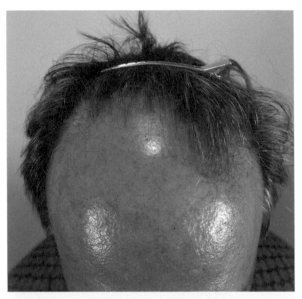

Fig. 5.6 Top view of a 67-year-old man with frontal fibrosing alopecia (FFA) demonstrating asymmetric hair loss.

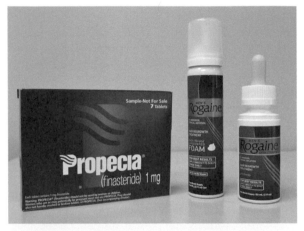

Fig. 5.7 Oral finasteride and topical minoxidil are Food and Drug Administration (FDA) approved treatments for male pattern hair loss (MPHL).

5.4 Treatment of Hair Loss

During initial consultation, it is helpful to explain to men that the two main approaches available to achieve hair regrowth are nonsurgical and surgical. Nonsurgical therapy includes medications that affect molecular signaling to stimulate the thinner, finer, hairs to cycle back as thicker, fuller versions of themselves. This approach will not only help stabilize ongoing hair loss but will also help slowly regrow hair starting as early as 6 months. By combining medical therapies, synergistic results can be achieved with maximum regrowth over 3 to 5 years.

5.4.1 Nonsurgical Options for Hair Loss

There are two Food and Drug Administration (FDA) approved medical therapies available to patients: oral finasteride and topical 5% minoxidil solution and foam (▶ Fig. 5.7). It is important to present these options first, as they exhibit the most robust data to support their use and are generally well tolerated. Other off-label therapies

for hair loss include oral dutasteride, topical finasteride, oral minoxidil, low-level light therapy (LLLT), and platelet-rich plasma (PRP). A number of supplements as well as plant-based 5-alpha reductase inhibitors such as saw palmetto and pumpkin seed oil are also currently available.

5.4.2 FDA-Approved Nonsurgical Options

Topical minoxidil was approved in the 1980s under the trade name Rogaine. It was initially studied as an oral antihypertensive medication, but was found to have the unwanted side effect of hypertrichosis. Johnson & Johnson subsequently conducted randomized clinical trials for a 5% solution that was ultimately approved for twice daily application in men. Now the foam vehicle is also FDA approved for twice daily application.

Minoxidil can be very effective, but as with any medical therapy, patients must be compliant for 4 to 6 months before they will start noticing results (▶ Fig. 5.8). Patients are encouraged to use it in an open-ended fashion, just as they would brush their teeth. Although rare, patients may develop an allergy to minoxidil, and should also be informed that the solution formulation contains the preservative propylene glycol, which is a known contact allergen.[2] Patients who report itching with the solution should switch to the foam before discontinuation of all topical minoxidil.

Oral finasteride became FDA approved in 1992 under the trade name Proscar at a 5-mg dose for benign prostatic hypertrophy (BPH). When it was observed that patients on this medication were experiencing hair regrowth, researchers began studying oral finasteride for its hair regenerative properties. Clinical trials demonstrated that a 1-mg daily dose was sufficient to help regrow hair. Whereas these trials evaluated the vertex scalp, this area was selected specifically for ease of standardization and imaging. Oral finasteride has since been shown to successfully grow hair in the frontal scalp as well (▶ Fig. 5.9).[3]

In 1997, the medication was approved by the FDA for hair loss, under the trade name Propecia. Finasteride works by blocking the conversion of testosterone to dihydrotestosterone (DHT), via type 2 5-alpha reductase. Some men worry that this treatment may cause unwanted facial hair or body hair growth. However, because the type 2 5-alpha reductase enzyme only exists in the scalp and the prostate, this is of little concern. As long as vellus hairs are intact on the scalp, darkening and thickening of such hair is possible. However, where hairs have fully involuted and the scalp appears shiny, there may be less opportunity for regrowth.

In a study from Japan, finasteride was found to be 80 to 90% effective for men in every decade of life.[4] We know from clinical trials that the degree of regrowth that can be achieved generally plateaus by around the fifth year of use. The drug can be taken either as a 1-mg pill or as one-fourth of a 5-mg pill daily. The latter option is generally less expensive but may result in less accurate dosing, depending on how well the patients are able to quarter the pill and how evenly the drug is distributed within the pill. Patients with BPH may benefit from the full 5-mg pill daily.

Finasteride can be taken with or without food, any time of day, and has not been reported to cause any allergies or known drug interactions. If patients are otherwise well with normal liver function tests, no laboratory monitoring is required. It is permissible for a man to start a family while he is taking finasteride. However, men who are taking finasteride are not permitted to donate blood due to the possibility of birth defects among pregnant women who are potential recipients. For the same reason, women of childbearing potential should not take or touch the drug. Taking finasteride can artificially lower a man's prostate-specific antigen (PSA) and interpreting physicians should double the PSA in order to obtain the true value.[5]

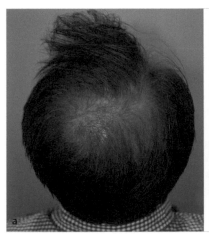
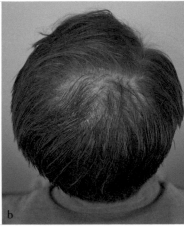

Fig. 5.8 (a) Vertex view of a 41-year-old man before treatment with topical 5% minoxidil. **(b)** Vertex view of the same patient 6 months after treatment with topical 5% minoxidil.

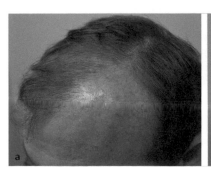
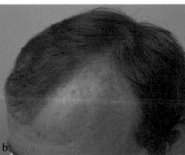

Fig. 5.9 (a) Side view of a 35-year-old man before treatment with oral finasteride 1 mg daily. **(b)** Side view of the same patient 6 months after treatment with oral finasteride 1 mg daily.

Subjects who participated in the clinical trials were found to have less than 2% chance of sexual side effects, including a decrease in desire, performance, or sperm volume. However, it is important to note that the half-life of the drug is very short, and abrupt cessation of the drug will result in clearance from the body in less than a week. Patients who are concerned about sexual side effects may choose to start at a dose of once a week, and slowly increase to two times per week, then three times per week until they feel comfortable taking it every day. Many men can experience stabilization of hair loss and some degree of regrowth at a thrice-a-week regimen.

Controversy exists regarding whether finasteride may cause long-term sexual side effects even after discontinuation of the medication.[6] Many studies have been limited by selection bias, recall bias, or lack of control for confounding variables—specifically causes of erectile dysfunction such as vascular disease, diabetes, depression, and smoking.[7] The term post-finasteride syndrome (PFS) has been used to describe a constellation of symptoms including depression and brain fog. As mentioned earlier, although it has not yet been determined that finasteride is the cause of such outcomes, the manufacturer has altered their packaging to reflect this possibility. Some hair loss specialists screen patients for preexisting anxiety, depression, or panic attacks with the concern that they may be at higher risk of developing PFS.

5.4.3 Off-Label Nonsurgical Options

Oral minoxidil has been used more recently as an alternative to the topical formulation as a means to improve compliance. When dosed as 10 or 20 mg under the trade name Loniten, it has been associated with a number of side effects including peripheral fluid retention and pericardial effusion. However, at lower doses of 0.1 to 0.625 mg (one-fourth of a 2.5-mg tablet), it can be helpful and well tolerated. Patients who are interested in the oral medication may want to first consult with their primary physicians, especially if they are already on other blood pressure–lowering agents. It is not FDA approved in this formulation for hair loss.

Dutasteride is a sister drug to finasteride, approved only for BPH. It blocks both type 2 and type 1 5-alpha reductase, making it theoretically even more effective than finasteride. However, it has a much longer half-life, lasting 170 to 300 hours in the body. As a result, the potential side effects of libido change or a reduction in sperm count may last for a much longer time. For this reason, it is not recommended for use in young men who may want to conceive and would not want the potential long-term effects of sperm reduction. It is still only FDA approved for hair loss in Korea.

Dutasteride has been used in combination with finasteride for men who have achieved a plateau in terms of hair regrowth. One published protocol that resulted in additional regrowth in the vertex scalp suggests a loading dose of 0.5 mg daily for 2 weeks, followed by weekly dosing in combination with 1-mg oral finasteride.[8] Other patients who suffer from BPH may consider going straight to dutasteride 0.5 mg daily and insurance may cover their drug cost.

LLLT involves the delivery of 600- to 700-nm infrared light via a hairbrush, headband, cap, or helmet. Many devices are now commercially available and some have received 510(k) FDA clearance as devices. They vary in their instructions for usage but generally require three to five treatments weekly, lasting 20 to 30 minutes each. The treatments are safe with no known side effects. The cost of these devices varies from $300 to $3,000, based on the number of diodes and intensity of light emitted. Unfortunately, we do not yet have any head-to-head studies showing the most effective device, but they all generally seem to have the same mechanism of action.

PRP has gained a lot of attention for its role in dental and orthopaedic medicine, specifically related to wound healing and in joints. More recently, dermatologists have investigated its ability to upregulate hair follicle growth and there is an increasing amount of basic science data to support this application. To obtain a sample of PRP for injection, venous blood is first collected from the patient and then spun down using a high-speed centrifuge to separate off the golden platelet-rich portion. Alpha granules within the platelets contain growth factors such as platelet-derived growth factor (PDGF), epidermal growth factor, and vascular endothelial growth factor (VEGF). The proposed hypothesis for PRP's effects is that when injected as aliquots of 0.1 to 0.5 mL over areas of hair thinning, plasma containing these growth factors can help enhance growth of hair follicles. Various protocols have been described in the medical literature, using the PRP alone, or adding various "activators" such a calcium gluconate or calcium chloride. A large number of commercially available PRP preparation kits are available.

Many questions remain with regard to the optimal protocol for PRP. What matters most: the concentration or absolute number of platelets injected? One recent publication demonstrated increased hair growth irrespective of platelet counts or quantification of growth factors.[9] How often should the PRP be administered? Does it need to be activated with exogenous agents such as calcium chloride or can the platelets become activated as a result of simple contact with collagen? What is the role of other additives such as matrices and can these products further improve PRP's efficacy?

Topical finasteride has been investigated as a means of delivering 5-alpha reductase blockade without the development of sexual side effects. One recent meta-analysis suggested that a 0.25% concentration could successfully lower scalp DHT levels without affecting serum DHT levels.[10] One possible setback is that this product must be formulated by a compound pharmacy; however, this can provide the opportunity to combine it with topical minoxidil for synergistic results. In addition to finasteride, there is also evidence that topical tretinoin may help enhance the efficacy of topical minoxidil.[11]

Many over-the-counter supplements are available for hair regrowth. Viviscal Pro contains the proprietary AminoMar complex containing marine proteins such as shark cartilage and oyster shell, as well as procyanidins, which have antioxidant effects.[12] Nutrafol is another commercially available hair supplement that contains newer antioxidant ingredients like ashwagandha and a proprietary biocurcumin.[13] Supplements advertised for prostate health contain the plant-based 5-alpha reductase inhibitors saw palmetto and pumpkin seed oil, which have some limited data to support their use.[14,15] Biotin is frequently used for hair loss but has no data to support its use for androgenetic alopecia.

5.5 Choice of Nonsurgical Therapy

Clinicians must carefully watch for verbal and nonverbal cues during the initial consultation with a male hair loss patient. Some men will express little to no interest whatsoever in medical therapy, either as a result of previous treatment failure, perceived inefficacy, or concerns about side effects. These men may be more amenable to other nonsurgical treatments such as LLLT or PRP, or they may directly express a preference for surgical options as definitive treatment. Still others may be excellent surgical candidates but are not prepared to pursue hair transplantation.

It is incumbent upon the surgeon to explain the risks, benefits, and alternatives—including no treatment—of the various treatment options for male pattern hair loss. Additionally, it is important to discuss and establish realistic expectations. As an example, the authors use the analogy of male pattern hair loss as a leaky bathtub. The patient presents for treatment because they are unhappy with the level of water in the tub. Hair transplantation moves hair from the back of the scalp to the front—like pouring a big bucket of water into the tub. Patients get a nice one-time rise in the level of water in the tub, but surgery alone does nothing to prevent ongoing hair thinning. It is helpful to explain that utilizing one or more nonsurgical medical therapies is the equivalent of plugging the leak in the bottom of the tub. Patients must understand it does not matter what type of medical therapy they use, just that they consider something to help stop the ongoing hair thinning.

5.6 Surgical Options for Hair Loss

Hair transplantation has evolved considerably over the years. In 1939, Dr. Shoji Okuda of Japan was one of the first to use punch grafts to treat hair loss due to alopecia areata, leprosy, and cicatricial alopecia. In 1959, Dr. Norman Orentreich began using punch grafts at NYU, ultimately establishing a successful private hair transplant practice in Manhattan.[16] Although the initial surgical transplantation of hair loss was a surgical success, it was considered a cosmetic failure by many based on the "plug" appearance of these punch grafts. Terms like "picket fence" and "doll hairs" evolved to describe the unnatural appearance of many of these early transplants.

Dr. O'Tar Norwood, a dermatologist from Oklahoma, worked tirelessly to advance the field of hair surgery. In 1990, he compiled the first Hair Transplant Forum publication. In 1993, Dr. Norwood, Dr. Dow Stough, and others founded the International Society of Hair Restoration Surgery, organizing the first and largest meeting devoted strictly to hair and scalp surgery. It was held in Dallas, and there were 430 attendees, 80 assistants. Since that time, the society has grown to over 1,100 members representing 70 countries worldwide.

In 1994, Dr. Bobby Limmer suggested the use of stereoscopic microscopes to separate the hairs into their native follicular groupings of one to four hairs each (▶ Fig. 5.10).[17] He modernized hair surgery by making the hair look more natural and better able to mimic the appearance of surrounding hairs. He also paid close attention to matching the existing hair angle in order to avoid placing hairs too perpendicularly, or in the vertex scalp where continued loss could result in an unnatural-looking island of transplanted hair.

5.6.1 Consultation and Candidate Selection

During the initial consultation, in addition to reviewing past medical and surgical history, medications, and known allergies, one must consider a patient's age, degree of hair loss, family history of hair loss, and current and past hair loss treatments and results. Furthermore, it is imperative to determine a patient's goals and expectations of therapy. If a patient is very young, 15 to 25 years

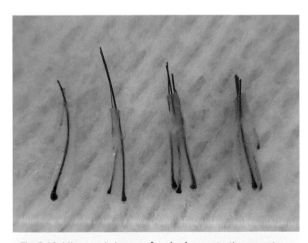

Fig. 5.10 Microscopic image of scalp demonstrating one- to four-hair follicular units.

old, with early hair loss, it is best to first stabilize their hair loss with medical therapy and observe how quickly they may be progressing. If they are very young with more advanced hair loss, they may consider surgery, but it is important to emphasize that additional hair surgery may be required if they do not also consider combination therapy with medical treatment. In those patients with a strong family history of hair loss, there is a greater likelihood of additional loss in the future.

Patients with balding or very advanced hair loss may require several surgeries in order to achieve their goals, and may still not achieve complete coverage due to limited availability of donor hair. For instance, if a patient has been wearing a hairpiece for many years and are considered to be a Norwood 7, they may be best served by continuing with this coverage option due to the limited donor zone and ability to adequately distribute over the rest of the scalp. However, if these patients agree with a plan to reframe the face by filling in the frontal one-third to two-thirds of the scalp, they may do very well with transplantation. It is helpful to remind men that the front of the face is what most of their friends, coworkers, and family will see, and that fewer people care about the back of the head as much as they do.

Patients who are transgender, specifically those individuals transitioning from male to female, can do very well with surgery. Additionally, patients of almost any ethnicity, if deemed an appropriate candidate, can achieve success with the procedure. Patients of African or Caribbean descent are at a higher risk for hypertrophic scarring or keloid formation, and should be counseled appropriately. If patients report a history of keloid formation, the surgeon may consider prophylactic triamcinolone injections in the donor zone. It is advised that, whenever possible, patients on anticoagulation discontinue it, such as warfarin and clopidogrel, 7 to 10 days prior to surgery. However, patients on low-dose aspirin (81 mg) or the newer blood thinners such as rivaroxaban may need less or no time off the drug. It is strongly advised that surgeons consult with the patient's prescribing physician, whenever necessary.

During the consultation, be vigilant about patients with unrealistic expectations. Encourage the creation of an age-appropriate hairline, which will look good in both 1 and 20 years. Explain that a rounded off hairline can be feminizing and that if the patient has ongoing recession of the temporal hairline, they may be left with awkward-looking hairs that do not belong there in the future.

5.6.2 Methods of Harvesting

There are two primary techniques used to harvest donor hairs. The first, which is still considered the gold standard by many, is the donor ellipse, or "strip," surgery. This technique, also known as follicular unit transplantation (FUT), allows the surgeon to harvest the largest numbers of hairs in the shortest amount of time with the least

amount of trauma, from the most permanent donor zone. However, it comes with the tradeoff of potentially leaving a linear scar. Depending on the age of the patient, technique used, and number of previous surgeries, this scar may be 1 to 5 mm wide and could be difficult to conceal with short haircuts.

The second harvesting technique is follicular unit excision (FUE). This procedure involves removing individual one- to four-hair follicular units (FUs), using a small 0.8- to 1-mm-wide manual or motorized punch device. The advantage of FUE is that it does not leave a linear scar, so men are still able to wear the hair very short. This technique is preferred by young men who are in the military or who prefer to wear their head shaved in the back. The term was recently changed from follicular unit *extraction* to *excision* in order to more accurately categorize this as a surgical procedure.

With either technique, it is essential to explain to patients that this is a surgical procedure that must be done by a medical professional. It cannot be delegated to non-medical personnel. The physician should perform not only the harvesting of the grafts but also the hairline design, creation of graft sites, and should closely supervise graft placement. Ultimately, it is the placement of the grafts back into the scalp that determines the cosmetic outcome.

5.6.3 Surgical Anesthesia

Hair surgery can be done while patients are awake and relaxed. Every aspect of the case can be performed with local anesthesia. Preoperative medications can include 2 mg oral lorazepam, 500 to 1,000 mg acetaminophen, and 25 to 50 mg diphenhydramine. The donor area is sprayed with a menthol-containing cooling spray, and gentle vibration is applied with a massaging device. A combination of short- and long-acting local anesthesia is helpful. We begin with buffered 0.5 to 1% lidocaine + 1:100,000 epinephrine, attached to 32-gauge needle, followed by a second pass with 2% lidocaine + 1:100,000 epinephrine and then a third pass with 0.25% bupivacaine. For FUT, it is helpful to tumesce the area with saline to help separate the follicles from the underlying vasculature, and from each other. Tumescence is generally avoided in the donor area with FUE harvesting because it can alter the natural direction of the follicles under the skin surface and increase the risk of transection.

5.6.4 Donor Ellipse Harvesting

The first step during harvesting of the ellipse is to pick up the overlying hairs in the occipital scalp and locate the occipital protuberance. This is generally a safe level from which to harvest the hair, given that hairs may recede from the vertex inferiorly, or at the neckline superiorly (retrograde miniaturization). By trimming a sample 1-cm area, the donor density in that area can be assessed in order to determine the required length of the donor strip

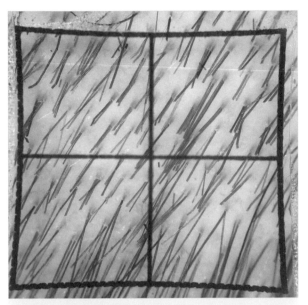

Fig. 5.11 View of scalp through a densitometer can help estimate donor density.

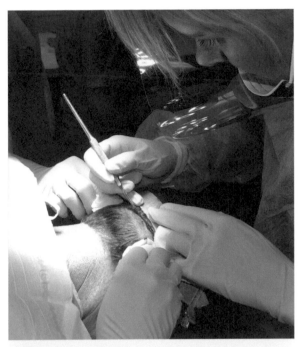

Fig. 5.12 Removal of donor strip using caudally oriented scalpel.

(▶ Fig. 5.11). For instance, if the surgical plan is to harvest 1,000 grafts and the donor density is 25 FUs per 0.25 cm² (100 FUs/cm²), then the donor strip would need to be 10 cm long × 1 cm wide.

A no. 10 or 15 blade can be used to harvest the strip. Care must be taken to angle the blade to match the exit angles of the hairs in the occipital scalp (▶ Fig. 5.12). If the blade is angled too inferiorly or superiorly, it may result in transection of the follicles. An initial scoring of the epidermis and upper dermis can be performed first, followed by tension dissection technique using opposing skin hooks (▶ Fig. 5.13). The strip is gently removed by separating along the subcutaneous plane, just below the follicles and well above the galea.

Optimal results can often be achieved using the trichophytic closure. This involves harvesting a small ledge of epidermis from one or both sides of the skin edge so that when apposed, the hair will "grow through" the resultant scar. It is also important not to make the donor strip too wide. If a width of more than 1.5 cm is excised, there may be unsightly widening of the donor scar. For patients who may require multiple surgeries, it can be helpful to offset the donor area from the central occiput to alternating sides of the scalp. However, caution must be used such that the donor scar is not readily visible in areas of thinning.

Skin edges can be brought together with staples or suture. Dissolving sutures are best for patients who live out of town and may not be able to return for suture removal. It is also helpful to keep the skin edges together for extended time, especially in the context of a nonvirgin scalp, which may stretch more, or for very physically

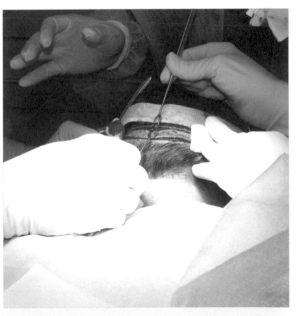

Fig. 5.13 Tension dissection is used to separate hair follicles.

active individuals. The authors use a running 4–0 poliglycaprone 25 suture with good results and high patient satisfaction. Patients appreciate that they can immediately cover the suture line with their overlying hair (▶ Fig. 5.14).

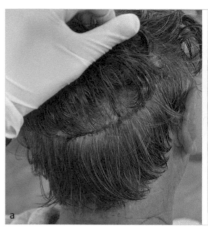
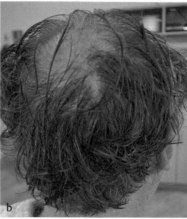

Fig. 5.14 (a) View of donor area immediately after suturing of skin edges. **(b)** Donor site is completely hidden by overlying hair.

With strip harvesting, the hair-bearing tissue is next bread-loafed into serial "slivers" one FU wide (▶ Fig. 5.15). Each sliver is then separated into individual one- to four-hair follicular groupings. The tissue can be separated using handheld single-edge blades or a no. 10 blade scalpel. The creation of grafts from a donor strip is greatly expedited with the use of high-power magnification. Attached to each FU is an arrector pili muscle and sebaceous gland. Optimal results are achieved by keeping each FU intact so that the stem cells derived from the bulb, bulge, and sebaceous glands can work cohesively to regenerate hair in their new location.

5.6.5 Follicular Unit Excision Harvesting

FUE harvesting can be more time and labor intensive than strip harvesting. However, it has gained popularity among young men who want to avoid the creation of a linear scar in the back of the scalp. It is also a more delicate procedure, as potential tethering and/or difficulty in graft extraction may lead to increased trauma to the grafts. Transection of follicles may also occur if the angle of the punch device does not exactly match the exit angle of the hairs. Thus, there can be a learning curve for novice hair surgeons. It is essential to gain proficiency in both FUE and strip surgery in order to be able to offer both techniques.

The best results are generally obtained by shaving the occipital donor hair to leave just 1 to 2 mm of growth. Patients can be placed in the prone position or may sit up facing forward depending on the surgeon's preference. Very high-power loupes (3.5-6X) are helpful to visualize the exit angle of the hairs from the occipital scalp. A number of devices are available to remove the grafts either manually or with motorized assistance (▶ Table 5.1). These devices vary considerably in their cost and functionality. Surgeons should be wary of companies that advocate delegation of graft harvesting to nonmedically trained

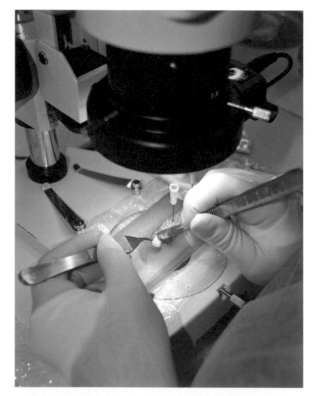

Fig. 5.15 Slivering of donor strip under microscope.

personnel. This is unethical and usually results in very poor outcomes.

There are also a variety of sizes and styles of tips available for each model of FUE device. Patients with fine donor hair in one- to two-hair groupings may undergo surgery with 0.8-mm-wide tips. Conversely, patients with coarser three- to four-hair FUs may require 1-mm-wide tips. Depending on the goals of surgery, the surgeon can choose relatively smaller or larger size follicular groupings. Tips with a flared or trumpet shape can help lower transection rates. Some tips are interchangeable among different FUE devices.

As the extracted grafts are counted, they should be carefully inspected for quality control. Petroleum jelly or antibiotic ointment can be applied to the site of extractions postoperatively. The surrounding hairs will generally regrow within a week to completely cover where the grafts were harvested (▶ Fig. 5.16). Tiny pink dots may remain in the donor sites for 1 to 4 weeks after surgery.

The donor sites are generally not visible so long as FUE tips are less than 1 mm in width.

Patients should understand that if they are not on medical therapy for hair loss, they may face a shrinking donor area over time. Thus, the hairs harvested and placed in their new location may not be permanent if they were otherwise programmed to undergo miniaturization at a later date. It is best to avoid harvesting too near the vertex or too near the neckline in the event that this may occur.

5.6.6 Graft Storage

As soon as the hair-bearing tissue is removed from the body, it and the resultant hair grafts must be stored in a moist Petri dish (▶ Fig. 5.17). Many physicians use simple saline as a holding solution, whereas others use more sophisticated holding solutions designed to provide pH buffering and reduce free radical formation at chilled temperatures. PRP has also been used to hold grafts while they are out of the body. Every effort should be made to place the grafts back in the body as quickly as possible. Graft survival time generally drops off after 12 to 24 hours outside the body, even under the best of conditions.

5.6.7 Hairline Design

Men generally benefit from the creation of a "regularly irregular" hairline. It is helpful to look for native, landmark, hairs. These can be a guide to reestablishing and fortifying the most age-appropriate hairline. Doctors new to hair surgery should be cautious about aggressively lowering the hairline on the first surgery. Remind patients that we can always lower the hairline with subsequent surgeries, but we cannot raise the hairline without removing grafts or using laser hair removal. Many doctors create small triangles or mounds along the hairline so that it does not appear to be a straight line.

Table 5.1 Devices for follicular unit excision (FUE)

Name of FUE device	Company/location
ARTAS™ ® Robotic Hair Restoration	Venus Concept, Toronto, Canada
Dr. Jack's E-FUE device	Robbins Instruments, Chatham, New Jersey, United States
Ertip	Ertip Hair Transplant Instruments, Istanbul, Turkey
Mamba FUE Device	Trivellini Instruments, Asuncion, Paraguay
Neograft™ ®	Venus Concept, Toronto, Canada
Smartgraft™ ®	Vision Medical, Glen Mills, Pennsylvania, United States
Safe System	Harris FUE Instruments, Greenwood Village, Colorado, United States
Powered Cole Isolation Device (PCID)	Cole Instruments, Atlanta, Georgia, United States
WAW FUE System	DeVroye Instruments, Brussels, Belgium
Dr.UGraft	Dr.UGraft, Redondo Beach, California, United States

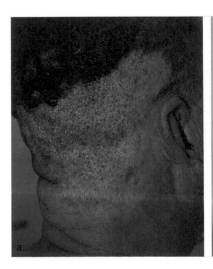
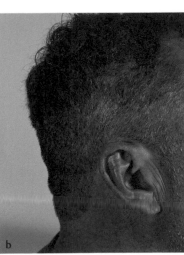

Fig. 5.16 (a) Donor area immediately after follicular unit excision (FUE) harvesting. **(b)** Donor area 1 week after FUE harvesting.

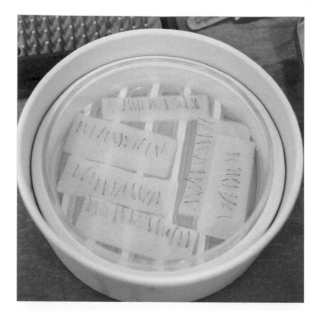

Fig. 5.17 Graft storage.

Table 5.2 Tools for recipient site creation

Tool	Width	Grafts selection
20-gauge needle	0.908 mm	1-hair Caucasian grafts
19-gauge needle	1.067 mm	2-hair Caucasian grafts
18 gauge needle	1.270 mm	3- to 4-hair Caucasian grafts; 1- to 2-hair African American grafts
16-gauge needle	1.651 mm	3- to 4-hair African American grafts

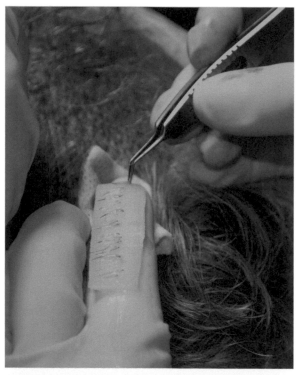

Fig. 5.18 Careful placement of grafts back into areas of hair thinning.

5.6.8 Creation of Graft Sites

Local anesthesia can be used to perform a ring block. A cooling spray, followed by local vibration can help reduce the pain associated with injection. Starting with 0.5% lidocaine with epinephrine is also helpful, followed by a second pass with 2% lidocaine with epinephrine. Some physicians perform nerve blocks targeting the supraorbital and supratrochlear nerves. Allow 5 to 10 minutes for the vasoconstrictive effects to take place and then tiny, needle-sized, incisions can be created. There are a wide variety of commercially available instruments that may be used for this purpose, but simple disposable needles work very well. ▶ Table 5.2 lists needles used to create graft sites, and their associated size grafts.

Correct recipient site angles will determine how natural the transplanted hair looks. The sites must be angled in such a way that they match the exit angle of the surrounding hairs. When in doubt, it is always safest to orient them slightly anteriorly and toward the midline. Disastrous results can occur when the grafts are oriented too radially, or too perpendicularly. Care should also be taken to avoid creating the appearance of a straight line in the transplanted hairline.

As the sites are created, the depth of the sites should correspond with the length of the follicles. For instance, if the donor follicles are short, such as 3 mm or less, they may sink down into sites that are too deep. It is important to ensure that the recipient site width is sufficient to allow the grafts to sit snugly. If the sites are too wide, there may be bleeding or popping during graft placement. If the sites are too narrow, the grafts may be crushed during the placement process. Test placement of a few grafts at the beginning can help prevent this from occurring.

5.6.9 Graft Placement

Specialized forceps are used to gently grasp the inferior portion of the bulb and carefully slide it into each recipient site (▶ Fig. 5.18). Great care should be taken not to crush, twist, or fold the grafts as they are inserted. It is helpful if there is a small bit of adipose tissue below the bulb to grasp the graft and pull it into position. Angled forceps are helpful with placing grafts on the left and central parts of the scalp. Straight forceps can be more helpful placing on the right side of the scalp.

Good lighting and ergonomics are an essential component of the graft placement procedure. One to two adjustable overhead light-emitting diode (LED) lamps are generally helpful, and do not generate too much heat. Patient positioning is also important, and they should be positioned in a way that is ergonomically optimal for those placing the grafts, limiting musculoskeletal discomfort and fatigue. High-power magnification, with either drug-store magnifiers or customized 3.5 to 5X loupes, allows for good graft visualization during placement.

Several challenges can be associated with graft placement. Poor hemostasis can slow the placement process and decrease visibility. Holding pressure, or using dilute epinephrine, can help control bleeding. Popping, its exact cause is unknown, occurs when the grafts extrude and need to be placed back into their graft sites. Asking the patients to stop all supplements 7 to 10 days prior to surgery can help avoid cases of bleeding due to fish oil, vitamin E, or other unknown blood thinners. Patients who are on low-dose (81-mg) aspirin do not have to stop unless otherwise directed by their primary care physician.

Many surgeons use implanters to help gently slide the grafts into place. Some physicians use them after the creation of donor sites, whereas others use sharp implanters to create the incision and place the graft in a single movement. These devices are made of metal or plastic and can be manual or spring loaded.

5.6.10 Post-Op Care

At the completion of hair surgery, antibiotic ointment is applied to the donor area. It is then covered by an abdominal (ABD) pad. Ointment is not applied to the grafted area to prevent the grafts from becoming dislodged or rearranged. A nonadhesive bandage is placed gently over the grafted area. Then, conforming gauze is wrapped around the entire head to cover the grafts and to secure it in place. Paper tape is then applied and a bandana or ski cap is gently placed over the bandage to hold it all in place.

The first night, patients are encouraged to rest, have a nice meal, and take pain medication as needed. We generally prescribe acetaminophen with a low-dose hydrocodone, but many patients have good pain control with acetaminophen alone. The next day, patients are instructed to remove the bandage, if it has not fallen off overnight, and gently spray the grafted area with a saline solution. They may gently run shower water over the grafts but are instructed to protect the transplanted area with a washcloth. They are asked to wait until the third postoperative day to shampoo the grafted area.

Scabs will form in the transplanted area, and patients are instructed not to pick or scratch at them. If the transplanted area is very itchy, they can apply over-the-counter hydrocortisone, moisturizing lotion, or gently shower water over the grafts several times per day. By day 6 or 7, patients may use a salicylic acid–based shampoo to help gently dissolve the scabs. The hair-bearing grafts will enter a resting phase and shed between 2 and 6 weeks after surgery. At 6 to 8 weeks, there may still be some faint

erythema, but it will otherwise look as if nothing was done. Then, slowly, the grafts will start to grow in between 4 to 8 months, with the final results between 12 and 18 months. ► Fig. 5.19 shows the transplanted area immediately post-op, 8 days later, at 5 months, and 12 months.

5.6.11 Special Situations

The early days of hair restoration have left many individuals with unfortunate pluggy-looking punch grafts. Reconstructive hair surgery can be used to harvest such grafts and place them back into the scalp as individual one- to four-hair groupings in appropriate, natural-appearing angles. They can also be harvested using FUE instrumentation when they occur individually but have angles that are too perpendicular or radially oriented. Patients who are unhappy with their linear donor scar can also undergo FUE transplantation, where hairs are harvested individually from above or below and placed back into the scar.

Men born with very limited beard or mustache growth can also benefit from hair transplantation. The hairs can be harvested from the occipital scalp via either strip or FUE and placed back into the necessary areas, just as they are placed in the scalp (► Fig. 5.20). Eyebrows can also be restored using hair from the back of the scalp. However, the patients must understand that the growth phase will be longer than the eyebrows and that these hairs will require trimming every few weeks.

Areas of previous scarring from cranial surgery, trauma, or radiation therapy can also benefit from hair transplantation, as grafts can grow very successfully in these areas. Likewise, patients with previous browlift surgery can benefit from grafting along the frontal hairline in order to cover the scar and soften its appearance. Men may also benefit from body hair transplantation if they are out of donor scalp follicles. Donor hair may be taken from the beard or the back or the chest. The latter can be more difficult, however, as body hairs are generally finer and grow at a more acute angle.

5.6.12 Camouflage

There are a number of camouflage products that can help instantly reduce the contrast between hair color and scalp color. They are available as sprays, fibers, compact applicators, tinted shampoos, and leave-in products. They do not make the hair grow but can increase confidence and help reduce self-consciousness while patients are waiting for their hair to grow in.

5.6.13 Scalp Micropigmentation

SMP is a relatively new option in the treatment of hair loss. It can be used to help camouflage linear donor scars, especially for men who want to wear their head shaved. It can also be used to enhance the appearance of density in

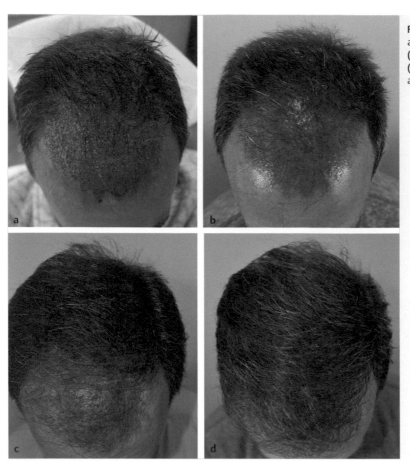

Fig. 5.19 **(a)** A 52-year-old man immediately status post placement of 1,800 grafts. **(b)** The same patient 8 days after surgery. **(c)** 4 months after surgery. **(d)** 12 months after surgery.

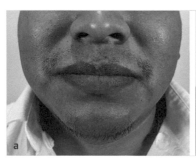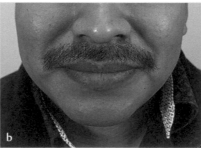

Fig. 5.20 **(a)** A 31-year-old man before mustache transplantation. **(b)** The same patient 7 months after placement of 550 grafts.

already transplanted areas. Tiny dots of pigment are placed very superficially in the skin to help reduce the contrast between scalp and hair color. Optimal results require between one to three sessions and can last for up to 5 years.

Caution must be used to avoid tattooing along an unstable frontal male hairline. If the person is still very young, and is not on medical therapy, their tattoo may over time become visible and look unnatural. Likewise, the inks must be carefully chosen to match the hair color. Inks deposited too deeply in the skin may bleed together or change color over time, leaving an unnatural greenish or bluish hue. Finally, patients must plan to keep their hair color the same for another 5 years, rather than letting it go gray or white, for example.

5.7 Conclusion

Hair restoration can provide dramatic and life-changing results for men affected by hair loss. Fortunately, there are a number of medical and surgical options that can regrow hair over 6 to 12 months. The choice of therapies is dependent on the patient's family history of hair loss, lifestyle preferences, and degree of hair loss.

5.8 Pearls

- Identify cause of hair loss prior to starting treatment.
- Stabilize male pattern hair loss using FDA approved therapies like minoxidil and finasteride.
- Consider patient's age, family history of hair loss, and hairstyle preference prior to planning surgery.
- Choose patients with good health and realistic expectations for surgery.
- Encourage open-ended use of medical therapy even after hair surgery to prevent ongoing hair thinning.

References

[1] Cheung EJ, Sink JR, English Iii JC. Vitamin and mineral deficiencies in patients with telogen effluvium: a retrospective cross-sectional study. J Drugs Dermatol. 2016; 15(10):1235–1237

[2] Friedman ES, Friedman PM, Cohen DE, Washenik K. Allergic contact dermatitis to topical minoxidil solution: etiology and treatment. J Am Acad Dermatol. 2002; 46(2):309–312

[3] Leyden J, Dunlap F, Miller B, et al. Finasteride in the treatment of men with frontal male pattern hair loss. J Am Acad Dermatol. 1999; 40(6, Pt 1):930–937

[4] Sato A, Takeda A. Evaluation of efficacy and safety of finasteride 1 mg in 3177 Japanese men with androgenetic alopecia. J Dermatol. 2012; 39(1):27–32

[5] D'Amico AV, Roehrborn CG. Effect of 1 mg/day finasteride on concentrations of serum prostate-specific antigen in men with androgenic alopecia: a randomised controlled trial. Lancet Oncol. 2007; 8(1):21–25

[6] Andy G, John M, Mirna S, et al. Controversies in the treatment of androgenetic alopecia: the history of finasteride. Dermatol Ther (Heidelb). 2019; 32(2):e12647

[7] Irwig MS, Kolukula S. Persistent sexual side effects of finasteride for male pattern hair loss. J Sex Med. 2011; 8(6):1747–1753

[8] Boyapati A, Sinclair R. Combination therapy with finasteride and low-dose dutasteride in the treatment of androgenetic alopecia. Australas J Dermatol. 2013; 54(1):49–51

[9] Rodrigues BL, Montalvão SAL, Cancela RBB, et al. Treatment of male pattern alopecia with platelet-rich plasma: a double-blind controlled study with analysis of platelet number and growth factor levels. J Am Acad Dermatol. 2019; 80(3):694–700

[10] Lee SW, Juhasz M, Mobasher P, Ekelem C, Mesinkovska NA. A systematic review of topical finasteride in the treatment of androgenetic alopecia in men and women. J Drugs Dermatol. 2018; 17(4):457–463

[11] Sharma A, Goren A, Dhurat R, et al. Tretinoin enhances minoxidil effect in androgenetic alopecia by upregulating folliucular sulfotransferase enzymes. Dermatol Ther. 2019; 32(3):e12915

[12] Ablon G. A 6-month, randomized, double-blind, placebo-controlled study evaluating the ability of a marine complex supplement to promote hair growth in men with thinning hair. J Cosmet Dermatol. 2016; 15(4):358–366

[13] Farris PK, Rogers N, McMichael A, Kogan S. A novel, multi-targeting approach to treating hair loss, using standardized nutraceuticals. J Drugs Dermatol. 2017; 16(11):s141–s148

[14] Rossi A, Mari E, Scarno M, et al. Comparitive effectiveness of finasteride vs Serenoa repens in male androgenetic alopecia: a two-year study. Int J Immunopathol Pharmacol. 2012; 25(4):1167–1173

[15] Cho YH, Lee SY, Jeong DW, et al. Effect of pumpkin seed oil on hair growth in men with androgenetic alopecia: a randomized, double-blind, placebo-controlled trial. Evid Based Complement Alternat Med. 2014; 2014:549721

[16] Singer N. Norman Orentreich, 96, Force Behind Hair Transplants, Dies. 2019. Available at: https://www.nytimes.com/2019/02/21/business/dr-norman-orentreich-dead.html?fbclid=IwAR2_mK12h8fnVKjKsCQY32pLcezObVvMettoL7Jc5LDy9J7XqyPhs21WKSY

[17] Limmer BL. Elliptical donor stereoscopically assisted micrografting as an approach to further refinement in hair transplantation. J Dermatol Surg Oncol. 1994; 20(12):789–793

6 Finding the Right Balance: Chemical Peels

Jeave Reserva, Rebecca Tung, and Seaver Soon

Summary

Chemical peels are a mainstay of aesthetic medicine and an increasingly popular cosmetic procedure performed in men. The approach to chemical peels in men includes consideration of intrinsic and extrinsic skin variables that affect various aspects of the peeling process. Owing to the increased sebaceous quality of their skin and thicker dermis, male patients, in general, may require a greater number of treatments, larger volumes of peeling agent, more aggressive degreasing and peel application, and/or higher concentration of peeling agent to achieve optimal results. Patient selection is of utmost importance as poor photoprotective behavior and nonadherence to pre- and postpeel regimens could jeopardize clinical outcomes. The aesthetic clinician with good understanding of men's cosmetic concerns and a solid foundation on basic and advanced peeling techniques can help the contemporary male patient achieve his desired aesthetics. Chemical peels are safe, cost-effective treatments that provide reliable outcomes and should be an integral part of the aesthetic practitioner's cosmetic repertoire.

Keywords: chemical peel, chemexfoliation, chemabrasion, male, aesthetics, trichloroacetic acid, phenol-croton oil, salicylic acid, glycolic acid

6.1 Background

Perhaps the oldest aesthetic procedure performed to date, chemical peeling dates back as early as 1550 BC with the Ancient Egyptians using sour milk, animal oils, salt, and alabaster to aesthetically improve their skin.[1,2] In the early 1870s, the first descriptions of chemical peeling in modern medical literature were reported by dermatologists, whose specialty continued to advance the technique throughout the century.[2,3]

The low-cost and reliable results of chemical peeling have made it a staple procedure in aesthetic medicine. The American Society for Dermatologic Surgery and the American Society for Aesthetic Plastic Surgery reported chemical peels as the fifth most common nonsurgical cosmetic procedure performed in 2017.[4,5] An increase of 15.9% compared to the prior year, between 457,409 and 485,371 chemical peel procedures were performed in 2017 totaling $64 million in expenditures.[4,5] Men account for only 5.5 and 9.3% of all chemical peel procedures performed in the United States and worldwide, respectively.[4,6] Given the growing men's aesthetic market, chemical peels' cost-effectiveness in addressing many of men's top cosmetic concerns make it an essential skill for physicians in aesthetic medicine to develop.[7,8,9,10]

6.2 Chemical Peels and the Male Skin

6.2.1 Peeling Mechanisms and Classification

Chemical peels induce all three stages of tissue replacement—destruction, elimination, and regeneration—all under controlled inflammation via mechanisms specifically dependent on the peeling agent.[11] These peeling mechanisms can be characterized as being primarily caustic, metabolic, or toxic.[11] Although a large majority of the medical literature on chemical peeling has regarded acidity as the sole mechanism for peel-induced skin modifications, it is helpful to know that this sole caustic effect only applies to trichloroacetic acid (TCA). As TCA becomes more concentrated, the more acidic it becomes and the deeper it penetrates.[11] In addition to dose-dependent cytotoxicity, multiple cellular pathways have been proposed in TCA's mechanism of action. Platelet-derived growth factor (PDGF) produced by keratinocytes, platelets, and monocytes stimulates wound tissue fibroblast proliferation and integrin expression, which promotes re-epithelialization.[12] An inflammatory response involving both proinflammatory cytokine (interleukin-1 [IL-1]) and anti-inflammatory cytokine (IL-10) is also observed. Finally, a local skin equivalent of the hypothalamic–pituitary–adrenal (HPA) axis, known as the skin stress response system (SSRS), has been shown to upregulate pro-opiomelanocortin (POMC) independently of corticotropin-releasing hormone. Apart from melanocyte stimulation, POMC may also be responsible for the controlled inflammation and keratinocyte and fibroblast proliferation after TCA application.[13]

It has been hypothesized that cellular metabolic effects are partly responsible for the peeling outcomes of alpha hydroxy acids (AHA), such as glycolic and lactic acid, and beta hydroxy acids (BHA), such as salicylic acid (SA). Glycolic acid (GA) at low concentration (< 30%) interferes with sulfotransferases and phosphotransferases on the surface of corneocytes causing corneocyte dyscohesion and subsequent epidermal exfoliation. When used in concentrations such as 30 to 70% free acid in aqueous solution, GA exerts its effect directly based on acidity, detaching cells from each other. Other common peeling substances, such as phenol and resorcinol, work primarily through toxic effects, which cause increased cellular permeability, enzymatic inactivation, and protein denaturation with production of insoluble proteinates. Peeling procedures aim to maintain strict localization of these toxic effects, as other cells distant from where the chemical has been applied can also be affected. Although SA peels work primarily via metabolic mechanisms that cause cells to shed more readily, thereby resulting in keratolysis, it has toxic effects when used in large quantities or large surface areas. Even though they are rarely seen in practice, remembering that SA is made from sodium phenolate, a sodium salt of phenol, may help ensure that the toxic effects of SA are kept in mind and hence potentially avoided.[11]

Phenol-croton oil's ability to rejuvenate severely photodamaged skin, surpassing results seen from fully ablative CO_2 resurfacing, warrants a brief discussion of its proposed mechanisms. Its active ingredient, croton oil, is derived from *Croton tiglium* seeds that contain vegetal matrix of 12-myristate-13-acetate and other phorbol esters capable of inducing accelerated deoxyribonucleic acid synthesis and activation of protein kinase C causing extreme inflammatory response.[14] Initially thought to be the active ingredient in phenol-croton oil peels, phenol acts a solvent for croton oil allowing penetration of the phorbol esters into dermis where it induces dense dermal neocollagenesis and formation of organized elastic fibers.[15,16] These dense neocollagen bands are thicker than those induced by fully ablative CO_2 laser and persist decades after the procedure.[15,17]

Peels that function primarily by metabolic effects generally fall under keratolytics, whereas those that exert their effects via caustic or toxic effects are largely considered protein denaturants.[11,18] With these mechanisms in mind, the rationale behind peel combinations and peel selection for specific indications becomes more intuitive. Superficial peels, which are subdivided into very light and light peels, respectively, destroy keratinocytes down to the level of stratum spinosum and stratum basale. Medium peels penetrate into the upper reticular dermis, whereas deep peels wound to the level of the mid-reticular dermis.[19] Combining keratolytics with protein denaturants facilitates deeper peel penetration. Classification of common chemical peeling agents and their corresponding depth of penetration is described in ▶ Table 6.1.

6.2.2 Gender-Linked Skin Differences Relevant to Chemical Peeling

The difference between good and excellent peeling outcomes in men may be attributed in part to a working knowledge of gender-linked differences in skin, as peeling procedures can be very operator dependent and their planning requires careful consideration of multiple factors. The Obagi Skin Classification assesses skin variables such as color, oiliness, thickness, laxity, and fragility to systematically plan pre- and postprocedure skin regimen, select optimal peeling agent, and stratify risks for complication.[18] Integrating current research regarding how these variables differ between the sexes may facilitate better peeling outcomes.

Although no gender-linked differences have been reported for melanocyte distribution, intra-ethnic group comparative studies of skin tone show men have darker

Table 6.1 Classification of common chemical peel agents and corresponding histologic depth of penetration

Chemical peel classification	Histologic depth of penetration
Very light superficial • TCA (10–20%) • Glycolic acid (10–50%) • Salicylic acid (20–30%) • Retinoic acid (1–10%)	Stratum spinosum
Light superficial • TCA (20–30%) • Jessner's solution[a] • Glycolic acid (70%)	Stratum basale
Medium depth • TCA (35–40%) • Solid CO_2–TCA (35%; Brody combination) • Jessner's solution–TCA (35%; Monheit combination) • Glycolic acid (70%)–TCA (35%; Coleman combination) • Phenol (88%)	Superficial reticular dermis
Deep • Baker–Gordon phenol-croton oil peel[b] • Hetter's phenol-croton oil peel • TCA (> 50%)	Mid-reticular dermis

Abbreviation: TCA: trichloroacetic acid.
[a]Jessner's solution: 14 g resorcinol, 14 g salicylic acid, 14 g lactic acid (85%), and 100 mL (quantity sufficient to make total) ethanol (95%).
[b]Baker–Gordon phenol-croton oil peel: croton oil, phenol, and hexachlorophene (0.25%).

and less reflective complexions possibly from more vascularized superficial dermis and more melanin.[20] Men's constitutive pigmentation and facultative pigmentation from sun exposure are more robust with longer pigment retention than women.[20,21] As will be discussed later, predictable peeling outcomes and common complications from peeling treatment can be anticipated by classifying patients into a genetico-racial skin classification system.[22] However, within individual genetico-racial skin groups, men may benefit from longer prepeel skin conditioning and more aggressive photoprotection. Additionally, chromacity studies assessing color differences between erythema and normal skin show higher basal values in men, which may have some implications when evaluating postprocedural erythema.[21]

Due to androgenic hormone stimulation, it is no surprise that men have higher sebum production that is associated with pore enlargement and predisposition to acne vulgaris.[20,21] This propensity for excess sebum production has been associated with impaired stratum corneum barrier function. The increased transepidermal water loss is believed to be related to sebum-induced alterations in intercellular lipid structure and poor corneocyte maturation. Further worsening the barrier function are the behavioral tendencies related to excess sebum in men that result in their avoidance of skin care products due to the perceived fear of exacerbating their already tacky-feeling skin.[23] Because of men's relative oilier skin, a longer or more aggressive prepeel conditioning regimen in the form of stronger topical retinoids and/or more aggressive degreasing may be warranted. Postprocedure acne flares may also be more likely. On the other hand, because men have significantly higher average number of appendageal structures including sebaceous glands, sweat glands, and blood vessels than women, wrinkles may be relatively less prominent in men particularly in the perioral area.[24] Because of their higher sebaceous gland density, incorporation of lipophilic peels such as SA and Jessner's solution (JS) into a male patient's peel regimen should be given strong consideration if within clinical indication. The higher sebum excretion in men also promotes the growth of *Malassezia restricta* and *M. globosa*, which may be indirectly diminished by chemical peeling, thus preventing development or flares of seborrheic dermatitis.[25] Facility in performing focal medium to deep peels for sebaceous hyperplasia may also be of value as men may be more likely to seek treatment for this condition.[9]

Although the extent of differences varies by anatomical region, dermal thickness is greater in men as a result of increased dermal collagen partly from androgen receptor activation.[26,27] Differences in study design, measurement tools, sample size, and genetic backgrounds of the subjects may have played a role in some conflicting findings in some studies, but forehead and neck skin are noted to be significantly thicker in men in several studies.[21] Similarly, epidermal thickness is greater in the cheeks and back of men. Hence, in order to achieve the intended depth of peel penetration, peeling procedures in men may require higher concentrations and higher volumes of peel solution as well as greater peel application pressure, more peeling sessions, and/or longer prepeel skin conditioning.

Although there are no significant differences in skin elasticity between men and women, lower eyelid sagging is significantly more severe in men starting middle age.[28] This finding highlights a potential role for segmental, or targeted, peeling of a specific cosmetic unit, as an early intervention for periorbital rejuvenation in men. Skin microcirculation dysfunction in healthy, middle-aged men in the setting of elevated homocysteine levels may possibly be explained by protective effects of estrogens against homocysteine-induced vascular dysfunction.[29] However, in general, higher skin perfusion is observed in men than in women.[30,31] The larger number of microvessels in the male face could in theory make men more susceptible to medium- and deep peel–associated persistent erythemas, which result from angiogenic factors stimulating

vasodilation. This is a sign of prolonged phase of fibroplasia, which may lead to scarring.[32] Although men may be more likely to tolerate pain from chemical resurfacing,[33,34] androgen-associated diminished re-epithelialization rates may extend their expected downtime for these procedures.[35,36] Furthermore, more robust histamine response is observed in men and older age patients.[37] This has clinically significant implications especially in periorbital rejuvenation via medium or deep peeling in men, where significant edema may cause the eyes to swell shut but may be mitigated by aggressive prophylaxis and treatment with antihistamines.[38] ▶ Table 6.2 summarizes male-specific intrinsic skin variables and relevant peeling considerations.

6.2.3 Men and Extrinsic Factors Relevant to Chemical Peeling

Men may be more likely to avoid healthy skin care practices, as previously alluded to when discussing men with higher skin sebum content having poor skin care regimen.[23] They may also participate in behaviors that contribute to signs of aging, with smoking and ultraviolet (UV) light exposure being of most significance.[39] Because of higher risks for suboptimal peeling outcomes and worse complications, peeling procedures in patients who fail to modify these behaviors should be approached with extreme caution or not be attempted at all.[40]

The latest age-standardized worldwide prevalence of daily smoking for men is 25% compared to 5% for women.[41] In the United States, the most recent prevalence estimates are 21.7% for men versus 18.4% for women.[42] Factors such as vasoconstriction, increased oxidative damage, inhibition of fibroblastic activity, and upregulation of matrix metalloproteinases have been proposed as potential mechanisms of how tobacco exposure accelerates skin aging.[43] As a well-known risk factor for wrinkle development,[44] strong emphasis should be placed on smoking cessation when counseling men prior to any peeling procedure. The potentially increased risks for scarring and poor wound healing associated with tobacco exposure may lead to disastrous peeling outcomes.[45]

Outdoor occupations are overwhelmingly comprised by men.[46] To add to this occupational risk factor for UV radiation skin damage, men, including those already at high risk of skin cancer, are less likely to practice sun protective behaviors despite male skin's reduced antioxidant capacity and increased tendency for UV-induced immunosuppression.[47,48,49,50] Although each patient is unique, in light of these findings, men may be at a higher risk of chemical peel-associated postinflammatory hyperpigmentation (PIH) and may require longer skin prepeel conditioning. Postprocedure skin care regimen, including possible work-related UV exposure restrictions, must be discussed explicitly. Considering chemical peels' proven benefit in actinic keratosis (AK) reduction

Table 6.2 Intrinsic skin variables in men and relevant peeling considerations

Gender-specific skin-related variables	Peeling considerations
Color • Robust facultative pigmentation after sun exposure	• May require longer pretreatment • Higher risk for PIH → need more aggressive photoprotection
Oiliness • Higher sebum production • Predisposition to acne vulgaris • Avoidance of face products due to fear of worsening tacky skin sensation	• May require longer pretreatment and more potent topical retinoids • Must aggressively degrease (hard "scrub" as opposed to "wipe") • Better candidates for lipophilic peeling agents (e.g., salicylic acid) • High risk for postpeel acne flare → consider continuing or restarting oral acne meds • Poor skin barrier function → need more counseling on consistent daily skin regimen
Thickness • Increased dermal collagen in men due to androgen receptor activation • Thicker epidermis	• May require longer pretreatment and more aggressive degreasing • Commonly need higher volumes and higher concentrations of peeling agent • Firmer peel application pressure • More treatment sessions needed
Elasticity • Lower eyelid sagging presents much earlier	• Discuss the role of segmental peels in periorbital rejuvenation and offer such intervention earlier and in combination with other minimally invasive procedures
Pain perception • Ablative CO_2 laser-evoke potentials are lower in amplitude than females suggesting better pain tolerance	• May require less aggressive pain management (although individual variation likely)
Re-epithelialization rate • Slower wound healing due to androgens	• Set realistic expectation regarding postprocedural downtime
Histamine response • More robust response in men and increasing age	• Aggressive antihistamine prophylaxis to mitigate postprocedural edema especially in periorbital rejuvenation with medium or deep peeling agent

Abbreviations: PCP, primary care provider; PIH, postinflammatory hyperpigmentation.

and skin cancer prevention,[51] careful patient selection is of utmost importance.

Finally, peeling practitioners should be familiar with current research on men's preferences regarding skin care products.[52] In general, gender does not play a significant role in treatment adherence in dermatology except for acne where males have a reportedly lower adherence rates.[53] However, knowledge of men's preferences toward particular skin care products may prove advantageous in increasing likelihood of product utilization. Men tend to be very aggressive when they scrub, a habit that men may regard as a physical cue that the product is working. In the United States, men gravitate toward products that create a perception of "refreshing and reviving tired skin."[52] Cleansers that run thin and are clear blue or green with suspended bubbles are well liked by men. Similarly, men prefer emollients with lighter, airy feel to the skin as opposed to thick, opaque creams.[52] Familiarity with new and existing skin care products that fit these general principles may improve peeling outcomes in male patients by having a framework to select effective pre- and postpeel skin care products that men are more likely to use.

▶ Table 6.3 summarizes male-specific extrinsic skin variables and relevant peeling considerations.

6.2.4 Peel Considerations in Sexual Minority Men

More than 10 million adults in the United States identify as lesbian, gay, bisexual, and transgender (LGBT), with 3.9% of men identifying as belonging to this group.[54] Ongoing efforts throughout medicine and within the dermatology specialty have been put forth to bridge the gap in LGBT health.[55,56] The literature specifically addressing chemical peel considerations in sexual minority men appears even more scant than their heterosexual or cisgendered counterparts. This subsection aims to synthesize known epidemiological, behavioral, and physiological data pertaining to sexual minority men that are relevant to chemical peeling procedures (▶ Table 6.4).

In comparison to their heterosexual counterparts, homosexual men are more likely to consider noninvasive and invasive cosmetic procedures and, in general, are more open to disclosing their experience with these procedures.[57] Indoor tanning is up to six times more

Table 6.3 Extrinsic skin variables in men and relevant peeling considerations.

Gender-specific skin-related variables	Peeling considerations
Smoking • More prevalent in men (25%) than in women (5%)	• Discuss resultant accelerated aging, poor wound healing, and increased scarring risks → counsel on smoking cessation • For deep peels, at least 1-y cessation recommended
Ultraviolet radiation exposure • Higher occupational risks • Inadequate photoprotective behavior • Reduced skin antioxidant capacity	• Increased skin cancer risks → discuss benefits of chemical peeling for actinic keratosis reduction/skin cancer prevention • May need additional counseling on photoprotective behavioral modification
Facial cleansing habits • Aggressive scrubbing quite common	• Counsel on gentle skin care practices • Emphasize high risks for scarring if aggressive exfoliation is performed postpeel
Skin care product preferences • Cleansers: thin, clear blue or green with suspended bubbles • Emollients: preference for less occlusive vehicles	• Always consider vehicle preferences when recommending pretreatment or other skin conditioning medication (e.g., adapalene 0.3% gel may be preferred to tretinoin 0.1% cream) • For medium or deep peel postprocedure emollients, explain the barrier function rationale for using occlusive vehicles, which may ensure adherence

Table 6.4 Peeling considerations in sexual minority men

Skin-related variables in sexual minority men	Peeling considerations
Transgender men on cross-hormone testosterone therapy • Acne vulgaris on face and trunk peak after 4–6 mo of therapy	• Consider serial salicylic acid peels as adjunct to standard acne treatment • For body peeling: consider salicylic acid in polyethylene glycol vehicle given lower absorption and decreased risks for salicylism
Gay and bisexual men *Ultraviolet (UV) exposure* • Indoor tanning 6 times more prevalent than heterosexual counterpart *Anabolic androgenic steroid use* • More prevalent among ethnic minority gay and bisexual men and adolescents • Unlikely for many to openly discuss steroid misuse	• Photoprotective behavior counseling should focus on concepts of UV-associated accelerated aging/wrinkle formation • Serial chemical peeling may circumvent need and associated risks from using oral antibiotics to improve acne in patients concomitantly on anabolic steroids

common in gay and bisexual men than in heterosexual men.[58,59] Those who perceive their skin tone as not matching their darker ideal skin tones were more likely to engage in indoor and outdoor tanning, the highest of which were among light-skinned individuals.[60] These findings may make sexual minority men more likely to seek out resurfacing procedures such as chemical peels while being at high risk of behaviors that could negatively impact peeling outcomes or even exclude them from being candidates for chemical peels. Discussion and implementation of UV exposure behavior modification may be more seamless in sexual minority men whose culture may value lighter skin, although future research into this is necessary. Nevertheless, emphasizing wrinkle and skin aging prevention may effectively deter sexual minority men from engaging in UV exposure[61] that could jeopardize their candidacy and/or the outcomes of their chemical peeling procedure.

Transgender men undergoing cross-sex hormone treatment with testosterone commonly develop acne vulgaris, with up to 94% of patients developing acne on the face, chest, and back within 4 to 6 months of testosterone initiation.[62,63] In most cases, acne decreases in severity a year after testosterone therapy initiation and a majority are responsive to topical retinoids and topical/oral antibiotics.[62,64] Face and/or body peeling using serial SA and other peels[65] should be considered as they can offer immediate and reliable improvement of comedonal and inflammatory acne.[65,66] Severe cases may require treatment with isotretinoin, which involves nuanced comprehension surrounding the need for contraception and pregnancy testing in this population.[56,63] Superficial peels such as SA or JS may still be safely performed in patients concomitantly on isotretinoin and may serve as an effective adjunctive treatment.[67,68]

A higher prevalence of anabolic androgenic steroid (AAS) use is reported among sexual minority men in comparison to their heterosexual counterparts.[69,70,71] Moreover, AAS misuse among sexual minority adolescent boys is three to four times higher than in heterosexual boys, especially among Black and Hispanic males.[72] Although addressing misuse of AAS in these populations is beyond the scope of this chapter, similar peeling recommendations as discussed in transgendered men apply to this group and may improve self-esteem.[73]

6.3 Approach

6.3.1 Indications

As with any aesthetic procedure, proper patient selection, preoperative consultation, and procedural planning is tantamount to positive outcomes. Indications for chemical peeling in men (▶ Table 6.5) is very similar to women although some conditions may be more commonly observed in men, such as pseudofolliculitis barbae. It is crucial to understand the histopathologic changes present in the condition to be treated and the depth at which they occur in the skin as peeling agent(s) can be tailored to specifically address these issues. UV light examination can further assist in determination of level of pigment deposition. Moreover, patient photography under this lighting can illustrate the severity of patient's photodamage and subsequent improvements after treatment.[74,75] In general, the more superficial the skin pathology, the more responsive it is to a chemical peel; hence, deep wrinkles, as commonly seen in men, do not respond to peels as adequately and as readily as fine, superficial wrinkles.[22]

Table 6.5 Summary of chemical peel indications for men and corresponding peel selection

Indication	Example of peel selection	Practical considerations
Acne vulgaris and scarring Comedonal and mild/moderate inflammatory Truncal acne or skin of color patients Rolling acne scars Ice pick and/or boxcar acne scars	Salicylic acid (20–30%) Glycolic acid (70%) Salicylic acid (30%) in polyethylene glycol Salicylic acid (30%) + TCA (10–20%) Combination medium-depth TCA peels (e.g., Brody combination) CROSS method TCA (50–100%) CROSS method phenol-croton oil (88 and 4%, respectively)	Combine with other modalities: microneedling, PDL, subcision, erbium glass laser Polyethylene glycol vehicle may decrease risk of salicylism and postinflammatory hyperpigmentation (PIH) prone "hot spots"
Rosacea Erythrosis Papulopustular	Salicylic acid (20%) Salicylic acid (20–30%)	1 application 2–3 applications
Keratosis pilaris	Glycolic acid (50–70%)	Daily maintenance therapy with glycolic acid lotion (12–20%) 48-h postpeel
Melasma, PIH	Salicylic acid (20–30%) ± TCA (10%) Glycolic acid (50–70%) TCA (10–30%) Phenol-croton oil peels (light or very light Hetter's formulation for resistant cases)	Perform at 2-wk intervals May start at lower glycolic acid concentrations (30%) for PIH
Actinic keratosis	Salicylic acid (30%) + TCA (10–35%) Jessner's solution + spot TCA (35%) Glycolic acid (70%)	May pretreat with 5-FU (5%) cream × 1 wk or perform as "pulse peels"
Dermatoheliosis/periorbital rejuvenation • Mild photoaging • Moderate to severe photoaging	Jessner's solution Glycolic acid (70%) Salicylic acid (30%) + TCA (10%) Jessner's-TCA (35%) Solid CO_2-TCA (35%) Glycolic acid (70%)-TCA (35%) Hetter's phenol-croton oil Phenol (88%) in micropunch blepharopeeling	Use in combination with other minimally invasive procedures including neurotoxins, fillers, microneedling, and/or skin-tightening devices Segmental peeling (not full face) recommended when using phenol-croton oil in men due to difficulty camouflaging postprocedural erythema without makeup
Pseudofolliculitis barbae	Salicylic acid (30%) Glycolic acid (50–70%) Jessner's solution	Repeat every 2–4 wk as needed

Abbreviations: 5-FU, 5-fluorouracil; CROSS, chemical reconstruction of skin scars; PDL, pulsed dye laser; TCA, trichloroacetic acid.

6.3.2 Prepeel Consultation

A comprehensive prepeel consultation is crucial to ensure that both the physician and patient have communicated their expectations and risks and benefits are appropriately discussed. A thorough history should be obtained with the aim of identifying factors that can impact wound healing. Any pathologic process or medication that alters the health or density of pilosebaceous units may impair proper skin re-epithelialization. Systemic illness or postoperative status affecting overall nutritional state, such as in the case of postbariatric surgery patients, should be assessed as these may limit proper wound healing. A history of PIH or hypertrophic or keloid scarring should be assessed. Prior history of herpetic infection or recurrent staphylococcal infection facilitates proper planning for prophylactic medications.

Although superficial chemical peels may be safely performed during or within 6 months after isotretinoin therapy, current evidence precludes recommendation on the use of medium or deep chemical peels while on isotretinoin.[67,68] The reported and potentials risks of concomitant isotretinoin and medium/deep peels should be discussed thoroughly with the patient. Patients with acne concurrently on oral antibiotics such as doxycycline may continue therapy, although discussion about photosensitivity should be emphasized. Similarly, increased risk of hyperpigmentation should be discussed in patients on minocycline. Concurrent exogenous testosterone use may portend the need for ongoing serial chemical peeling procedures.

Psychiatric disorders such as depression, body dysmorphic disorder, or obsessive compulsive disorders should be screened, as adequate management by mental health specialists is necessary prior to proceeding with a chemical peeling procedure. Even when outcomes are successful objectively, patients undergoing a peel for barely noticeable skin anomalies are likely to be unhappy with postoperative results.[18] As extensively discussed in the prior sections, gender-specific extrinsic factors relevant to peeling such as UV radiation (recreational outdoor, occupational, or indoor tanning) exposure should be thoroughly assessed.

General absolute contraindications to chemical peels in men include active infection and allergic contact dermatitis to peel ingredient(s). Relative contraindications include smoking, regular indoor or outdoor tanning, history of PIH, history of poor wound healing, history of high-dose iatrogenic immunosuppression (e.g., for treatment of autoimmune disease or transplant rejection), active inflammatory dermatoses, cardiac, renal, or hepatic disease (for phenol-based peels), and habitual excoriation. Absolute contraindications to phenol-based peels include history of hypertrophic scarring or keloid formation, Fitzpatrick skin type VI, and recent surgical rhytidectomy, as vascular compromise and scar formation can occur when deep peel is applied to recently undermined skin.[75] No more than 5% body surface area (BSA) should be treated with phenol in a single session. The recommended

single-session phenol peeling maximum total BSA treated is 2% in those with underlying cardiovascular disease.[76] Transient rate-corrected QT interval (QTc) prolongation may occur during phenol-croton oil peel; thus, medications known to prolong QTc should be discontinued especially in those undergoing full-face or multiple segmental phenol-croton oil peel.[16,77] In addition, some peeling experts recommend smoking cessation for at least 12 months prior to any deep peeling procedure.[76] A summary of absolute and relative contraindications to chemical peels in men is listed in ▶ Table 6.6.

Ideal peel candidates should be both willing and actually adherent to pre- and postpeel care regimen. Poor adherence to prepeel skin conditioning could be a telltale sign of inability to closely follow postoperative instructions. Men who work or regularly exercise outdoors may present a relative contraindication depending on the patient's ability and/or willingness to avoid sun exposure of the treated area postpeel. Although there are no absolute contraindications for periorbital peeling, unless corrected prior to the chemical peel, preexisting ectropion or moderate to severe lower lid laxity are relative contraindications for lower eyelid peeling.[78] If a lag or ectropion is observed after the lower lid is pulled down away from the globe for several seconds (snap back test), deep peeling the lower eyelid with phenol-croton oil can lead to an ectropion.[75,76]

Skin type assessment is an integral part of the prepeel consultation. Common classification has been primarily based on degree of skin pigmentation and tanning/burning

Table 6.6 Contraindications to chemical peeling in men

Absolute contraindications	Relative Contraindications
Active infection at the treatment area	Active rosacea and other inflammatory dermatoses
History of keloid at the treatment area	Vitiligo
Allergic contact dermatitis to peeling agent to be used	Nutritional deficiencies (e.g., from bariatric surgery)
	Diabetes
Ehlers–Danlos syndrome	Isotretinoin use within 6–12 mo[a]
Habitual excoriation, emotional instability, or mental illness	History of radiation to treatment area
	Iatrogenic immunosuppression
Inability to follow instructions	Scleroderma or other collagen vascular disease
Unrealistic expectations	History of herpetic infections
	Significant hepatic/renal/cardiac disease[a]
	Recent rhytidectomy[a]
	Darker skin types (Fitzpatrick skin type VI)[a]
	Smoking/vaping/nicotine use
	Job- or recreation-related anticipation of inadequate photoprotection

[a]More relevant when performing deep peeling.

susceptibility. However, more reliable skin type classification for chemical peeling has been proposed by Fanous and Zari that utilizes a genetico-racial category (▸ Table 6.7).[22] Inhabitants from the three ancient continents—Europe, Africa, and Asia—exhibit predictably lighter, thinner skin and smaller features as one moves north, and gradually display darker, thicker skin with larger features as one moves south. In this classification, Europe and Africa run in a parallel vertical fashion to Asia and is divided into six total categories. By using this genetico-racial classification, peel outcomes can be reliably predicted, and complications are more likely to be prevented. For example, despite their Fitzpatrick phototype, it may not be advisable to proceed with a deep peel in Nordics (e.g., Scandinavian, Irish, or Scottish) as their thin skin may make them prone to scarring. A useful peeling guideline that incorporates this genetico-racial classification is as follows: (1) medium to deep peels for mid-Europeans and southern Europeans (Mediterraneans), (2) medium and light to medium peels for northern Europeans (Nordics) and Asians, (3) light peels for southern Caucasians (Indo-Pakistanis), and (4) very light peels for Africans.

6.3.3 Prepeel Skin Conditioning

Proper skin conditioning prior to a peel, also called skin priming, is essential to a successful chemical peeling outcome. The overall goal of skin priming is restoration of skin back to a normal state prior to wounding it.[79] This is achieved by thinning the stratum corneum, melanocyte regulation, and dermal collagen production. These processes facilitate uniform peeling agent penetration, prevention of postinflammatory dyspigmentation, and predictable and more rapid re-epithelialization.

Skin priming may be divided into two phases: pretreatment and preparation.[80] Pretreatment includes the days up to months before the peeling procedure. Preparation consists of the steps performed immediately before the peeling procedure, which include degreasing and application of topical anesthesia, as needed. Due to various intrinsic and extrinsic factors previously discussed, men may require longer pretreatment regimen as well as more aggressive skin preparation. Agents used during the pretreatment phase can include topical retinoids (tretinoin, retinaldehyde, adapalene, or tazarotene), keratolytics (lactic acid, SA, kojic acid, or GA), and lightening agents (hydroquinone or azelaic acid; ▸ Table 6.8). Because men gravitate toward simple, quick therapeutic strategies, their adherence to regimens that entail multistep daily routines may be dismal.[81] Since convenience and simplicity are key for men, agents already commercially available in combination or an individually compounded topical prescription may be more ideal. Typical pretreatment begins 4 to 6 weeks prior to planned chemical peeling; however, skin of color patients may require 8 to 12 weeks.[74] A common skin priming regimen involves compounded hydroquinone (8%), tretinoin (0.025%), and hydrocortisone (1%; modified Kligman's formula) at night for the entire pretreatment period.[80] For genetico-racial groups at risk of postpeel hyperpigmentation (▸ Table 6.7), as well as those with history of dyschromia, expert consensus recommends cessation of topical retinoid 1 week prior to chemical peel in order to prevent potential peel overpenetration.[82-84] Particularly for GA peeling, there may be value to incorporating a topical cream or lotion containing 8 to 10% GA in the patient's at home priming regimen, as unusual sensitivity to GA may be unmasked, allowing the peeling practitioner an opportunity to select a more appropriate peeling agent.[85] In contrast, there are differing views among peeling experts regarding the importance of pretreatment prior to deep peeling with phenol-croton oil.[40]

Pretreatment of the entire face should be performed with a topical retinoid or GA cream, including the upper eyelids, which should be treated once to twice a week[74] especially if periorbital rejuvenation is planned. Pretreatment feathering into the hairline, jawline, and preauricular areas is also recommended, noting that the hairline may extend significantly into the scalp in some men. Daily regimen should include a broad-spectrum UVA/UVB sunscreen with a minimum sun protection factor 30 (SPF 30). Visible light protection, present in tinted sunscreens, should be strongly considered in skin of color patients and is a must for those with dyschromia, as visible light has been shown to induce pigment darkening in these individuals.[86,87,88]

Another very important goal of pretreatment, albeit an indirect one, is it facilitates "natural selection" among prospective peeling candidates. Instituting a typical prepeel skin regimen by itself can improve a patient's appearance.[74] Those uncertain about their decision to proceed with the peeling procedure who were adherent to the prepeel regimen may be more motivated to move forward after seeing initial improvements. Conversely, those unable to adhere to the prepeel regimen are more likely to have suboptimal peeling outcomes and may be more likely to have challenges in adhering to postoperative instructions.[80] A change in skin color that shows a medium pink hue may be observed after 4 to 12 weeks of pretreatment and is a reliable indicator of a successful prepeel treatment, which can be detected even in skin of color patients.[22]

The preparation phase of skin priming is the immediate period prior to the peeling procedure and involves degreasing and administration of topical anesthesia, sedative, and/or antihistamines. Regarding degreasers, there is no difference between the efficacy of alcohol, acetone, or chlorhexidine gluconate.[89] However, because of its relatively low flash point and high risk of combustion, use of acetone for degreasing should be avoided in the vicinity of any potential ignitors especially when ventilation is inadequate.[89] Interestingly, some peeling experts have

Table 6.7 Genetico-racial skin classification categories and trichloroacetic acid (TCA)[a] peel outcomes

	Central and Southern Africans	Southern Caucasians/Indo-Pakistanis (e.g., Indian, Egyptian, or Saudi Arabian)	Northern, Central, and Southern Asians (e.g., Chinese, Japanese, or Filipino)	Northern Europeans/Nordics (e.g., Scandinavian, Irish, or Scottish)	Southern Europeans/Mediterraneans (e.g., Spanish, Greek, Italian, or Turkish)	Mid-Europeans (e.g., French, German, or English)
Geographic origin	Central and Southern Africa	Northern Africa and Western Asia	Eastern Asia	Northern Europe	Southern Europe, Northern Africa, and Western Asia	Central Europe
Facial features	Large	Moderately large	Moderately large	Fine	Slightly large	Medium
Skin characteristics	Thick, with black to deep black	Thick, with a deep tan to dark brown	Thick, with light medium, or dark brown	Thin white, with a pink element	Slightly thick, with a medium tan	Average thickness, white, or light tan
TCA peel outcomes	Acceptable (with very light peels)	Acceptable to good (with light peels)	Good (with light and medium peels)	Good (with light to medium peels)	Good to very good (with medium and deep peels)	Excellent (with all peels)
Hyperpigmentation	+++	+++	++	+/−	++	+
Hypopigmentation	(if deep peel)	(if deep peel)	(rare with deep peel)	−	−	−
Erythema	+/−	+/−	++ (later turns into hyperpigmentation)	+++	++	+

[a]Very light peels with TCA is less than 30%, light is 30–35%, medium is 35–40%, and deep is 40–45%.

Table 6.8 Pretreatment regimen[a]

Indication	Medication and dosing
PIH prevention and peel absorption optimization	**Topical retinoids** Start at least 4–6 wk prior to peel (8–12 wk in skin of color); stop 1–2 wk if treating PIH or melasma; 1–2 d for photoaging Tretinoin 0.02–0.1% cream or gel every night at bedtime Adapalene 0.3% gel every night at bedtime *For more sensitive skin, consider:* Glycolic acid 8–10% lotion/cream Adapalene 0.1% lotion or cream *For patients with moderate to severe acne scars, consider:* Tazarotene 0.05% cream every night at bedtime **Lightening agents:** Start 4–6 wk prior to peel; stop 1–2 d prior to peel Hydroquinone 4–10% twice a day Azelaic acid 15% gel or 20% cream twice a day
Preexisting melasma or PIH	Fluocinolone cream (0.01–0.025%) twice a day for 2–12 wk Tinted sunscreen for visible light protection
UV radiation protection	Broad-spectrum SPF (titanium dioxide- and zinc oxide-based sunscreen preferable)

Abbreviations: PIH, postinflammatory hyperpigmentation; SPF, sun protection factor; UV, ultraviolet.
[a]Consider having pretreatment agents compounded together to potentially improve adherence.

discontinued degreasing with alcohol all together, citing the unnecessary irritation it often causes that may affect homogenous peel absoprtion.[22] Degreasing typically takes less than 2 minutes and may be performed as either a "wipe" in a unidirectional motion or a "scrub" with bidirectional motion and greater friction.[90] In general, men will require more vigorous scrubs given the higher sebaceous quality of their skin and higher prevalence of deeper rhytids. Skin preparation may also involve application of topical anesthesia and administration of mild sedative. Various topical anesthetics may also be applied to the skin 30 minutes prior to the procedure with or without occlusion.[22,80] There is literature recommending against the use of topical anesthetics when performing medium-depth peels citing unpredictable increases in peel penetration and insufficient pain relief as deterrents.[18,74] Some peeling experts recommend using it after the initial peeling agent in a combination peel has been applied, that is, prior to the application of TCA.[91] Nonsedating antihistamine may also be administered prior to the procedure to minimize edema and may be continued after the procedure to manage pruritus.

Patients with a history of herpes simplex or herpes zoster infection are at an increased risk for viral reactivation due to skin trauma from chemical peeling. Most literature on chemical peeling recommend herpes prophylaxis for all medium and deep peel candidates beginning the day before or the day of the procedure, as the scarring could be devastating and the infection could easily disseminate.[18,74,75,92] Common prophylactic regimens include 200 to 400 mg of acyclovir three times daily or valacyclovir 500 mg twice daily until full re-epithelialization occurs (typically 7–10 days for medium peels and up to 14 days for deep peels). A herpetic outbreak may happen in patients without prior history of occurrence; however, in those with history of frequent herpes simplex infection, valacyclovir may be started 7 days prior to the procedure at 1 g twice daily and continued for 14 days postpeel. Although most chemical peel experts do not use empiric antibiotic or anti-*Candida* agent on every patient, some do recommend topical mupirocin ointment applied to the nares three times daily beginning 7 days before medium or deep peel and continued until full re-epithelialization.[74] For patients undergoing medium and deep peels, the authors (R.T./J.R.) recommend doxycycline 100 mg twice daily for 7 to 10 days beginning from the day of the procedure, with the patient understanding that photoprotection becomes even more crucial. Other published antibiotic prophylaxis for chemical peels suggests cephalexin 500 mg twice daily starting the day before the procedure and continued for 7 days.[93]

6.3.4 Postpeel Skin Care

Immediate postpeel skin care, which occurs up until full re-epithelialization, may vary based on chemical peel depth. For superficial peels, this simply involves gentle soap-free cleansers twice daily and abundant use of fragrance-free emollient cream.

Mild burning sensations and pruritus in medium-depth peels may improve with oral analgesics and antihistamines, as well as diluted white vinegar (1 tablespoon in 1 cup of water) compresses followed by thorough water rinses two to four times daily. Liberal application of white petrolatum three times daily is recommended. Thereafter, the patient may switch to an emollient cream (fragrance free) or continue using petrolatum until re-epithelialization is complete.[82]

Deep peels require avoidance of facial shower or bathing for at least 2 days.[76] Frequent sterile saline washes or sterile saline compresses is recommended, as well as the application of pure petrolatum every 2 to 6 hours, with the goal of maintaining skin crusts soft. Manipulation of crusts should be avoided by patients. Current literature lacks comparative human studies on postpeel care after deep peels[94]; however, some peeling experts favor waterproof zinc oxide tape occlusion, which is removed by the physician 24 to 48 hour after application.[76] For phenol-croton oil periorbital rejuvenation, the authors of this chapter do not tape occlude the eyelids. Bismuth subgallate powder, which has antiseptic and anti-inflammatory properties, may then be applied to the treated areas, which dry up and form a protective "green cocoon." This protective layer separates from the underlying epidermis after a week and is gently removed after soaking overnight in petrolatum.[95]

The authors recommend that male patients avoid shaving of the treated area until fully re-epithelialized. Postprocedure erythema may be addressed with green-tinted cosmetic products or topical α-adrenergic receptor agonists, though in one author's (S.S.) experience effectiveness is unpredictable in the latter. Postpeel skin care regimen should be initiated immediately upon full re-epithelialization, which may begin as early as 3 days for superficial peels to as late as 14 days for deep peels. Once again, keeping regimens simple may promote better adherence in men; hence, restarting the same pretreatment combination topical formulation that the patient previously used may be a wise recommendation.

6.4 Procedures

There are a handful of chemical peel agents with various combinations, concentrations, and formulations. Those who have developed a mastery of the art and science of chemical peels tend to limit their peeling repertoire to a select number of agents.[75] In-depth clinical experience using a few peeling agents is more likely to deliver outstanding outcomes as one becomes intimately familiar with all aspects of such peels.

A broad knowledge of men's cosmetic concerns may allow peeling practitioners to identify peeling regimens best suited for those particular indications. In a recent study of 600 men, the periorbital region was at the top of men's concerns, including crow's feet, tear troughs, and dark circles and bags under the eyes.[8] These and other common presenting concerns by men, such dyschromias, acne scars, and pseudofolliculitis,[10,96] can all be improved by a variety of peeling techniques alone or in combination with other minimally invasive interventions (▸ Table 6.5). Because men tend to be more direct when discussing their desired outcomes and have very specific self-perceived cosmetic flaw, evaluation of each cosmetic unit and selecting peels best suited to treat the pathology in that specific facial area, also known as combination segmental peeling, can be very effective.[97,98]

6.4.1 Salicylic Acid Peel

This lipophilic BHA is known for its efficacy in treating inflammatory and noninflammatory acne lesions and its safety profile in all skin types.[99] Most commonly used formulations are SA 20 to 30% in ethanol, which crystallizes upon ethanol evaporation. This leaves a pseudofrost that can be a visual aid that facilitates uniform peel application (▸ Fig. 6.1). This pseudofrost, composed of SA crystals, should not be confused with frosting observed when

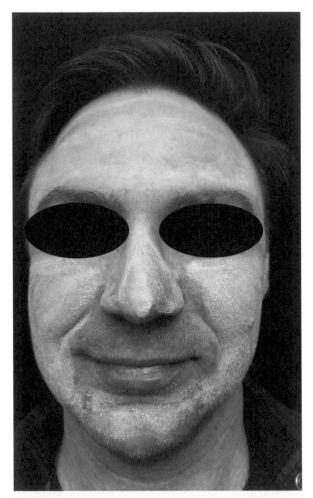

Fig. 6.1 Pseudofrost after two applications of salicylic acid (30%) peel.

proteins coagulate. Burning and stinging should be expected immediately after each application, which may be significantly alleviated with a portable hand-held fan. An anesthetic effect may be observed a minute or so after peel application.

It is best to begin with SA 20% to assess patient's sensitivity and reactivity. After degreasing, large cotton-tip applicators or gauze sponges are used to evenly apply peeling agent, with multiple applications to more problematic areas. The peel is left on for 3 to 5 minutes, and the face is carefully blotted with a cold, wet wash cloth to remove as much of pseudofrost prior to rinsing the area with tap water. In patients at high risk of PIH, a thin layer of mid-potency topical steroid may be applied to the treated areas after gently patting dry with wash cloth. Thereafter, a mineral-based broad-spectrum sunscreen is liberally applied. SA peels should be repeated in 2- to 4-week intervals, with optimal results seen after a series of three to six sessions (▸ Fig. 6.2).[99]

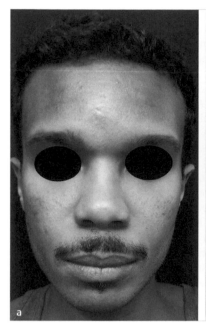
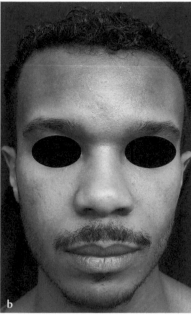

Fig. 6.2 (a,b) Improvement of mild acne scarring and postinflammatory hyperpigmentation (PIH) after a series of three salicylic acid (20–30%) peels performed at 2-week intervals in a Fitzpatrick phototype V.

SA 30% in polyethylene glycol (SA-PEG) vehicle is a newer SA formulation that is associated with minimal to no discomfort after application. SA-PEG causes minimal desquamation and little to no risk of PIH often associated with "hot spots" of ethanolic SA overpenetration.[82,100] It has shown superior results in improving acne when compared with SA in ethanol with minimal peel absorption beyond the cornified layer but greater follicular penetration.[100] Because it may significantly diminish the risk of salicylism,[101] this formulation may be of clinical value when performing body peeling in those with propensity to develop truncal acne, such as cis- or transgender men on exogenous testosterone therapy. SA-PEG must have at least 5 minutes of contact time and requires thorough rinsing after application due to its occlusive vehicle.[82] When performing body peeling for truncal acne, three to five sessions of SA-PEG or ethanolic SA peels may be performed at 2- to 4-week intervals for optimal results.

Jessner's Solution

JS consists of SA (14 g), resorcinol (14 g), lactic acid 85% (14 g), and ethanol (sufficient quantity to make 100 mL).[102] The skin-lightening effect of resorcinol (a phenol derivative), combined with the keratolytic effect of SA and lactic acid, makes this a good agent for milder cases of acne, melasma, PIH, lentigo, freckles, and photodamage. A modified JS, in which citric acid is substituted for resorcinol, circumvents the potential risk for allergic contact dermatitis and increased hyperpigmentation in Fitzpatrick VI phototypes.[103] At least two coats are needed to achieve a superficial peel, whereas additional coats increase the depth of peeling. A patchy pseudofrosting from the component SA can be observed. Neutralization is not necessary, although some peeling experts recommend washing off the peeling agent after 6 minutes.[18,102]

6.4.2 Glycolic Acid Peel

GA is the most commonly used AHA used as single peeling agent.[85] This "lunch time peel" has grown in popularity among men owing to its relatively mild postprocedural erythema and desquamation.[85,104] Peeling agent contact time with subsequent neutralization is quintessential for this AHA peel as GA left on the skin for 15 minutes can wound the dermis to a depth identical to that of 35 to 50% TCA.[105] GA peels are available in a variety of delivery systems, which include free acid, partially neutralized, buffered, and esterified.[85] The practical benefits of buffered, partially neutralized, and esterified GA peels have been questioned,[85] although there is some literature suggesting that these delivery systems may be safer than GA peel as free acid.[106] Although the GA concentration in general indicates its potency, the pH of the GA peel dictates its wounding potential.[107,108] For example, a buffered or partially neutralized 70% GA at pH 5 is far less potent than a 20% GA at pH 3.[107]

A series of GA peels is almost always required to achieve the desired clinical outcomes. It is advisable to begin with GA peels containing 20 to 30% free acids, with increasing concentration and application time over subsequent peeling sessions repeated every 2 to 4 weeks.[85,108] The desired clinical endpoint is uniform erythema; areas with frosting or blanching designate epidermolysis and should be immediately neutralized.[85] Neutralization often results in initial stinging sensation that quickly subsides.[85] Water or basic solutions, such as ammonium salts, sodium bicarbonate, or sodium hydroxide, are common neutralizers used in GA peeling and cause a foaming reaction, which marks the desired neutralization.[85,108] GA peels with 20 or 30% free acids typically will cause an even erythema when left on the skin for 2 to 5 minutes. Subsequent GA peels should be performed at higher concentrations for each time that no visible erythema is achieved at 5 minutes of contact time.[85] Because of the added required step of neutralization and its central role in the safety of the procedure, there may be an argument for some peeling practitioners to prefer other superficial peeling agents over GA. Combining topical 5-fluorouracil (5-FU; 5%) with GA (70%) peel increases the efficacy for treating AK when performed as "pulse peels" every 1 to 2 weeks.[109,110] Hence, physicians should consider facility in performing GA peels at least for specific indications such as AKs.

6.4.3 Trichloroacetic Acid and Combination Medium-Depth Peels

Considered as the "workhorse" of chemical peels, TCA can be used as a superficial, medium, or deep peeling agent. Although it may be helpful to classify TCA peels as very light (< 30%), light (30–35%), medium (35–40%), and deep (> 40%), it is important to understand that larger volumes (i.e., multiple peel applications and/or a wetter gauze or cotton-tip applicator) and deeper application pressure of even very light TCA peels can cause enough protein coagulation to reach the superficial reticular dermis. The key concept underlying chemical peeling, however, is efficient and controlled wounding of the skin at the intended depth. This is the rationale behind combination medium-depth peels that utilize a superficial peeling agent such as solid CO_2 (Brody's combination), GA (70%; Coleman's combination), or JS (Monheit's combination) prior to the application of TCA (35%), thereby allowing TCA to more quickly reach the dermis. Otherwise, TCA needs to coagulate epidermal proteins before it can reach its intended dermal depth, thus lengthening the procedure time and potential discomfort. Conversely, TCA concentrations greater than 35% are capable of significantly more rapid protein coagulation—even an additional small volume coat can lead to dermal wounding much deeper than intended, which may result in scarring. Thus, TCA ≥ 40% are generally utilized in deliberate destruction of discrete isolated lesions or reconstruction of scars.[111]

The clinical endpoint for a light, medium, or deep peel with TCA is based on frosting. A light peel should only have scattered, nonorganized light white frost (level I frost) designating predominantly epidermal wounding. Additional coats of TCA result in an even white frost with a diffuse pink background (level II frost), which correlates with papillary dermal protein coagulation. Continued TCA application results in TCA penetration into the upper reticular dermis, which clinically appears as a solid white frost without any pink background (level III frost). A "grayish" frost signals penetration into the mid-reticular

dermis, which is associated with increased risk of scarring and hypopigmentation. Thus, level III frost is the maximum endpoint recommended for most TCA peels.[18,74,91,111]

Skin priming should be performed prior to TCA peeling as previously discussed. A practical way to approach TCA peeling is to use the genetico-racial classification (▶ Table 6.7) for TCA peel and to carefully limit frosting to level I for light peels, level II for medium peels, and level III for deep peels. A series of light TCA peels performed at 2- to 4-week intervals can be effective for mild epidermal pathologies such as mild photoaging, superficial melasma, or PIH. Again, although this can be achieved faster with TCA 35%,[22] or slower with more coats using TCA 10%, the ease of achieving level II frosting with higher TCA concentration should be kept in mind especially in genetico-racial categories in which medium peels are not reliably safe. For hypertrophic AKs, absorption of the peeling solution may be facilitated by curettage of the hyperkeratosis prior to targeted vigorous chemical peel application using a cotton-tipped applicator (▶ Fig. 6.3).[91]

Solid CO_2 and TCA 35% (Brody's Combination)

A block of solid CO_2 applied to the skin at varying durations allows for quicker penetration of TCA 35% into the dermis resulting in a medium-depth peel. Solid CO_2 may be purchased at a local hardware and broken into a shape that can be conveniently manually handled, dipped into acetone, and applied with mild (3–5 seconds), moderate (5–8 seconds), or hard pressure (8–15 seconds) to the entire face. Application of solid CO_2 to the skin is painless. The skin is wiped dry and topical anesthesia may be applied prior to applying TCA 35%. Among the three most common combination medium-depth peels, solid CO_2–TCA combination has been reported to result in the greatest improvement in treating more advanced photoaging, thicker epidermal lesions, and acne scarring.[91]

Glycolic Acid 70% and TCA 35% (Coleman's Combination)

GA 70% unbuffered free acid is applied onto the skin and neutralized immediately after 2 minutes of contact time.[18,74,91] The use of water as a neutralizer may make this combination peel more efficient, since using a base as a neutralizer may alter the pH of the skin, thereby affecting the pH of the TCA when it is applied. Once neutralization is complete, the area is cleansed with water and wiped dry prior to application of TCA 35%.

Jessner's Solution and TCA 35% (Monheit's Combination)

JS is applied to the areas to be treated in one or two coats, which should cause mild pseudofrosting. A Wood lamp

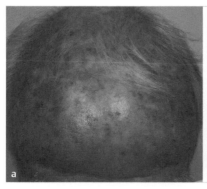
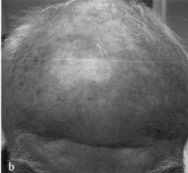

Fig. 6.3 (a,b) Actinic keratoses treated with Jessner's solution and spot trichloroacetic acid (TCA; 35%).

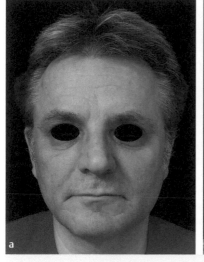
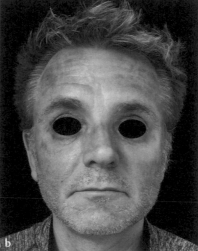
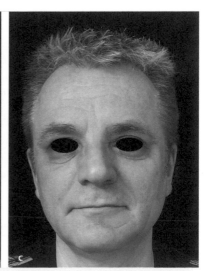

Fig. 6.4 Solid CO_2–trichloroacetic acid (TCA; 35%) combination peel. **(a)** Prepeel, **(b)** 4 days postpeel, and **(c)** 14 days postpeel.

may be used to ensure that an even layer of JS is applied on to the skin, which appears as an even fluorescent green layer. This is important because an even JS facilitates even penetration of TCA 35% into the dermis.[91] TCA (35%) alone or preceded by solid CO_2, GA (70%), or JS can be repeated every 12 weeks as needed to achieve desired results (▶ Fig. 6.4a-c).[112]

6.4.4 Chemical Reconstruction of Skin Scars Technique

The chemical reconstruction of skin scars (CROSS) method involves the firm and focal application of TCA at high concentrations (50–100%) deep into the depressed area of atrophic acne scars.[113,114] Its pioneers recommend against skin pretreatment with retinoid due to the risk of unpredictable and excessive TCA penetration, although pretreatment with hydroquinone or other lightening agents is safe and may further decrease the low rates of postinflammatory pigmentary changes associated with this procedure.[114] The CROSS technique activates fibroblasts deep within atrophic scars, leading to localized scar formation and remodeling. This technique has also been used to improve the appearance of enlarged pores.[114,115]

Depending on the peeling practitioner's preference and/or experience, a sharpened wooden applicator, or a 31-gauge, 8-mm straight or bent needle on a 1-mL insulin syringe is used to firmly apply TCA onto the atrophic scar on stretch.[114,116] Box car and ice pick acne scars are the acne scar types most responsive to CROSS technique.[117] Approximately 10 seconds after application, level II or III frosting is observed within the treated area, with development of mild edema in its immediate surroundings. Prickling and burning sensation may be felt during the procedure and is tolerated by most patients without need for anesthesia. The treated areas are then washed with a gentle cleanser with subsequent application of a topical antibiotic ointment once[114] and plain fragrance-free emollient cream thereafter. Discrete crusts develop in the treated areas and should be allowed to detach on their own (usually in 7 days), a process that may be inadvertently impeded if occlusive dressings are used.[114] Optimal

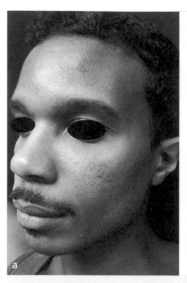 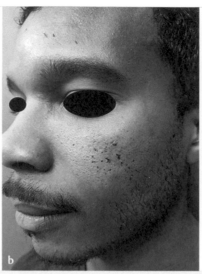 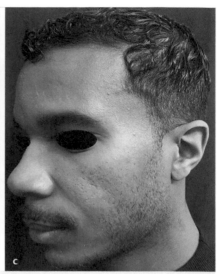

Fig. 6.5 Chemical reconstruction of skin scars (CROSS) technique using trichloroacetic acid (TCA; 100%). **(a)** Before, **(b)** 5 days after the second treatment, and **(c)** 4 weeks after the third treatment.

results are observed after five or six treatment sessions spaced 2 to 6 weeks apart, although clinical improvement may be seen even after just two or three sessions (▶ Fig. 6.5).[113,114,116]

6.4.5 Phenol Croton-Oil peel

Phenol-croton oil peels can induce dermal neocollagenesis and elastic fiber formation that result in skin rejuvenation surpassing that observed after fully ablative CO_2 resurfacing. Erythema designates reticular dermal collagen formation and is expected for 3 to 6 months after undergoing phenol-croton oil peel.[16] Use of makeup to camouflage this erythema is a normal part of postpeel management in these patients particularly in full face phenol-croton oil peels, which have predominantly been performed in females.[76] Although there may be ongoing shifts in cultural norms making it more acceptable for men to use makeup,[118,119,120] the majority of male patients likely to present in clinic who are ideal candidates for phenol-croton oil peels (e.g., fair-skinned with significant photoaging) most likely would be put off by the anticipatory need for postprocedure erythema cosmetic camouflage. Hence, the role of phenol-croton oil peels in men tends to revolve primarily around segmental peeling techniques for specific indications such as periorbital rejuvenation. These segmental deep peels can address the most bothersome facial cosmetic concerns in men and circumvent the need for cardiac monitoring or intravenous hydration typical of phenol-croton oil peeling of larger surface areas.[16] Other indications for phenol-croton oil peel in men include acne scars by the CROSS technique, AK, actinic cheilitis, and lip rejuvenation.[76]

The face can be divided into six cosmetic units: forehead, nose, periocular, left cheek, right cheek, and perioral area. Each unit can be treated at different peeling depths based on each subunit's typical skin characteristics and clinical severity of photoaging (▶ Fig. 6.6).[16] The boundaries of these cosmetic units should be marked to ensure that the phenol-croton oil formulation is applied to its corresponding recommended location and/or photoaging severity. The use of the traditional Baker–Gordon peel has fallen out of favor due to its unacceptably high rates of permanent hypopigmentation.[16,40] Newer formulations by Hetter (▶ Table 6.9) have allowed for phenol-croton oil peels to be used in the treatment of mild to moderate photoaging and acne scarring.[16,18,74] The light and very light Hetter's Heresy formulas are considered appropriate for the periorbital areas.[16,121] For example, the very light formulation can provide significant tightening of the anterior lamella for younger male patients who show only textural changes and mild fat protrusion and are not yet seeking surgical interventions.[78]

Alternatively, periorbital rejuvenation may include micropunch blepharopeeling performed using straight phenol (89%). This peeling agent is applied to the area between the upper eyelid's superior tarsal plate border and the eyebrow's inferior border, as well as within 1 to 2 mm of the lower eyelid margin. Immediately after frosting, multiple (between 5 and 20) 3- to 5-mm snip excisions arranged in a random gridlike pattern are performed on the central and lateral areas of the upper eyelid, which are allowed to heal by secondary intention.[122,123] This procedure has shown excellent aesthetic outcomes in treating periocular rhytids without the associated volume loss and linear scarring seen in conventional surgical blepharolplasty.[122,123]

Cardiac safety considerations arise especially when performing phenol peels in more than one cosmetic unit (area of palm without finger) or greater than 0.5% of the BSA. Continuous electrocardiographic monitoring and hydration (PO or IV) are recommended when total BSA to be peeled exceeds 1%.[16] After one cosmetic unit is treated (forehead, nose, periocular, right cheek, left cheek, perioral), air circulation and safety pauses of 15 to 20 minutes are recommended to facilitate adequate phenol excretion.[16,124] For segmental peel of only one cosmetic unit, hydration involves patient oral intake of a minimum of 1 liter of water throughout the procedure.[16]

Neoprene gloves must be worn when performing phenol peeling, especially if gauze pads will be used to apply the agent or catch any inadvertent drip, as phenol can penetrate into latex and nitrile gloves.[16,125] Use of activated carbon-containing masks, such as reusable acid gases and organic vapor masks or disposable organic vapor masks, is recommended to mitigate any acute inhalation adverse effects to medical personnel.[126] Once appropriate personnel protective equipment is worn and skin preparation is completed, croton oil is mixed with 88% phenol, followed by soap and water (▶ Video 6.1). The solution separates into two phases after 1 minute; hence, the mixture must be swirled prior to each coat.[18,74] The authors prefer using cotton-tipped applicators when rubbing the solution onto the skin, whereas the nondominant hand holds a gauze for any inadvertent drips and stabilizes the treated area. A solid white frost immediately forms on the treated skin, which also quickly dissipates and thus may falsely signal the need for additional peel application, leading to inadvertently deeper wounding.[18,74]

6.4.6 Combination of Chemical Peeling with Other Minimally Invasive Procedures

Combining chemical peels with other minimally invasive procedure continues to be common practice.[127,128] A retrospective review of 114 patients (39 men) with predominantly rolling acne scars treated with a single session that combined TCA (20%), extensive subcision, and fractional

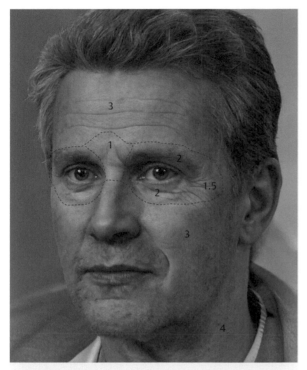

Fig. 6.6 Segmental combination chemical peel in men. Phenol–croton oil for the periorbital area with varying penetration depth depending on cosmetic subunits; Jessner's solution for the neck; and solid CO_2–trichloroacetic acid (TCA; 35%) for the rest of the face with feathering into the hairline, preauricular/tragus, and mandible (1 = deepest, 4 = light application). (Photo by Generated Photos.)

Table 6.9 Hetter's Heresy phenol-croton oil formulations[121]

	Very light	Light	Medium	Heavy	Very heavy
Indication	Eyelids, neck	Periocular	Forehead, cheeks	Perioral, nose	Perioral, chin
Croton oil concentration (%)	0.12	0.4	0.8	1.2	1.6
Phenol concentration (%)	27.5	35	35	35	35
Hetter's stock croton oil[a]	0.25 ml	1 ml	2 ml	3 ml	4 ml
Phenol (88%)	3.75 ml	3 ml	2 ml	1 ml	0 ml
Septisol	0.5 ml	0.5 ml	0.5 ml	0.5 ml	0.5 ml
Water	5.5 ml	5.5 ml	5.5 ml	5.5 ml	5.5 ml

[a]Hetter's croton oil stock solution is comprised of 1 mL of croton oil mixed with 24 mL of 88% phenol. This stock solution contains 4% croton oil in phenol. One drop of croton oil from a Delasco dropper is equal to 0.04 mL of croton oil.[16]

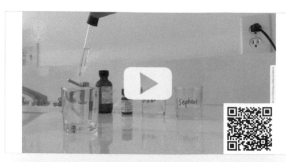

Video 6.1 Mixing Hetter formula.

CO_2 laser revealed significant scar improvement and high patient satisfaction with treatment results.[128] Other reports have suggested prepeel treatment with botulinum toxin and/or hyaluronic acid filler has a synergistic effect in the treatment of rhytids.[129,130] In patients previously treated with neurotoxin, injection of neurotoxin 2 to 3 weeks prior to a medium or deep chemical peel has been posited to facilitate healing due to diminished facial movement.[76] For treatment-naive patients, neurotoxin injection 10 to 14 days after a phenol-croton oil peel may prolong desired neuromuscular blockade.[76] Although same-day neurotoxin treatment and chemical peeling are generally not recommended due to potential neurotoxin diffusion from edema, soft-tissue augmentation may be performed on the same day if superficial or medium-depth peels are used or different areas are treated. Otherwise, treatment should be performed 4 to 6 months after a deep chemical peel.[76]

6.5 Complications

As previously discussed, intrinsic and extrinsic male skin variables can predispose men to slower re-epithelialization rates, more exuberant postprocedural edema, and bruising. Complications from chemical peels are very similar to other resurfacing modalities discussed in this book.[45] Although early identification, treatment, and prevention of chemical peel complications (▶ Table 6.10) is not gender specific, special circumstances are worthy of discussion. In an atrophic bald scalp with multiple AKs, chemexfoliated areas showing delayed re-epithelialization may be a consequence of diminished adnexal structures or actinically damaged skin itself.[131] In these patients, adherence to postoperative wound care should be further emphasized while maintaining a high index of suspicion for infection or erosive pustular dermatosis of the scalp. Certain areas are prone to hypertrophic scarring from medium or deep peels and should be peeled less vigorously even in men. These areas are the medial upper eyelids, lateral lower eyelids, zygomatic arch, preauricular area, and the neck. Medium-depth peels have unpredictable outcomes on the neck and a tendency to cause scarring; superficial

peels in combination with skin tightening devices, neurotoxin, and/or biostimulatory fillers should be considered instead.

6.6 Conclusion

Amid new laser technologies and other minimally invasive devices, there is a resurgence of interest in chemical peeling given its reliable and cost-effective aesthetic outcomes. A good comprehension of men's most common cosmetic concerns as well as intrinsic and extrinsic variables that affect their skin helps the aesthetic practitioner create a successful treatment plan most fitting to the patient's desires. Although over 70% dermatology residents in the United States plan to perform chemical peels in their future clinical practices, a large majority have not had primary hands-on experience in chemical peeling.[132] Hands-on workshops, such as those offered by the International Peeling Society (https://www.peelingsociety.com), provide invaluable exposure to chemical peeling techniques that can help fill gaps in cosmetic training.[98] Facility in performing chemical peels and understanding gender-specific nuances of this technique may be well rewarded in today's growing aesthetic market.

6.7 Pearls

- Limit your chemical peeling repertoire to a few peeling agents. Extensive experience in using only a select number of peels tends to produce desired outcomes consistently and is central to avoiding complications.
- Medium-depth peels typically utilize a keratolytic prior to application of a protein denaturant, with the former facilitating efficient dermal penetration of the latter. Solid CO_2-TCA (35%) combination tends to result in the greatest skin improvement when treating advanced photoaging.
- Lipophilic peels such as SA and JS may result in a more pronounced skin improvement in men given their skin's higher sebaceous gland density than women's. Strongly consider incorporating these peels when selecting peeling agents for men.
- Due to intrinsic male skin characteristics, peeling procedures in men often require higher concentrations and higher volumes of peel solution, greater peel application pressure, more peeling sessions, and/or longer prepeel skin conditioning to achieve the intended depth of peel penetration.
- Optimize convenience and simplicity when selecting pre- and postpeel skin care regimen for men. Choose agents that are already commercially available in combination or consider having the individual agents combined in a compounded formulation, ideally in "lighter" vehicles.

Table 6.10 Management and prevention of chemical peeling complications

Sequelae	Pearls	Management Tips
Painful erosions or ulcerations	• Painful skin lesions occurring postpeel should be treated as herpetic infection	• Polymerase chain reaction–based testing, direct fluorescent antibody test, and/or viral culture for herpes simplex virus (HSV) or varicella-zoster virus (VZV) • Empiric valacyclovir 1 g thrice a day × 10 d

Hypertrophic scarring	• Early signs of scar formation: persistent erythema, induration, pruritus, and delayed healing
	• Initiate treatment at earliest recognition of scarring
		• Silicone gel sheeting
		• Scar massage
		• Topical, intralesional, or oral steroids:
		  ○ Class I topical steroid twice a day
		  ○ Intralesional triamcinolone acetonide injections (10–20 mg/mL tailored to scar thickness) performed monthly
		• Pulsed dye laser (PDL)
		• 5-fluorouracil injections may be used in combination with intralesional steroids and/or PDL treatments

Postinflammatory hyperpigmentation (PIH)	• Fitzpatrick skin types III–VI at highest risk
	• Consider performing test spot in at-risk patients
	• Initiate treatment once re-epithelialized
		• Sunscreen with physical blocking ingredient (titanium dioxide or zinc oxide) and visible light protection (tinted versions)
		• Hydroquinone 4% or higher twice a day:
		  ○ ±topical retinoid and low-potency steroid (or combination product with hydroquinone/retinoid/steroid)
		  ○ May alternate months with azelaic acid 15% gel or 20% cream to diminish risk of ochronosis
		• Topical immunomodulator (tacrolimus 0.1% ointment) may be added to treat residual inflammation
		• Glycolic acid peels (10–30%) every other week

Allergic contact dermatitis	• Most commonly due to resorcinol	• Topical steroids • If severe/persistent: methylprednisolone dose pack
Pustule formation	• Bacterial or *Candida* infection	• Swab for Gram stain, culture, and sensitivities • Empiric fluconazole 150 mg oral × 1 dose • Consider addition of oral antibiotic (e.g., doxycycline) while awaiting culture results
Acneiform eruption	• Associated with medium depth peels	• Unroof pustules • Tetracycline class oral antibiotic × 2 wk • Intralesional triamcinolone acetonide injection (2.5 mg/mL)

- Cardiac safety considerations arise especially when performing phenol peels in more than one cosmetic unit (area of palm without finger) or greater than 0.5% BSA.
- The use of light or very light Hetter's formula for peri-orbital rejuvenation during a segmental combination chemical peeling can successfully address a top cosmetic concern in men.
- When combining chemical peels with other minimally invasive procedures, consider the target depths of the different procedures (same depths may increase risk of scar), how the inflammation or edema from chemical peeling may alter the outcomes of the other procedure(s) (e.g., neurotoxin diffusion), or how the other procedure may alter the penetration of the peeling agent (e.g., microneedling, nonablative fractional resurfacing).

References

[1] Weissler JM, Carney MJ, Carreras Tartak JA, Bensimon RH, Percec I. The evolution of chemical peeling and modern-day applications. Plast Reconstr Surg. 2017; 140(5):920–929

[2] Brody HJ, Monheit GD, Resnik SS, Alt TH. A history of chemical peeling. Dermatol Surg. 2000; 26(5):405–409

[3] Bangash HK, Eisen DB, Armstrong AW, et al. Who are the pioneers? A critical analysis of innovation and expertise in cutaneous noninvasive and minimally invasive cosmetic and surgical procedures. Dermatol Surg. 2016; 42(3):335–351

[4] American Society for Aesthetic Plastic Surgery. 2017 Cosmetic Surgery National Data Bank Statistics. Available at: https://www.surgery.org/media/statistics. Updated 2018. Accessed Dec 15, 2018

[5] American Socitey for Dermatologic Surgery. ASDS Survey on Dermatologic Procedures: Report of 2017 Procedures. Available at: https://www.asds.net/medical-professionals/practice-resources/asds-survey-on-dermatologic-procedures. Updated 2018. Accessed Dec 15, 2018

[6] International Society of Aesthetic Plastic Surgery. ISAPS International Survey on Aesthetic/Cosmetic Procedures Performed in 2017. Available at: https://www.isaps.org/wp-content/uploads/

2018/10/ISAPS_2017_International_Study_Cosmetic_Procedures.pdf. Updated 2018. Accessed December 15, 2018

[7] Keaney T. Male aesthetics. Skin Therapy Lett. 2015; 20(2):5–7

[8] Jagdeo J, Keaney T, Narurkar V, Kolodziejczyk J, Gallagher CJ. Facial treatment preferences among aesthetically oriented men. Dermatol Surg. 2016; 42(10):1155–1163

[9] Frucht CS, Ortiz AE. Nonsurgical cosmetic procedures for men: trends and technique considerations. J Clin Aesthet Dermatol. 2016; 9(12):33–43

[10] Handler MZ, Goldberg DJ. Cosmetic concerns among men. Dermatol Clin. 2018; 36(1):5–10

[11] Dewandre L, Tenenbaum A. The chemistry of peels: a hypothesis of action mechanisms and a proposal of a new classification of chemical peelings. In: Tung RC, Rubin MG, eds. Procedures in Cosmetic Dermatology Series: Chemical Peels. 2nd ed. Philadelphia, PA: Saunders; 2011:1–16

[12] Yonei N, Kanazawa N, Ohtani T, Furukawa F, Yamamoto Y. Induction of PDGF-B in TCA-treated epidermal keratinocytes. Arch Dermatol Res. 2007; 299(9):433–440

[13] Kimura A, Kanazawa N, Li HJ, Yonei N, Yamamoto Y, Furukawa F. Influence of chemical peeling on the skin stress response system. Exp Dermatol. 2012; 21 Suppl 1:8–10

[14] Bertolini TM. Is the phenol-croton oil peel safe? Plast Reconstr Surg. 2002; 110(2):715–717

[15] Kligman AM, Baker TJ, Gordon HL. Long-term histologic follow-up of phenol face peels. Plast Reconstr Surg. 1985; 75(5):652–659

[16] Wambier CG, Lee KC, Soon SL, et al. Advanced chemical peels: phenol-croton oil peel. J Am Acad Dermatol. 2019; 81(2):327–336

[17] Moy LS, Kotler R, Lesser T. The histologic evaluation of pulsed carbon dioxide laser resurfacing versus phenol chemical peels in vivo. Dermatol Surg. 1999; 25(8):597–600

[18] Obagi S. Injectables and resurfacing techniques: chemical peels. In: Rubin JP, ed. Plastic Surgery. Vol. 2. 4th ed. London: Elsevier; 2018:86–96

[19] Khunger N. Choosing the right peeling agent. In: Khunger N, ed. Chemical peels. 2nd ed. New Delhi, India: Jaypee Brothers Medical Publishers; 2014:40

[20] Giacomoni PU, Mammone T, Teri M. Gender-linked differences in human skin. J Dermatol Sci. 2009; 55(3):144–149

[21] Rahrovan S, Fanian F, Mehryan P, Humbert P, Firooz A. Male versus female skin: what dermatologists and cosmeticians should know. Int J Womens Dermatol. 2018; 4(3):122–130

[22] Fanous N, Zari S. Universal trichloroacetic acid peel technique for light and dark skin. JAMA Facial Plast Surg. 2017; 19(3):212–219

[23] Mizukoshi K, Akamatsu H. The investigation of the skin characteristics of males focusing on gender differences, skin perception, and skin care habits. Skin Res Technol. 2013; 19(2):91–99

[24] Paes EC, Teepen HJ, Koop WA, Kon M. Perioral wrinkles: histologic differences between men and women. Aesthet Surg J. 2009; 29(6):467–472

[25] Draelos ZD. Cosmeceuticals for male skin. Dermatol Clin. 2018; 36(1):17–20

[26] Sandby-Møller J, Poulsen T, Wulf HC. Epidermal thickness at different body sites: relationship to age, gender, pigmentation, blood content, skin type and smoking habits. Acta Derm Venereol. 2003; 83(6):410–413

[27] Markova MS, Zeskand J, McEntee B, Rothstein J, Jimenez SA, Siracusa LD. A role for the androgen receptor in collagen content of the skin. J Invest Dermatol. 2004; 123(6):1052–1056

[28] Ezure T, Yagi E, Kunizawa N, Hirao T, Amano S. Comparison of sagging at the cheek and lower eyelid between male and female faces. Skin Res Technol. 2011; 17(4):510–515

[29] Hornstra JM, Hoekstra T, Serné EH, et al. Homocysteine levels are inversely associated with capillary density in men, not in premenopausal women. Eur J Clin Invest. 2014; 44(3):333–340

[30] Fei W, Xu S, Ma J, et al. Fundamental supply of skin blood flow in the Chinese Han population: measurements by a full-field laser perfusion imager. Skin Res Technol. 2018; 24(4):656–662

[31] Stücker M, Steinberg J, Memmel U, Avermaete A, Hoffmann K, Altmeyer P. Differences in the two-dimensionally measured laser Doppler flow at different skin localisations. Skin Pharmacol Appl Skin Physiol. 2001; 14(1):44–51

[32] Nikalji N, Godse K, Sakhiya J, Patil S, Nadkarni N. Complications of medium depth and deep chemical peels. J Cutan Aesthet Surg. 2012; 5(4):254–260

[33] Staikou C, Kokotis P, Kyrozis A, et al. Differences in pain perception between men and women of reproductive age: a laser-evoked potentials study. Pain Med. 2017; 18(2):316–321

[34] Bulls HW, Freeman EL, Anderson AJ, Robbins MT, Ness TJ, Goodin BR. Sex differences in experimental measures of pain sensitivity and endogenous pain inhibition. J Pain Res. 2015; 8:311–320

[35] Gilliver SC, Ruckshanthi JP, Hardman MJ, Zeef LA, Ashcroft GS. 5alpha-dihydrotestosterone (DHT) retards wound closure by inhibiting re-epithelialization. J Pathol. 2009; 217(1):73–82

[36] Gilliver SC, Ashworth JJ, Ashcroft GS. The hormonal regulation of cutaneous wound healing. Clin Dermatol. 2007; 25(1):56–62

[37] Bordignon V, Burastero SE. Age, gender and reactivity to allergens independently influence skin reactivity to histamine. J Investig Allergol Clin Immunol. 2006; 16(2):129–135

[38] Costa IMC, Damasceno PS, Costa MC, Gomes KGP. Review in peeling complications. J Cosmet Dermatol. 2017; 16(3):319–326

[39] Keaney TC. Aging in the male face: intrinsic and extrinsic factors. Dermatol Surg. 2016; 42(7):797–803

[40] Kass LG, Kass KS. The lost art of chemical peeling: my fifteen year experience with croton oil peel. Adv Ophthalmol Optom. 2017; 2(1):391–407

[41] GBD 2015 Tobacco Collaborators. Smoking prevalence and attributable disease burden in 195 countries and territories, 1990–2015: a systematic analysis from the Global Burden of Disease Study 2015. Lancet. 2017; 389(10082):1885–1906

[42] Peters SAE, Muntner P, Woodward M. Sex differences in the prevalence of, and trends in, cardiovascular risk factors, treatment, and control in the united states, 2001 to 2016. Circulation. 2019; 139(8):1025–1035

[43] Gill JF, Yu SS, Neuhaus IM. Tobacco smoking and dermatologic surgery. J Am Acad Dermatol. 2013; 68(1):167–172

[44] Manríquez JJ, Cataldo K, Vera-Kellet C, Harz-Fresno I. Wrinkles. BMJ Clin Evid. 2014; 2014:1711

[45] Vanaman M, Fabi SG, Carruthers J. Complications in the cosmetic dermatology patient: a review and our experience (part 2). Dermatol Surg. 2016; 42(1):12–20

[46] Bureau of Labor Statistics. 2018 Employed Persons by Detailed Occupation, Sex, Race, and Hispanic or Latino Ethnicity. United States Department of Labor. Available at: https://www.bls.gov/cps/cpsaat10.htm. Accessed February 23, 2019

[47] Bertolin M, Cercato MC, Requena C, et al. Awareness, attitude, and adherence to preventive measures in patients at high risk of melanoma. A cross-sectional study on 185 patients. J Cancer Educ. 2015; 30 (3):552–566

[48] Damian DL, Patterson CR, Stapelberg M, Park J, Barnetson RS, Halliday GM. UV radiation-induced immunosuppression is greater in men and prevented by topical nicotinamide. J Invest Dermatol. 2008; 128(2):447–454

[49] Ide T, Tsutsui H, Ohashi N, et al. Greater oxidative stress in healthy young men compared with premenopausal women. Arterioscler Thromb Vasc Biol. 2002; 22(3):438–442

[50] Falk M, Anderson CD. Influence of age, gender, educational level and self-estimation of skin type on sun exposure habits and readiness to increase sun protection. Cancer Epidemiol. 2013; 37(2):127–132

[51] Hantash BM, Stewart DB, Cooper ZA, Rehmus WE, Koch RJ, Swetter SM. Facial resurfacing for nonmelanoma skin cancer prophylaxis. Arch Dermatol. 2006; 142(8):976–982

[52] Crudele J, Kim E, Murray K, Regan J. The importance of understanding consumer preferences for dermatologist recommended skin cleansing and care products. J Drugs Dermatol. 2019; 18 1s:s75–s79

[53] Blair R, Gupta G. Impact of demographic and treatment-related factors. In: Davis SA, ed. Adherence in Dermatology. Cham: Springer International; 2016:17–28

[54] Newport F. In U.S., estimate of LGBT population rises to 4.5%. Available at: https://news.gallup.com/poll/234863/estimate-lgbt-population-rises.aspx. Accessed February 23, 2019

[55] Yeung H, Luk KM, Chen SC, Ginsberg BA, Katz KA. Dermatologic care for lesbian, gay, bisexual, and transgender persons: terminology, demographics, health disparities, and approaches to care. J Am Acad Dermatol. 2019; 80(3):581–589

[56] Yeung H, Luk KM, Chen SC, Ginsberg BA, Katz KA. Dermatologic care for lesbian, gay, bisexual, and transgender persons: epidemiology, screening, and disease prevention. J Am Acad Dermatol. 2019; 80(3):591–602

[57] Montes JR, Santos E. Evaluation of men's trends and experiences in aesthetic treatment. J Drugs Dermatol. 2018; 17(9):941–946

[58] Yeung H, Chen SC. Sexual orientation and indoor tanning device use: a population-based study. JAMA Dermatol. 2016; 152(1):99–101

[59] Mansh M, Katz KA, Linos E, Chren MM, Arron S. Association of skin cancer and indoor tanning in sexual minority men and women. JAMA Dermatol. 2015; 151(12):1308–1316

[60] Klimek P, Lamb KM, Nogg KA, Rooney BM, Blashill AJ. Current and ideal skin tone: associations with tanning behavior among sexual minority men. Body Image. 2018; 25:31–34

[61] Admassu N, Pimentel MA, Halley MC, et al. Motivations among sexual-minority men for starting and stopping indoor tanning. Br J Dermatol. 2019; 180(6):1529–1530

[62] Wierckx K, Van de Peer F, Verhaeghe E, et al. Short- and long-term clinical skin effects of testosterone treatment in trans men. J Sex Med. 2014; 11(1):222–229

[63] Motosko CC, Zakhem GA, Pomeranz MK, Hazen A. Acne: a side-effect of masculinizing hormonal therapy in transgender patients. Br J Dermatol. 2019; 180(1):26–30

[64] Nakamura A, Watanabe M, Sugimoto M, et al. Dose-response analysis of testosterone replacement therapy in patients with female to male gender identity disorder. Endocr J. 2013; 60(3):275–281

[65] Kontochristopoulos G, Platsidaki E. Chemical peels in active acne and acne scars. Clin Dermatol. 2017; 35(2):179–182

[66] Tung R, Sato M, Kim N, Brenner FM. Body peeling. In: Tung RC, Rubin MG, eds. Procedures in Cosmetic Dermatology Series: Chemical Peels. 2nd ed. Philadelphia, PA: Saunders; 2011:117–122

[67] Spring LK, Krakowski AC, Alam M, et al. Isotretinoin and timing of procedural interventions: a systematic review with consensus recommendations. JAMA Dermatol. 2017; 153(8):802–809

[68] Waldman A, Bolotin D, Arndt KA, et al. ASDS guidelines task force: consensus recommendations regarding the safety of lasers, dermabrasion, chemical peels, energy devices, and skin surgery during and after isotretinoin use. Dermatol Surg. 2017; 43(10):1249–1262

[69] Griffiths S, Murray SB, Dunn M, Blashill AJ. Anabolic steroid use among gay and bisexual men living in Australia and New Zealand: associations with demographics, body dissatisfaction, eating disorder psychopathology, and quality of life. Drug Alcohol Depend. 2017; 181:170–176

[70] Ip EJ, Yadao MA, Shah BM, et al. Polypharmacy, infectious diseases, sexual behavior, and psychophysical health among anabolic steroid-using homosexual and heterosexual gym patrons in san francisco's castro district. Subst Use Misuse. 2017; 52(7):959–968

[71] Ip EJ, Barnett MJ, Tenerowicz MJ, Perry PJ. The anabolic 500 survey: characteristics of male users versus nonusers of anabolic-androgenic steroids for strength training. Pharmacotherapy. 2011; 31(8):757–766

[72] Blashill AJ, Calzo JP, Griffiths S, Murray SB. Anabolic steroid misuse among US adolescent boys: disparities by sexual orientation and race/ethnicity. Am J Public Health. 2017; 107(2):319–321

[73] Kouris A, Platsidaki E, Christodoulou C, et al. Patients' self-esteem before and after chemical peeling procedure. J Cosmet Laser Ther. 2018; 20(4):220–222

[74] Obagi S, Niamtu J. Chemical peel. In: Joe Niamtu, ed. Cosmetic Facial Surgery. 2nd ed. Philadelphia, PA: Elsevier; 2018:732–755

[75] Duffy DM. Avoiding complications. In: Tung RC, Rubin MG, eds. Procedures in Cosmetic Dermatology Series: Chemical Peels. 2nd ed. Philadelphia, PA: Saunders; 2011:151–172

[76] Wambier CG, de Freitas FP. Combining phenol-croton oil peel. In: Issa MCA, Tamura B, eds. Chemical and Physical Procedures. Cham: Springer International Publishing; 2018:101–113

[77] Landau M. Cardiac complications in deep chemical peels. Dermatol Surg. 2007; 33(2):190–193, discussion 193

[78] Landau M, Bensimon RH. Chemical peels. In: Cantisano-Zilkha M, Haddad A, eds. Aesthetic Oculofacial Rejuvenation. New York, NY: Elsevier; 2010:29–37

[79] Obagi S. Niamtu J. Chemical peel. In: Niamtu J, ed. Cosmetic Facial Surgery. 2nd ed. Beijing, China: Elsevier; 2018:732–755

[80] Resnik BI. The role of priming the skin for peels. In: Tung R, Rubin M, eds. Procedures in Cosmetic Dermatology Series: Chemical Peels. Philadelphia, PA: Saunders; 2011:23–25

[81] Henry M. Cosmetic concerns among ethnic men. Dermatol Clin. 2018; 36(1):11–16

[82] Lee KC, Wambier CG, Soon SL, et al. Basic chemical peeling: superficial and medium-depth peels. J Am Acad Dermatol. 2018; 81(2):313–324

[83] Committee for Guidelines of Care for Chemical Peeling. Guidelines for chemical peeling in japan (3rd edition). J Dermatol. 2012; 39 4:321–325

[84] Khunger N, IADVL Task Force. Standard guidelines of care for chemical peels. Indian J Dermatol Venereol Leprol. 2008; 74 Suppl:S5–S12

[85] Ditre CM. Alpha-hydroxy acid peels. In: Tung RC, Rubin MG, eds. Procedures in Cosmetic Dermatology Series: Chemical Peels. 2nd ed. Philadelphia, PA: Saunders; 2011:27–40

[86] Singer S, Karrer S, Berneburg M. Modern sun protection. Curr Opin Pharmacol. 2019; 46:24–28

[87] Sarkar R, Gokhale N, Godse K, et al. Medical management of melasma: a review with consensus recommendations by Indian pigmentary expert group. Indian J Dermatol. 2017; 62(6):558–577

[88] Mancuso JB, Maruthi R, Wang SQ, Lim HW. Sunscreens: an update. Am J Clin Dermatol. 2017; 18(5):643–650

[89] Peikert JM, Krywonis NA, Rest EB, Zachary CB. The efficacy of various degreasing agents used in trichloroacetic acid peels. J Dermatol Surg Oncol. 1994; 20(11):724–728

[90] Leonhardt JM, Rossy KM, Lawrence N. Trichloroacetic acid (TCA) peels. In: Tung RC, Rubin MG, eds. Procedures in Cosmetic Dermatology Series: Chemical Peels. 2nd ed. Philadelphia, PA: Saunders; 2011: 64.

[91] Leonhardt JM, Rossy KM, Lawrence N. Trichloroacetic acid (TCA) peels. In: Tung RC, Rubin MG, eds. Procedures in Cosmetic Dermatology Series: Chemical Peels. 2nd ed. Philadelphia, PA: Saunders; 2011: 66–67.

[92] Coleman KM, Coleman WP. Complications. In: Tung RC, Rubin MG, eds. Procedures in Cosmetic Dermatology Series: Chemical Peels. 2nd ed. Philadelphia, PA: Saunders; 2011:173–182

[93] Perkins SW, Waters HH. Management of aging skin. In: Flint PW, Haughey BH, Lund V, et al., eds. Cummings Otolaryngology: Head and Neck Surgery. 6th ed. Philadelphia, PA: Saunders; 2015:391–408

[94] Hetter GP. An examination of the phenol-croton oil peel: part IV. Face peel results with different concentrations of phenol and croton oil. Plast Reconstr Surg. 2000; 105(3):1061–1083, discussion 1084–1087

[95] Rullan P, Karam AM. Chemical peels for darker skin types. Facial Plast Surg Clin North Am. 2010; 18(1):111–131

[96] Ross EV. Nonablative laser rejuvenation in men. Dermatol Ther. 2007; 20(6):414–429

[97] Reserva J, Champlain A, Soon SL, Tung R. Chemical peels: indications and special considerations for the male patient. Dermatol Surg. 2017; 43 Suppl 2:S163–S173

[98] Brody HJ. Commentary on chemical peels in men. Dermatol Surg. 2017; 43 Suppl 2:S174–S175

[99] Grimes PE. Salicylic acid peels. In: Tung R, Rubin M, eds. Procedures in Cosmetic Dermatology Series: Chemical Peels. Philadelphia, PA: Saunders; 2011:41–47

[100] Dainichi T, Ueda S, Imayama S, Furue M. Excellent clinical results with a new preparation for chemical peeling in acne: 30% salicylic acid in polyethylene glycol vehicle. Dermatol Surg. 2008; 34(7):891–899, discussion 899

[101] Dainichi T, Amano S, Matsunaga Y, et al. Chemical peeling by SA-PEG remodels photo-damaged skin: suppressing p53 expression and normalizing keratinocyte differentiation. J Invest Dermatol. 2006; 126 (2):416–421

[102] Grimes PE. Jessner's solution. In: Tosti A, Grimes PE, De Padova MP, eds. Color Atlas of Chemical Peels. Berlin: Springer; 2006:23–29

[103] Ghersetich I, Brazzini B, Lotti T, De Padova MP, Tosti A. Resorcinol. In: Tosti A, Grimes PE, De Padova MP, eds. Color of Atlas of Chemical Peels. Berlin: Springer; 2006:41–47

[104] Rubin C. Are you man enough for a peel? The New York Times. January 22, 2015;E; Style Desk; SKIN DEEP:4

[105] Moy LS, Peace S, Moy RL. Comparison of the effect of various chemical peeling agents in a mini-pig model. Dermatol Surg. 1996; 22(5):429–432

[106] Becker FF, Langford FP, Rubin MG, Speelman P. A histological comparison of 50% and 70% glycolic acid peels using solutions with various pHs. Dermatol Surg. 1996; 22(5):463–465

[107] Cohen BJ. The value of pH. Aesthetics. 2014. Available at: https://aestheticsjournal.com/feature/the-value-of-ph. Accessed February 24, 2019

[108] Sharad J. Glycolic acid peel therapy: a current review. Clin Cosmet Investig Dermatol. 2013; 6:281–288

[109] Bagatin E, Teixeira SP, Hassun KM, Pereira T, Michalany NS, Talarico S. 5-Fluorouracil superficial peel for multiple actinic keratoses. Int J Dermatol. 2009; 48(8):902–907

[110] Marrero GM, Katz BE. The new fluor-hydroxy pulse peel. A combination of 5-fluorouracil and glycolic acid. Dermatol Surg. 1998; 24(9):973–978

[111] Harmon CB, Hadley M, Tristani P. Tricholoroacetic acid. In: Tosti A, Grimes PE, De Padova MP, eds. Color atlas of Chemical Peels. Berlin: Springer; 2006:59–67

[112] Brody HJ. Do chemical peels tighten the skin? Dermatol Surg. 2014; 40 Suppl 12:S129–S133

[113] Fabbrocini G, De Padova MP, Tosti A. Superficial to medium-depth peels: a personal experience. In: Tung RC, Rubin MG, eds. Procedures in Cosmetic Dermatology Series: Chemical Peels. 2nd ed. Philadelphia, PA: Saunders; 2011:123–132

[114] Cho SB, Chung KY, Lee KH, Lee JB. Chemical reconstruction of skin scars (CROSS) technique. In: Tung RC, Rubin MG, eds. Procedures in Cosmetic Dermatology Series: Chemical Peels. Philadelphia, PA: Saunders; 2011:101–107

[115] Lee JB, Chung WG, Kwahck H, Lee KH. Focal treatment of acne scars with trichloroacetic acid: chemical reconstruction of skin scars method. Dermatol Surg. 2002; 28(11):1017–1021, discussion 1021

[116] Khunger N, Bhardwaj D, Khunger M. Evaluation of CROSS technique with 100% TCA in the management of ice pick acne scars in darker skin types. J Cosmet Dermatol. 2011; 10(1):51–57

[117] Leheta T, El Tawdy A, Abdel Hay R, Farid S. Percutaneous collagen induction versus full-concentration trichloroacetic acid in the treatment of atrophic acne scars. Dermatol Surg. 2011; 37(2):207–216

[118] Jacobs B. Is men's make-up going mainstream? Available at: http://www.bbc.com/culture/story/20190206-is-mens-make-up-going-mainstream. Updated 2019. Accessed March 12, 2019

[119] Wolfson S. Face time: is makeup for men the next big beauty trend? The Guardian Web site. Available at: https://www.theguardian.com/fashion/2018/oct/13/makeup-for-men-beauty-trend. Updated 2018. Accessed March 12, 2019

[120] Jung K, Choi M, Hong S, et al. Realistic and aggregated exposure assessment of Korean men and women to color make-up products. Food Chem Toxicol. 2018; 118:382–389

[121] Hetter GP. An examination of the phenol-croton oil peel: part I. Dissecting the formula. Plast Reconstr Surg. 2000; 105(1):227–239, discussion 249–251

[122] Sterling JB. Micropunch blepharopeeling of the upper eyelids: a combination approach for periorbital rejuvenation–a pilot study. Dermatol Surg. 2014; 40(4):436–440

[123] Hetter GP, Brody HJ, Monheit GD, Landau M. Interactive peeling session. Proceedings from the International Peeling Society's Chemical Peel Course: International Day at the American Academy of Dermatology Annual Meeting. Orlando, FL, March 2, 2017

[124] Chisaki C, Horn G, Noriega LF. Phenol solutions for deep peels. In: Issa MCA, Tamura B, eds. Chemical and Physical Procedures. Cham: Springer International Publishing; 2018:73–99

[125] Office of Environmental Health & Safety. Phenol safety fact sheet. Available at: https://ehs.usc.edu/files/phenol-fact-sheet.pdf. Updated 2018. Accessed March 12, 2019

[126] Wambier CG, Beltrame FL. Air safety and personal protective equipment for phenol-croton oil peels. Dermatol Surg. 2018; 44(7):1035–1037

[127] Linder J. Chemical peels and combination therapies. Plast Surg Nurs. 2013; 33(2):88–91, quiz 92–93

[128] Taylor MB, Zaleski-Larsen L, McGraw TA. Single session treatment of rolling acne scars using tumescent anesthesia, 20% trichloracetic acid extensive subcision, and fractional CO2 laser. Dermatol Surg. 2017; 43 Suppl 1:S70–S74

[129] Tung R, Mahoney AM, Novice K, et al. Treatment of lateral canthal rhytides with a medium depth chemical peel with or without pretreatment with onabotulinum toxin type A: a randomized control trial. Int J Womens Dermatol. 2016; 2(1):31–34

[130] Landau M. Combination of chemical peelings with botulinum toxin injections and dermal fillers. J Cosmet Dermatol. 2006; 5(2):121–126

[131] Quaedvlieg PJF, Ostertag JU, Krekels GA, Neumann HAM. Delayed wound healing after three different treatments for widespread actinic keratosis on the atrophic bald scalp. Dermatol Surg. 2003; 29 (10):1052–1056, discussion 1056

[132] Champlain A, Reserva J, Webb K, et al. Cosmetic dermatology training during residency: outcomes of a resident-reported survey. Dermatol Surg. 2018; 44(9):1216–1219

7 The Tech Sector: Lasers, Light, and Energy Devices

Yiping Xing, Derek Hsu, Murad Alam, and Jeremy A. Brauer

Summary

Lasers and light-based therapies are powerful and versatile nonsurgical tools that can be used to treat a wide range of cosmetic and medical dermatologic conditions, including several that are more prevalent in men. As the number of male patients seeking non-invasive cosmetic procedures continue to increase, tailoring treatment methodologies to account for gender-specific anatomical variances and preferences will be essential in optimizing cosmetic outcomes and increasing patient satisfaction. Herein this chapter we will review the major classes of lasers by clinical indication, with particular focus on their use in men.

Keywords: lasers, lasers in men, laser hair removal, laser tattoo removal, laser resurfacing, vascular lasers.

7.1 Background

The demand for surgical and nonsurgical cosmetic procedures has increased dramatically in the past decade, with an estimated 18,100,000 procedures performed in 2019 alone.[1] Although the total number of yearly cosmetic procedures has risen by 44.8% since 2009, minimally invasive procedures account for 94.6% of this increase, with laser and light-based treatments encompassing a significant portion of this growth.[1,2]

Although the demographic landscape of the cosmetic market is comprised mostly of female patients, interest in cosmetic procedures has also been steadily increasing among male patients, with 1,300,000 total cosmetic procedures performed in 2019 according to the American Society of Plastic Surgeons.[1] Minimally invasive procedures accounted for the vast majority of this volume (83.7%), with laser hair removal (LHR) and laser skin resurfacing ranking as the second and sixth most popular procedures among male patients, respectively.[1]

A multitude of factors contribute to the rising interest in laser and light-based therapies among male patients. Advancements in the field of lasers and light-based therapies have provided aesthetic patients a minimally invasive option for treating a large breadth of cutaneous cosmetic concerns, including several conditions that are more prevalent or severe in the male population such as acne scarring, rhytids, pseudofolliculitis barbae (PFB), and rhinophyma.[3] These procedures can often deliver meaningful yet subtle natural results while also offering minimal downtime and reduced risk—characteristics that have been highlighted in recent research as important considerations for male aesthetic patients.[4,5] Furthermore, it is the opinion of the authors that laser and light-based therapies carry a lower risk of feminizing the face compared to other minimally invasive modalities, such as injectable dermal fillers.

As awareness and social acceptability of cosmetic procedures continue to rise among male patients, it is essential that health care professinals understand not only the capabilities and limitations of different treatment options available but also the distinct nuances of male facial anatomy. Adapting treatment protocols to account for these differences and appreciating the varied treatment goals of different patient demographics will lead to improved cosmetic outcomes and patient satisfaction.[6] Herein this chapter we will review these topics as they pertain to laser and light-based therapies.

7.2 Anatomy and Physiology

As the largest organ in the human body, the skin is comprised of multiple layers and complex adnexal structures that serve various barrier, immunologic, thermoregulatory, and sensory functions.[7,8] It is well established that genetics and hormonal differences contribute to underlying sex-related biophysical differences in cutaneous structure and function.[9] These differences can have implications not only in the prevalence and pathogenesis of certain skin diseases but also in terms of treatment protocols and cosmetic interventions. Knowledge of these underlying gender-linked differences is essential when performing laser and light-based therapies on men.

Multiple studies have demonstrated that dermal skin thickness is increased in men compared to women across all ages and anatomical regions.[8,10,11] Additionally, whereas skin thickness decreases linearly over time in men, it has been shown to remain constant in women up until the fifth decade, after which it steadily declines.[10] These observations have been attributed to the influence of sex hormones on collagen production, which has been shown to directly correlate with skin thickness in both animal models and humans.[8,11-13] On the contrary, men tend to have less subcutaneous adipose, which, combined with stronger muscles of facial expression, may lead to more severe, dynamic wrinkles in certain locations such as the forehead.[5,14,15] Additionally, men may initially present with deeper wrinkles because they tend to pursue cosmetic treatment at later stages compared to women.[5] In order to achieve a comparable cosmetic result in men, more aggressive protocols or greater number of laser and light-based treatments may be required.

Men also have a greater density of dermal microvessels, resulting in greater baseline facial skin arterial perfusion. This perfusion is especially increased in the lower face, which is highly vascularized to support the coarse terminal hairs in the beard region.[5,6,16] Consequently, male patients experience a higher rate of postoperative bleeding complications after undergoing plastic facial surgical procedures such as rhytidectomy.[17] Likewise, they may be at increased risk of bruising after certain laser procedures.

There are also gender-related differences in hair characteristics and distribution. The effect of androgens on hair growth in men can vary according to anatomic region.[9] Men typically will have an increased density of coarse terminal hairs on the face and neck compared to women. Thus, physicians should be cognizant of the potential risk to inadvertently damage hair follicles when performing laser and light-based procedures on the face and neck.

As with the other features of male cutaneous anatomy discussed earlier, the sebaceous and eccrine glands on the face are also hormone dependent. Adult male patients generally exhibit larger pore sizes and secrete significantly greater amounts of sebum compared to age matched female patients, which may explain why males are more prone to certain diseases, such as rhinophyma or more severe acne resulting in more severe scarring.[8,11,18,19]

Awareness of these anatomical and physiologic gender-related differences is important when counseling male cosmetic patients and constructing problem-based treatment plans that optimize cosmesis and minimize potential adverse outcomes.

7.3 Introduction to Lasers

Most modern-day lasers in clinical dermatology employ the theory of selective photothermolysis, which was introduced by Anderson and Parrish in 1983.[20] This theory details how pulsed laser energy can be applied to preferentially target specific structures in the skin for thermally mediated injury while minimizing damage to surrounding tissues. This process involves a combination of selective light absorption by specific chromophores present in the skin and applying a pulse duration equal to shorter than the thermal relaxation time (TRT) of the target tissue so that thermal injury is confined to the desired regions, minimizing the potential for adverse effects.[20] Additionally, the fluence, or energy density, must be adequate to destroy the intended target.[21]

Clinically relevant chromophores can be endogenous or exogenous. The principle endogenous chromophores in the skin include water, melanin, and hemoglobin. Exogenous chromophores most often include tattoo pigment. The majority of lasers available today emits energy at specific wavelengths that correspond to the absorption spectrum of one or more of these chromophores.[22] Importantly, the laser–skin interaction is complex and depends on several additional factors such as the size, depth, and surrounding environment of the target tissue.[23] These anatomic elements, which can vary significantly with gender, must also be considered when selecting laser parameters such as wavelength, pulse duration, spot size, and fluence.

Lasers can be broadly categorized based on their intended targets and clinical applications. In the following sections, we will review the major classes of lasers and their common clinical applications in male aesthetic patients.

7.3.1 Resurfacing Lasers

Advances in laser resurfacing technology have provided laser surgeons powerful nonsurgical tools to address a wide range of cosmetic cutaneous concerns, such as photoaging, rhytids, dyspigmentation, scarring—including hypertrophic scars and keloids, and superficial skin growths. Modern-day resurfacing lasers can be broadly categorized into two main classes—ablative and nonablative, both of which can be subdivided further into fractionated and traditional, or full field, forms.[24] In general, ablative resurfacing techniques vaporize the epidermis, leading to prolonged recovery times, but in many cases yielding more dramatic cosmetic results. Nonablative techniques preserve the epidermis and thus are associated with shortened recovery times and fewer side effects.

7.3.2 Ablative Resurfacing Lasers

Traditional ablative resurfacing lasers include the 10,600-nm carbon dioxide (CO_2) lasers and the 2,940-nm erbium:yttrium aluminum garnet (Er:YAG) laser. CO_2 lasers emit light at a wavelength absorbed by water in skin tissue, triggering water superheating and destruction of the entire epidermis and a variable part of the dermis to a controlled depth.[25] Thermal injury is also extended to the adjacent tissue causing coagulation necrosis in the area directly bordering the ablated tissue.[26] Further away from the direct interaction, there is reversible thermal damage, which causes heat-induced collagen shrinkage and leads to tighter and smoother skin during the healing process.[26,27]

Traditional full-field ablative CO_2 lasers were highly efficacious for treatment of photodamaged skin; however, they carried notable risk for posttreatment side effects such as edema, prolonged erythema, burning discomfort, pigmentary alteration—including delayed-onset permanent hypopigmentation—infection, and scarring.[27–30] In a retrospective analysis of 500 patients who underwent cutaneous laser resurfacing with a CO_2 laser by a single operator, 100% of patients developed postoperative erythema lasting on average several months, and 37% of patients developed hyperpigmentation lasting on average 32 days postoperatively.[28] The risk of postprocedure pigment alteration is greater in patients with Fitzpatrick skin type IV or greater (► Fig. 7.1).[28,31]

The Er:YAG laser was developed after CO_2 lasers in an attempt to retain the benefits of ablative CO_2 laser resurfacing while decreasing side effects. Er:YAG laser emits near-infrared light at a wavelength of 2,940 nm, which yields an absorption coefficient of water 16 times that of

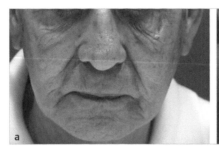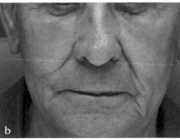

Fig. 7.1 (a) Lower eyelid laxity and photo-damage (pre-treatment). **(b)** Post-treatment after one session with ablative full field 10,600 nm CO_2 laser. (Courtesy of Jose Raul Montes, MD).

the CO_2 laser.[32] As the epidermis is composed predominantly of water, the vast majority of the laser energy is absorbed superficially. This corresponds to more superficial ablation with less surrounding thermal damage in the dermis. Therefore, the Er:YAG laser results in less dermal coagulation, and may be associated with poorer intraoperative hemostasis.[25] Although the Er:YAG laser was effective for superficial targets and offered faster recovery time, it was less effective than CO_2 lasers when targeting deep rhytids and skin laxity, controlling for fluence per pulse and number of passes.[26] Consequently, increasing the pulse duration or number of passes is often needed to achieve the desired depth of thermal damage and clinical outcome.[33,34] A retrospective study found similar side effect profiles and comparable healing times in 100 patients who underwent laser skin resurfacing with either single-pass CO_2 or multipass long-pulsed Er:YAG.[33]

Fractional ablative technology has largely replaced the traditional full-field ablative resurfacing lasers, which, although very effective, were undermined by their significant posttreatment morbidity and side effect profiles. Fractionated ablative resurfacing employs the concept of fractional photothermolysis, which involves creation of vertical columns of epidermal and dermal ablation, also known as microscopic treatment zones (MTZs), surrounded by uninjured tissue at regularly spaced intervals.[35] Only a fraction of the skin is treated in an individual session, and the presence of adjacent unaffected tissue offers a viable reservoir of cutaneous stem cells, which can facilitate rapid re-epithelialization.[36] As a result, fractional ablative methods tend to have fewer posttreatment side effects and less downtime compared to traditional full-field ablative laser resurfacing, while still offering meaningful cosmetic outcomes.[24,37,38] Skin resurfacing with fractional ablative CO_2 or Er:YAG lasers can therefore be an option for men with deeper rhytids, significant solar elastosis, or skin laxity. However, it is important to note that although fractionated ablative lasers are safer than their nonfractionated counterparts, they still carry increased risk and recovery time compared to nonablative fractionated lasers, which have become the contemporary standard for skin resurfacing.[39] Notably, prolonged erythema of up to 2 months have been reported, which may be particularly challenging for male patients, who do not typically wear makeup to camouflage skin.[36]

Beyond photorejuvenation, ablative lasers can be used to treat rhinophyma, a cosmetically disfiguring complication of rosacea that almost exclusively affects male patients at a ratio of 30:1 compared to female patients.[40] Rhinophyma is characterized by progressive bulbous enlargement of the nose, sebaceous gland hyperplasia, enlarged pores, hypervascularity, and fibrosis.[41] Although a benign entity in of itself, rhinophyma can often be psychologically distressing and cause functional impairment such as nasal obstruction in the late stages.[42] Management can be difficult and usually necessitates surgical or destructive procedures. Full-field and fractionated ablative CO_2 and Er:YAG lasers have all been shown to be tolerable, effective, and provide comparable results to electrosurgery (▶ Fig. 7.2).[43,44,45,46]

7.3.3 Nonablative Resurfacing Lasers

The original nonablative resurfacing lasers entered the clinical arena in the late 1990s in response to concerns regarding prolonged recovery time and posttreatment complications associated with traditional full-field ablative lasers.[24,29] Nonablative resurfacing is based on the premise that dermal thermal injury is the catalyst for collagen formation, remodeling, and contraction, and thus the basis for the clinical improvement seen with ablative resurfacing lasers.[47] Nonablative lasers that were traditionally used for resurfacing purposes emitted light at wavelengths that were either absorbed by oxyhemoglobin in dermal vasculature (585–595 nm) or dermal water (1,000–1,500 nm)[21,47] or 585- and 595-nm pulse dye lasers have been trialed for skin resurfacing purposes, and although well tolerated, their use in this capacity is limited due to overall inconsistent and unimpressive results.[48,49] The long-pulsed 1,320-nm neodymium:yttrium aluminum garnet (Nd:YAG) laser was the first laser marketed exclusively for nonablative skin resurfacing.[50] At this infrared wavelength, absorption by superficial epidermal tissue is relatively weak, which allows for energy penetration deeper into the dermis. Nonablative systems also utilize concomitant cooling devices to further prevent epidermal heating and damage. Because the epidermis is preserved, downtime and risk of side effects are minimal. Although several studies have demonstrated clinical improvement in the appearance of mild to moderate winkles and acne scarring with the 1,320-nm Nd:YAG laser, the effects are

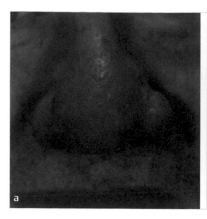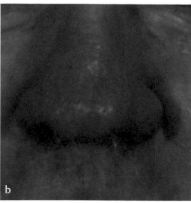

Fig. 7.2 **(a)** Rhinophyma (pre-treatment). **(b)** Post-treatment after one session with ablative full field 10,600 nm CO_2 laser. (Courtesy of Jennifer L. MacGregor, MD).

generally mild compared to their ablative counterparts and require multiple sessions to achieve.[51,52,53] Other infrared lasers that have been used for nonablative skin resurfacing include the 1,064-nm Nd:YAG, 1,450-nm diode, and 1,540-nm erbium:glass lasers. These systems also exhibit similar side effect profiles and limitations in efficacy.

The first commercially available fractional resurfacing device was the nonablative fractionated laser, which has since become the most popular and widely utilized class of resurfacing lasers, especially in male patients.[54] Nonablative fractionated lasers are more effective than their nonablative predecessors while concomitantly offering faster recovery and a more tolerable side effect profile compared to ablative resurfacing.[32]

Men and women may seek resurfacing laser treatments for different reasons. A retrospective review of a single dermatologist's experience over a 14-month period found that the most popular concern among men seeking nonablative fractional resurfacing was acne scarring, accounting for 44% of male patients compared to only 14% of female patients.[54] This correlates with the greater prevalence of severe nodulocystic acne in men, likely due to the effects of androgens on the skin.[55] Several studies have corroborated the safety and efficacy of the 1,550-nm erbium fiber fractional laser in the treatment of acne scarring, including patients of Fitzpatrick skin types IV to VI.[56,57]

Improving the appearance of photoaged skin is another common reason why both the male and female patient may pursue resurfacing treatments.[54] Multiple wavelengths utilized within nonablative fractional devices, such as 1,470, 1,540, 1,550, and 1,927 nm, have been shown to be effective for men who wish to improve the texture, tone, and pigmentation of photodamaged skin. One device offers both the 1,550- and 1,927-nm wavelengths, as the 1,550-nm wavelength is more effective at targeting solar elastosis and stimulating neocollagensis as it penetrates deeper in the dermis while the 1,927-nm wavelength targets superficial structures of the skin and has been shown to improve pigmentation as well as treat

actinic keratoses.[58,59] Actinic damage is significantly more prevalent in men, especially among elderly men with androgenetic alopecia.[60] Results of a prospective, multicenter study suggest that the combination of wavelengths in a single treatment is a safe and effective treatment to address both the deeper and superficial sequelae of photodamaged skin.[58]

Picosecond pulse duration lasers such as the 755-nm alexandrite laser with a diffractive lens array, and the dual 532 and 1,064 nm with holographic beam splitter, have also been shown to be a safe and effective option for the treatment of facial acne scarring and photoaging, even in darker skin tones.[61,62,63,64] Although picosecond pulse duration lasers were originally developed with removal of tattoo and pigmentation in mind, the combination with a diffractive lens array allows the picosecond pulse to be distributed into few highly concentrated beams surrounded by background areas with low-level heat energy. The unique action of these high-energy beams promotes neocollagenesis without ablation with minimal side effects and downtime, with posttreatment erythema lasting only for several hours.[62,63,65]

7.4 Pigmentation

7.4.1 Laser Hair Removal

In 2019, LHR was the second most popular noninvasive cosmetic procedure among men, with more than 170,000 procedures performed.[1] This represents a 100% increase from 2000.[1,66] For men, the most commonly treated areas include the neck, chest, and back. The targeted chromophore in LHR is melanin in the hair shaft, which, upon absorption of sufficient laser energy, will induce thermal injury to nearby hair stem cells in the hair bulge and bulb.[67]

Melanin does not exhibit a single absorption peak. Rather, it absorbs wavelengths from 400 to 1,200 nm, with greater absorption at the lower end of this spectrum.[68] Consequently, lasers that emit light at lower wavelengths carry higher risk for epidermal damage and subsequent dyspigmentation or scarring, especially in individuals of darker skin types.[69] Although the ideal LHR candidate may be a patient with fair skin and dark terminal hairs, utilizing longer wavelength lasers and concomitant epidermal contact cooling can diminish the risk for epidermal injury in patients with darker skin types. Conversely, longer wavelength lasers are less effective at destroying lightly pigmented or thinner hair due to relatively weaker melanin absorption.

Several lasers and light-based therapies across a broad range of wavelengths have been used successfully in the photothermal destruction of the follicular unit, including long-pulsed 694-nm ruby, 755-nm alexandrite, 810-nm diode, 1,064-nm Nd:YAG, and intense pulsed light (IPL). The benefit–risk profile of these lasers varies and depends on the specific characteristics of each individual patient. Importantly, because men tend to have thicker terminal hairs as well as increased hair density, they may be at increased risk of side effects due to overall increased energy absorption in the treated areas.

Although used less in practice today, the long-pulsed ruby laser was one of the first lasers approved for hair removal. At an emission wavelength of 694 nm, light from the ruby laser is avidly absorbed by melanin and does not penetrate deeply into the skin, limiting its use in patients with darker skin types, especially during the summer months, given high risk of blistering, burns, and pigmentary alteration.[70]

The 755-nm alexandrite laser is a popular and effective option for patients with Fitzpatrick skin types I to III. At 755 nm, the alexandrite laser penetrates deeper than the 694-nm ruby and thus is theoretically safer in darker skin types; however, a retrospective study looking at the side effect profiles of different hair removal lasers in Fitzpatrick skin types I to V found that the 755-nm alexandrite laser was associated with higher risk of side effects compared to the 1,064-nm Nd:YAG laser.[70] Thus, caution is still advised in patients with darker skin types.

The 810-nm diode laser is also a popular and effective option for LHR.[71,72] In head-to-head comparative study of patients undergoing LHR with diode, Nd:YAG, and alexandrite lasers, the diode laser and alexandrite were more effective than Nd:YAG, a finding that was statistically significant.[73] Meanwhile, there was no statistically significant difference between the diode and alexandrite lasers.[73] Newer versions of the diode laser offer larger spot sizes resulting in brisk treatment of larger surface areas such as the chest and back.[74] Although diode lasers are generally thought to be safer than its lower wavelength counterparts, some of the same concerns regarding unwanted collateral epidermal damage in darker skin individuals remain (▶ Fig. 7.3).

The 1,064-nm Nd:YAG is safe for patients of all Fitzpatrick skin types, having been specifically developed for patients with darker skin.[75] The Nd:YAG is an effective laser for hair removal; however, although it may possess a more benign side effect profile, as noted earlier, it may not be quite as efficacious as the diode or alexandrite laser.[70,73]

Although many men may seek LHR for cosmetic removal of unwanted hair, LHR can also be an effective treatment for medical conditions that predominantly affect men, such as PFB and acne keloidalis nuchae (AKN). PFB is a common, chronic, inflammatory condition that affects between 45 and 83% of men of African ancestry.[76] The disorder is characterized by inflammatory papules and pustules that form as a result of cutaneous entrapment of recently cut, coarse, curly hairs. Over time, chronic inflammation can cause significant scarring and hyperpigmentation.[77] In many cases, medical management may not be adequate, especially when behavioral modifications in shaving habits are not feasible. Similarly, AKN is another chronic inflammatory condition in which follicular-based papules and pustules develop in the occipital scalp and posterior neck predominantly in men of African descent, which, if left untreated, result in formation of keloidal plaques.[78,79] As both PFB and AKN are more common in patients with darker skin types, longer wavelength lasers are the LHR device of choice.

7.4.2 Tattoo Removal

Although tattoos are often intended to be permanent, some patients desire removal as personal or professional circumstances change. Laser tattoo removal is a common procedure in the United States, with over 160,000 procedures performed in 2019.[1] In tattoo removal, exogenously placed tattoo pigment acts as the target chromophore. Thus, removal can be a complex process as tattoos are often polychromatic, and potential side effects include allergic reactions, dyspigmentation, and scarring.[80] Depending on the color of the targeted pigment and its

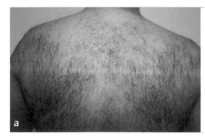
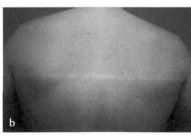

Fig. 7.3 (a) Unwanted hair (pre-treatment). **(b)** Post-treatment after six sessions with a 1064-nm Nd:YAG. (Courtesy of Shino Bay Aguilera, DO).

Table 7.1 Lasers corresponding to different tattoo pigments

Colors	Lasers
Black, blue	QS/PS alexandrite, QS/PS 1,064-nm Nd:YAG, QS ruby
Green	QS/PS alexandrite, QS ruby
Red, orange, yellow	QS/PS 532-nm Nd:YAG
White	CO_2, Er:YAG

Abbreviations: Er:YAG, erbium:yttrium aluminum garnet; Nd:YAG, neodymium:yttrium aluminum garnet; PS, picosecond; QS, Q-switched.

associated absorption peak, different wavelengths and types of lasers are used. In general, the lasers used to target commonly encountered colors are discussed in detail below (▶ Table 7.1).

The historical standard for tattoo removal has been the nanosecond, Q-switched (QS) laser, which uses an internal mirror to generate a very short pulse.[81] However, newer picosecond (PS) pulse duration lasers are now preferred due to their increased efficiency and efficacy over their nanosecond predecessors.[82,83,84] In a systematic review evaluating eight trials with 160 participants, 69 to 100% of tattoos showed over 70% of clearance of pigment after 1 to 10 laser treatments with the picosecond laser.[81] Although mild transient effects such as erythema and pinpoint bleeding were often reported, no permanent scarring was noted in any of the trials.[82] Other studies have demonstrated higher clearance rates of difficult-to-treat blue, green, and yellow tattoos with picosecond lasers.[85,86]

It is also important to be aware of challenges and complications that may arise with laser tattoo removal. In general, professional tattoos are harder to remove due to the deeper placement of the pigment.[80] Additionally, pigments used in tattoos can be impure, and can be an amalgam of different substances and colors, which makes their response to laser removal procedures somewhat unpredictable.[87]

A complication to be aware of when treating certain tattoo colors is paradoxical darkening.[88] This phenomenon has been partially attributed to laser-induced reduction of ferric oxide or titanium dioxide used in certain tattoo dyes.[89] Ferric oxide is a rust color and commonly used in red-, pink-, and flesh-colored tattoos.[89] However, it becomes jet black when reduced to ferrous oxide.[89] Similarly, titanium dioxide, a compound frequently seen in white or flesh-colored tattoos, turns blue in its reduced form.[90] These reactions are irreversible and may cause treatment-resistant pigmentary alteration. However, a recent case series demonstrated efficacy in treating paradoxical darkening with the 532- and 1,064-nm picosecond lasers.[91]

Certain tattoo dyes may contain metal salts that can elicit allergic reactions, necessitating tattoo removal.[92] Red inks are commonly implicated as they frequently contain mercuric sulfide though allergic reactions to other colors have been reported.[92,93] Tattoo dye allergies pose notable therapeutic challenges, especially with larger tattoos that cannot be easily excised. Although Q-switched lasers have been used successfully in the removal of allergic tattoos, there have been reports of generalized allergic reactions following laser treatment.[94,95,96] Recently, ablative fractional resurfacing has been shown to be effective, standalone or in combination with Q-switched lasers, in removing tattoo inks and alleviating allergic symptoms.[93] Additionally, the combination of ablative fractional resurfacing with Q-switch lasers may be synergistic in clearing tattoo pigment that traditionally are more difficult to eliminate, such as white.[97]

Multiple treatments over many months may be needed for successful tattoo removal. Since some tattoos may never completely fade, it is imperative that realistic expectations and understanding of potential complications and outcomes are discussed at initial consultation.

7.5 Pigmented Lesions

Male patients may also seek laser treatment for epidermal and dermal melanin-containing lesions. Common indications include lentigines and ephelides and both congenital and acquired forms of dermal melanocytosis.

For more superficial epidermal-based pigmented lesions such as lentigines and ephelides, lasers that emit wavelengths at the lower end of the melanin absorption spectrum, such as the 532-nm frequency-doubled Nd:YAG (normal mode or Q-switched), have been shown to be effective and well tolerated for patients with Fitzpatrick skin types I to IV.[98,99] The 694-nm Q-switched ruby laser is another option for treating solar lentigines and has been shown to be superior to medical management with triple combination therapy in comparative studies.[100]

For deeper melanin-containing lesions such as nevus of Ota and nevus of Ito, longer wavelength lasers are more effective as they penetrate deeper into the skin and can affect the target chromophore in the dermis. The Q-switched 694-nm ruby, 755-nm alexandrite, and 1,064-nm Nd:YAG lasers have all been used successfully for the treatment of dermal melanin-containing lesions, with the Q-switched 1,064-nm Nd:YAG as the most studied device to date.[101] However, a recent meta-analysis noted that the newer picosecond alexandrite laser may be more efficacious than the traditional Q-switched lasers for the treatment of nevus of Ota though further studies are needed to corroborate the success noted in early reports.[101,102]

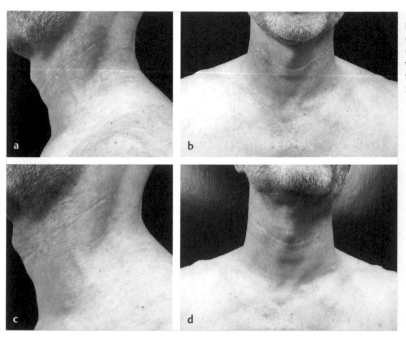

Fig. 7.4 (a) and **(b)** Poikiloderma, photodamage and scarring (pre-treatment). **(c)** and **(d)** post-treatment after one session with non-ablative fractional 1927 nm thulium laser followed by one session of 595 nm pulsed dye laser.

7.6 Vascular Lasers

Lasers used for the treatment of vascular lesions target oxyhemoglobin, which has absorption peaks in both visible light (418, 542, and 577 nm) and the infrared spectrum (700–1,100 nm).[103] The goal of vascular lasers is to induce intravascular thrombosis while minimizing collateral effects, leading to blood vessel damage and contraction.[104] Male patients may frequently seek treatment for facial erythema or telangiectasias, which may be secondary to chronic actinic damage, genetics, or underlying conditions such as erythematotelangiectatic rosacea or collagen vascular disease.[105] Other common indications include poikiloderma, angiomas, superficial hemangiomas, port wine stains, erythematous or hypertrophic scars, and keloids (▶ Fig. 7.4).[103]

Notably, many wavelengths utilized in the treatment of pigmented lesions are also used for vascular lesions; therefore, additional care must be taken to avoid unintended absorption by melanin, especially at the shorter wavelengths. Thus, epidermal cooling by way of cryogen spray or chilled sapphire plates is employed to minimize this risk. Additionally, vascular lasers that emit longer wavelengths are preferred, especially in patients with Fitzpatrick skin types IV to VI where the risk of epidermal damage and dyspigmentation is higher.[106] Additionally, longer wavelengths are associated with deeper penetration and therefore may be more appropriate for deeper vascular lesions, whereas superficial vascular lesions may be more effectively targeted with shorter wavelengths.[107]

The pulsed dye laser (PDL), primarily at a wavelength of 595 nm, is considered the gold standard for treatment of many of the aforementioned conditions and one of the most popular vascular lasers. It has a strong track record of efficacy and safety across a broad range of cutaneous vascular lesions and even in pediatric populations.[108] Laser parameters can be altered depending on the target lesion's size, location, and the patient's Fitzpatrick skin type. Notably, short pulse durations tend to induce bruising. Whereas this may speed response time and decrease the overall number of treatments needed, bruising may not be cosmetically acceptable for certain patients, especially male patients who prefer minimal downtime and may not wish to reveal that they have undergone a cosmetic procedure.[5]

Other options for the treatment of vascular lesions include the potassium-titanyl phosphate (KTP laser), which emits a wavelength of 532 nm. In a study of 647 patients with a variety of vascular lesions, primarily telangiectasias or spider angiomas, 77.6% were "cleared" or "markedly improved" at 6 weeks after one to two treatments. Only 5.8% patients experienced adverse effects, mostly temporary swelling.[109] Because bruising is generally avoided with KTP lasers, it may be an attractive option for patients with facial telangiectasias even if more treatment sessions are needed to achieve a desired cosmetic outcome.[105]

The 1,064-nm wavelength of the Nd:YAG laser is not as avidly absorbed by oxyhemoglobin; however, its melanin absorption is also limited, making it a safer option for patients with darker skin types. The Nd:YAG laser is particularly effective for treating deeper vascular lesions, including leg veins, venous lakes, reticular blue veins, and the blebs and deeper component of port wine stains, that may not be adequately addressed by PDL or KTP laser.[110]

7.7 Intense Pulsed Light

IPL is a nonlaser flash lamp that emits polychromatic light with a broad spectrum of wavelengths (500–1,200 nm) that can target multiple chromophores.[111] Thus, filtration is necessary to select the proper wavelengths to ensure the correct chromophore is targeted. Whereas IPL has been reported to be modestly effective for repairing photodamage and rhytids on both clinical and histological levels,[111,112] it is generally used for treatment of erythema and dyspigmentation. For example, IPL is particularly effective in the treatment of both vascular and pigmented components of poikiloderma. In a study of 135 patients who underwent IPL treatment for poikiloderma of Civatte, 82% of patients saw at least a 75% reduction in poikiloderma changes.[113] IPL can also be an effective treatment for hair removal when used properly[114,115] though generally it is considered less effective than lasers for this indication.

7.8 Conclusion

Male patients represent an important, expanding segment of the aesthetic practice. Laser and light-based therapies are attractive treatment modalities for male patients, who generally prefer nonsurgical cosmetic procedures that are quick, efficient, and carry minimal recovery time. As described earlier, laser and light-based therapies have demonstrated efficacy in addressing a broad range of cosmetic indications and conditions that are of particular concern to men. Knowledge of the capabilities and limitations of existing technology, gender-specific anatomical distinctions, and the varied treatment goals of different patient populations is essential in improving cosmetic outcome and patient satisfaction.

7.9 Pearls

- Laser–skin interaction is complex and depends on several anatomic factors such as the size, depth, and surrounding environment of the target tissue. These can vary significantly with gender and must also be considered when selecting laser parameters such as wavelength, pulse duration, spot size, and fluence.
- Resurfacing lasers are powerful nonsurgical tools that can be used to address a wide range of cosmetic cutaneous concerns in men, such as photoaging, rhytids, dyspigmentation, acne scarring, and superficial skin growths.
- Given its balance between efficacy and recovery time, the nonablative fractionated laser has become the most popular and widely utilized class of resurfacing lasers, especially in male patients.
- As men tend to have thicker terminal hairs as well as increased hair density, they may be at increased risk of side effects due to overall increased energy absorption in the treated areas

- While many men may seek LHR for cosmetic removal of unwanted hair, LHR can also be an effective treatment for medical conditions that predominantly affect men, such as PFB and AKN.
- Successful tattoo removal may require multiple treatments over many months. As some tattoos may never completely fade, it is crucial that realistic expectations and understanding of potential complications and outcomes are discussed at initial consultation.
- PDL is considered the gold standard for treatment of many of these conditions and one of the most popular vascular lasers in male patients.
- Since many wavelengths utilized in the treatment of pigmented lesions and vascular lesions overlap, additional care must be taken to avoid unintended absorption by melanin, especially at the shorter wavelengths. To minimize this risk, vascular lasers that emit longer wavelengths are preferred (especially in patients with Fitzpatrick skin types IV to VI) and epidermal cooling by way of cryogen spray or chilled sapphire plates should be employed.
- Unlike lasers, IPL emits polychromatic light with a broad spectrum of wavelengths that can target multiple chromophores and is particularly effective at treating poikiloderma, which has both vascular and pigmented components.

References

[1] American Society of Plastic Surgeons. Plastic Surgery Statistics Report. ASPS National Clearinghouse of Plastic Surgery Procedural Statistics. American Society of Plastic Surgeons: Arlington Heights, IL; 2019
[2] American Society of Plastic Surgeons. Plastic Surgery Statistics Report. ASPS National Clearinghouse of Plastic Surgery Procedural Statistics. American Society of Plastic Surgeons: Arlington Heights, IL; 2009
[3] Cohen BE, Bashey S, Wysong A. Literature review of cosmetic procedures in men: approaches and techniques are gender specific. Am J Clin Dermatol. 2017; 18(1):87–96
[4] Montes JR, Santos E. Evaluation of men's trends and experiences in aesthetic treatment. J Drugs Dermatol. 2018; 17(9):941–946
[5] Keaney TC, Anolik R, Braz A, et al. The male aesthetic patient: facial anatomy, concepts of attractiveness, and treatment patterns. J Drugs Dermatol. 2018; 17(1):19–28
[6] Farhadian JA, Bloom BS, Brauer JA. Male aesthetics: a review of facial anatomy and pertinent clinical implications. J Drugs Dermatol. 2015; 14(9):1029–1034
[7] Boer M, Duchnik E, Maleszka R, Marchlewicz M. Structural and biophysical characteristics of human skin in maintaining proper epidermal barrier function. Postepy Dermatol Alergol. 2016; 33(1):1–5
[8] Rahrovan S, Fanian F, Mehryan P, Humbert P, Firooz A. Male versus female skin: what dermatologists and cosmeticians should know. Int J Womens Dermatol. 2018; 4(3):122–130
[9] Tur E. Physiology of the skin: differences between women and men. Clin Dermatol. 1997; 15(1):5–16
[10] Shuster S, Black MM, McVitie E. The influence of age and sex on skin thickness, skin collagen and density. Br J Dermatol. 1975; 93(6):639–643
[11] Bailey SH, Oni G, Brown SA, et al. The use of non-invasive instruments in characterizing human facial and abdominal skin. Lasers Surg Med. 2012; 44(2):131–142

[12] Brincat M, Kabalan S, Studd JW, Moniz CF, de Trafford J, Montgomery J. A study of the decrease of skin collagen content, skin thickness, and bone mass in the postmenopausal woman. Obstet Gynecol. 1987; 70 (6):840–845

[13] Markova MS, Zeskand J, McEntee B, Rothstein J, Jimenez SA, Siracusa LD. A role for the androgen receptor in collagen content of the skin. J Invest Dermatol. 2004; 123(6):1052–1056

[14] Tsukahara K, Hotta M, Osanai O, Kawada H, Kitahara T, Takema Y. Gender-dependent differences in degree of facial wrinkles. Skin Res Technol. 2013; 19(1):e65–e71

[15] Keaney TC, Alster TS. Botulinum toxin in men: review of relevant anatomy and clinical trial data. Dermatol Surg. 2013; 39(10): 1434–1443

[16] Mayrovitz HN, Regan MB. Gender differences in facial skin blood perfusion during basal and heated conditions determined by laser Doppler flowmetry. Microvasc Res. 1993; 45(2):211–218

[17] Baker DC, Stefani WA, Chiu ES. Reducing the incidence of hematoma requiring surgical evacuation following male rhytidectomy: a 30-year review of 985 cases. Plast Reconstr Surg. 2005; 116(7):1973–1985, discussion 1986–1987

[18] Pochi PE, Strauss JS. Endocrinologic control of the development and activity of the human sebaceous gland. J Invest Dermatol. 1974; 62 (3):191–201

[19] Cribier B. Rosacea under the microscope: characteristic histological findings. J Eur Acad Dermatol Venereol. 2013; 27(11):1336–1343

[20] Anderson RR, Parrish JA. Selective photothermolysis: precise microsurgery by selective absorption of pulsed radiation. Science. 1983; 220(4596):524–527

[21] Tanzi EL, Lupton JR, Alster TS. Lasers in dermatology: four decades of progress. J Am Acad Dermatol. 2003; 49(1):1–31, quiz 31–34

[22] Alster TS, Lupton JR. Lasers in dermatology. An overview of types and indications. Am J Clin Dermatol. 2001; 2(5):291–303

[23] Carroll L, Humphreys TR. LASER-tissue interactions. Clin Dermatol. 2006; 24(1):2–7

[24] Preissig J, Hamilton K, Markus R. Current laser resurfacing technologies: a review that delves beneath the surface. Semin Plast Surg. 2012; 26(3):109–116

[25] Khatri KA, Ross V, Grevelink JM, Magro CM, Anderson RR. Comparison of erbium:YAG and carbon dioxide lasers in resurfacing of facial rhytids. Arch Dermatol. 1999; 135(4):391–397

[26] Fitzpatrick RE, Goldman MP, Satur NM, Tope WD. Pulsed carbon dioxide laser resurfacing of photo-aged facial skin. Arch Dermatol. 1996; 132(4):395–402

[27] Hruza GJ, Dover JS. Laser skin resurfacing. Arch Dermatol. 1996; 132 (4):451–455

[28] Nanni CA, Alster TS. Complications of carbon dioxide laser resurfacing. An evaluation of 500 patients. Dermatol Surg. 1998; 24 (3):315–320

[29] Geronemus RG. Fractional photothermolysis: current and future applications. Lasers Surg Med. 2006; 38(3):169–176

[30] Alster TS, Garg S. Treatment of facial rhytids with a high-energy pulsed carbon dioxide laser. Plast Reconstr Surg. 1996; 98(5): 791–794

[31] Omi T, Numano K. The role of the CO_2 laser and fractional CO_2 laser in dermatology. Laser Ther. 2014; 23(1):49–60

[32] Alexiades-Armenakas MR, Dover JS, Arndt KA. The spectrum of laser skin resurfacing: nonablative, fractional, and ablative laser resurfacing. J Am Acad Dermatol. 2008; 58(5):719–737, quiz 738–740

[33] Tanzi EL, Alster TS. Single-pass carbon dioxide versus multiple-pass Er:YAG laser skin resurfacing: a comparison of postoperative wound healing and side-effect rates. Dermatol Surg. 2003; 29(1): 80–84

[34] Ross EV, McKinlay JR, Sajben FP, et al. Use of a novel erbium laser in a Yucatan minipig: a study of residual thermal damage, ablation, and wound healing as a function of pulse duration. Lasers Surg Med. 2002; 30(2):93–100

[35] Manstein D, Herron GS, Sink RK, Tanner H, Anderson RR. Fractional photothermolysis: a new concept for cutaneous remodeling using microscopic patterns of thermal injury. Lasers Surg Med. 2004; 34 (5):426–438

[36] Waibel J, Beer K, Narurkar V, Alster T. Preliminary observations on fractional ablative resurfacing devices: clinical impressions. J Drugs Dermatol. 2009; 8(5):481–485

[37] Christiansen K, Bjerring P. Low density, non-ablative fractional CO_2 laser rejuvenation. Lasers Surg Med. 2008; 40(7):454–460

[38] Trelles MA, Mordon S, Velez M, Urdiales F, Levy JL. Results of fractional ablative facial skin resurfacing with the erbium:yttrium-aluminium-garnet laser 1 week and 2 months after one single treatment in 30 patients. Lasers Med Sci. 2009; 24(2):186–194

[39] Fife DJ, Fitzpatrick RE, Zachary CB. Complications of fractional CO_2 laser resurfacing: four cases. Lasers Surg Med. 2009; 41(3):179–184

[40] Rohrich RJ, Griffin JR, Adams WP, Jr. Rhinophyma: review and update. Plast Reconstr Surg. 2002; 110(3):860–869, quiz 870

[41] Madan V, Ferguson JE, August PJ. Carbon dioxide laser treatment of rhinophyma: a review of 124 patients. Br J Dermatol. 2009; 161(4): 814–818

[42] Sadick H, Goepel B, Bersch C, Goessler U, Hoermann K, Riedel F. Rhinophyma: diagnosis and treatment options for a disfiguring tumor of the nose. Ann Plast Surg. 2008; 61(1):114–120

[43] Greenbaum SS, Krull EA, Watnick K. Comparison of CO_2 laser and electrosurgery in the treatment of rhinophyma. J Am Acad Dermatol. 1988; 18(2, Pt 1):363–368

[44] Gjuric M, Rettinger G. Comparison of carbon dioxide laser and electrosurgery in the treatment of rhinophyma. Rhinology. 1993; 31(1): 37–39

[45] Comeau V, Goodman M, Kober MM, Buckley C. Fractionated carbon dioxide laser resurfacing as an ideal treatment option for severe rhinophyma: a case report and discussion. J Clin Aesthet Dermatol. 2019; 12(1):24–27

[46] Orenstein A, Haik J, Tamir J, et al. Treatment of rhinophyma with Er:YAG laser. Lasers Surg Med. 2001; 29(3):230–235

[47] Goldberg DJ. Nonablative dermal remodeling: does it really work? Arch Dermatol. 2002; 138(10):1366–1368

[48] Hohenleutner S, Hohenleutner U, Landthaler M. Nonablative wrinkle reduction: treatment results with a 585-nm laser. Arch Dermatol. 2002; 138(10):1380–1381

[49] Bjerring P, Clement M, Heickendorff L, Egevist H, Kiernan M. Selective non-ablative wrinkle reduction by laser. J Cutan Laser Ther. 2000; 2 (1):9–15

[50] Goldberg DJ. Non-ablative subsurface remodeling: clinical and histologic evaluation of a 1320-nm Nd:YAG laser. J Cutan Laser Ther. 1999; 1(3):153–157

[51] Bhatia AC, Dover JS, Arndt KA, Stewart B, Alam M. Patient satisfaction and reported long-term therapeutic efficacy associated with 1,320 nm Nd:YAG laser treatment of acne scarring and photoaging. Dermatol Surg. 2006; 32(3):346–352

[52] Trelles MA, Allones I, Luna R. Facial rejuvenation with a nonablative 1320 nm Nd:YAG laser: a preliminary clinical and histologic evaluation. Dermatol Surg. 2001; 27(2):111–116

[53] Chan HH, Lam LK, Wong DS, Kono T, Trendell-Smith N. Use of 1,320 nm Nd:YAG laser for wrinkle reduction and the treatment of atrophic acne scarring in Asians. Lasers Surg Med. 2004; 34(2): 98–103

[54] Narurkar VA. Nonablative fractional resurfacing in the male patient. Dermatol Ther. 2007; 20(6):430–435

[55] Tan JK, Bhate K. A global perspective on the epidemiology of acne. Br J Dermatol. 2015; 172 Suppl 1:3–12

[56] Kaushik SB, Alexis AF. Nonablative fractional laser resurfacing in skin of color: evidence-based review. J Clin Aesthet Dermatol. 2017; 10 (6):51–67

[57] Cho SB, Lee SJ, Cho S, et al. Non-ablative 1550-nm erbium-glass and ablative 10 600-nm carbon dioxide fractional lasers for acne scars: a randomized split-face study with blinded response evaluation. J Eur Acad Dermatol Venereol. 2010; 24(8):921–925

[58] Narurkar VA, Alster TS, Bernstein EF, Lin TJ, Loncaric A. Safety and efficacy of a 1550 nm/1927 nm dual wavelength laser for the treatment of photodamaged skin. J Drugs Dermatol. 2018; 17(1):41–46

[59] Weiss ET, Brauer JA, Anolik R, et al. 1927-nm fractional resurfacing of facial actinic keratoses: a promising new therapeutic option. J Am Acad Dermatol. 2013; 68(1):98–102

[60] Flohil SC, van der Leest RJ, Dowlatshahi EA, Hofman A, de Vries E, Nijsten T. Prevalence of actinic keratosis and its risk factors in the general population: the Rotterdam Study. J Invest Dermatol. 2013; 133(8):1971–1978

[61] Brauer JA, Kazlouskaya V, Alabdulrazzaq H, et al. Use of a picosecond pulse duration laser with specialized optic for treatment of facial acne scarring. JAMA Dermatol. 2015; 151(3):278–284

[62] Wat H, Yee-Nam Shek S, Yeung CK, Chan HH. Efficacy and safety of picosecond 755-nm alexandrite laser with diffractive lens array for non-ablative rejuvenation in Chinese skin. Lasers Surg Med. 2019; 51 (1):8–13

[63] Weiss RA, McDaniel DH, Weiss MA, Mahoney AM, Beasley KL, Halvorson CR. Safety and efficacy of a novel diffractive lens array using a picosecond 755 nm alexandrite laser for treatment of wrinkles. Lasers Surg Med. 2017; 49(1):40–44

[64] Bernstein EF, Schomacker KT, Basilavecchio LD, Plugis JM, Bhawalkar JD. Treatment of acne scarring with a novel fractionated, dual-wavelength, picosecond-domain laser incorporating a novel holographic beam-splitter. Lasers Surg Med. 2017; 49(9):796–802

[65] Dierickx C. Using normal and high pulse coverage with picosecond laser treatment of wrinkles and acne scarring: long term clinical observations. Lasers Surg Med. 2018; 50(1):51–55

[66] American Society of Plastic Surgeons. Plastic Surgery Statistics Report. ASPS National Clearinghouse of Plastic Surgery Procedural Statistics. Arlington Heights, IL: American Society of Plastic Surgeons; 2000

[67] Cotsarelis G, Sun TT, Lavker RM. Label-retaining cells reside in the bulge area of pilosebaceous unit: implications for follicular stem cells, hair cycle, and skin carcinogenesis. Cell. 1990; 61(7):1329–1337

[68] Margolis RJ, Dover JS, Polla LL, et al. Visible action spectrum for melanin-specific selective photothermolysis. Lasers Surg Med. 1989; 9(4):389–397

[69] Ibrahimi OA, Avram MM, Hanke CW, Kilmer SL, Anderson RR. Laser hair removal. Dermatol Ther (Heidelb). 2011; 24(1):94–107

[70] Nanni CA, Alster TS. Laser-assisted hair removal: side effects of Q-switched Nd:YAG, long-pulsed ruby, and alexandrite lasers. J Am Acad Dermatol. 1999; 41(2, Pt 1):165–171

[71] Campos VB, Dierickx CC, Farinelli WA, Lin TY, Manuskiatti W, Anderson RR. Hair removal with an 800-nm pulsed diode laser. J Am Acad Dermatol. 2000; 43(3):442–447

[72] Lou WW, Quintana AT, Geronemus RG, Grossman MC. Prospective study of hair reduction by diode laser (800 nm) with long-term follow-up. Dermatol Surg. 2000; 26(5):428–432

[73] Bouzari N, Tabatabai H, Abbasi Z, Firooz A, Dowlati Y. Laser hair removal: comparison of long-pulsed Nd:YAG, long-pulsed alexandrite, and long-pulsed diode lasers. Dermatol Surg. 2004; 30(4, Pt 1):498–502

[74] Puri N. Comparative study of diode laser versus neodymium-yttrium aluminum: garnet laser versus intense pulsed light for the treatment of hirsutism. J Cutan Aesthet Surg. 2015; 8(2):97–101

[75] Alster TS, Bryan H, Williams CM. Long-pulsed Nd:YAG laser-assisted hair removal in pigmented skin: a clinical and histological evaluation. Arch Dermatol. 2001; 137(7):885–889

[76] McMichael AJ. Hair and scalp disorders in ethnic populations. Dermatol Clin. 2003; 21(4):629–644

[77] Nussbaum D, Friedman A. Pseudofolliculitis barbae: a review of current treatment options. J Drugs Dermatol. 2019; 18(3):246–250

[78] Dinehart SM, Herzberg AJ, Kerns BJ, Pollack SV. Acne keloidalis: a review. J Dermatol Surg Oncol. 1989; 15(6):642–647

[79] Goette DK, Berger TG. Acne keloidalis nuchae. A transepithelial elimination disorder. Int J Dermatol. 1987; 26(7):442–444

[80] Khunger N, Molpariya A, Khunger A. Complications of tattoos and tattoo removal: stop and think before you ink. J Cutan Aesthet Surg. 2015; 8(1):30–36

[81] Reiter O, Atzmony L, Akerman L, et al. Picosecond lasers for tattoo removal: a systematic review. Lasers Med Sci. 2016; 31(7):1397–1405

[82] Ross V, Naseef G, Lin G, et al. Comparison of responses of tattoos to picosecond and nanosecond Q-switched neodymium: YAG lasers. Arch Dermatol. 1998; 134(2):167–171

[83] Lorgeou A, Perrillat Y, Gral N, Lagrange S, Lacour JP, Passeron T. Comparison of two picosecond lasers to a nanosecond laser for treating tattoos: a prospective randomized study on 49 patients. J Eur Acad Dermatol Venereol. 2018; 32(2):265–270

[84] Herd RM, Alora MB, Smoller B, Arndt KA, Dover JS. A clinical and histologic prospective controlled comparative study of the picosecond titanium:sapphire (795 nm) laser versus the Q-switched alexandrite (752 nm) laser for removing tattoo pigment. J Am Acad Dermatol. 1999; 40(4):603–606

[85] Brauer JA, Reddy KK, Anolik R, et al. Successful and rapid treatment of blue and green tattoo pigment with a novel picosecond laser. Arch Dermatol. 2012; 148(7):820–823

[86] Alabdulrazzaq H, Brauer JA, Bae YS, Geronemus RG. Clearance of yellow tattoo ink with a novel 532-nm picosecond laser. Lasers Surg Med. 2015; 47(4):285–288

[87] Tope WD. State and territorial regulation of tattooing in the United States. J Am Acad Dermatol. 1995; 32(5, Pt 1):791–799

[88] Kirby W, Chen CL, Desai A, Desai T. Causes and recommendations for unanticipated ink retention following tattoo removal treatment. J Clin Aesthet Dermatol. 2013; 6(7):27–31

[89] Anderson RR, Geronemus R, Kilmer SL, Farinelli W, Fitzpatrick RE. Cosmetic tattoo ink darkening. A complication of Q-switched and pulsed-laser treatment. Arch Dermatol. 1993; 129(8):1010–1014

[90] Ross EV, Yashar S, Michaud N, et al. Tattoo darkening and non-response after laser treatment: a possible role for titanium dioxide. Arch Dermatol. 2001; 137(1):33–37

[91] Bae YS, Alabdulrazzaq H, Brauer J, Geronemus R. Successful treatment of paradoxical darkening. Lasers Surg Med. 2016; 48(5): 471–473

[92] Kazandjieva J, Tsankov N. Tattoos: dermatological complications. Clin Dermatol. 2007; 25(4):375–382

[93] Ibrahimi OA, Syed Z, Sakamoto FH, Avram MM, Anderson RR. Treatment of tattoo allergy with ablative fractional resurfacing: a novel paradigm for tattoo removal. J Am Acad Dermatol. 2011; 64 (6):1111–1114

[94] Ashinoff R, Levine VJ, Soter NA. Allergic reactions to tattoo pigment after laser treatment. Dermatol Surg. 1995; 21(4):291–294

[95] Izikson L, Avram M, Anderson RR. Transient immunoreactivity after laser tattoo removal: report of two cases. Lasers Surg Med. 2008; 40 (4):231–232

[96] Antony FC, Harland CC. Red ink tattoo reactions: successful treatment with the Q-switched 532 nm Nd:YAG laser. Br J Dermatol. 2003; 149 (1):94–98

[97] Weiss ET, Geronemus RG. Combining fractional resurfacing and Q-switched ruby laser for tattoo removal. Dermatol Surg. 2011; 37(1): 97–99

[98] Rashid T, Hussain I, Haider M, Haroon TS. Laser therapy of freckles and lentigines with quasi-continuous, frequency-doubled, Nd:YAG (532 nm) laser in Fitzpatrick skin type IV: a 24-month follow-up. J Cosmet Laser Ther. 2002; 4(3–4):81–85

[99] Kilmer SL, Wheeland RG, Goldberg DJ, Anderson RR. Treatment of epidermal pigmented lesions with the frequency-doubled Q-switched Nd:YAG laser. A controlled, single-impact, dose-response, multicenter trial. Arch Dermatol. 1994; 130(12):1515–1519

[100] Imhof L, Dummer R, Dreier J, Kolm I, Barysch MJ. A prospective trial comparing Q-switched ruby laser and a triple combination skin-lightening cream in the treatment of solar lentigines. Dermatol Surg. 2016; 42(7):853–857

[101] Williams NM, Gurnani P, Long J, et al. Comparing the efficacy and safety of Q-switched and picosecond lasers in the treatment of nevus of Ota: a systematic review and meta-analysis. Lasers Med Sci. 2021; 36(4):723–733

[102] Ge Y, Yang Y, Guo L, et al. Comparison of a picosecond alexandrite laser versus a Q-switched alexandrite laser for the treatment of nevus of Ota: a randomized, split-lesion, controlled trial. J Am Acad Dermatol. 2020; 83(2):397–403

[103] Wall TL. Current concepts: laser treatment of adult vascular lesions. Semin Plast Surg. 2007; 21(3):147–158

[104] Garden JM, Tan OT, Kerschmann R, et al. Effect of dye laser pulse duration on selective cutaneous vascular injury. J Invest Dermatol. 1986; 87(5):653–657

[105] West TB, Alster TS. Comparison of the long-pulse dye (590–595 nm) and KTP (532 nm) lasers in the treatment of facial and leg telangiectasias. Dermatol Surg. 1998; 24(2):221–226

[106] Shah S, Alster TS. Laser treatment of dark skin: an updated review. Am J Clin Dermatol. 2010; 11(6):389–397

[107] Stier MF, Glick SA, Hirsch RJ. Laser treatment of pediatric vascular lesions: port wine stains and hemangiomas. J Am Acad Dermatol. 2008; 58(2):261–285

[108] Garden JM, Bakus AD. Clinical efficacy of the pulsed dye laser in the treatment of vascular lesions. J Dermatol Surg Oncol. 1993; 19(4): 321–326

[109] Becher GL, Cameron H, Moseley H. Treatment of superficial vascular lesions with the KTP 532-nm laser: experience with 647 patients. Lasers Med Sci. 2014; 29(1):267–271

[110] Ozyurt K, Colgecen E, Baykan H, Ozturk P, Ozkose M. Treatment of superficial cutaneous vascular lesions: experience with the long-pulsed 1064 nm Nd:YAG laser. ScientificWorldJournal. 2012; 2012:197139

[111] Hernández-Pérez E, Ibiett EV. Gross and microscopic findings in patients submitted to nonablative full-face resurfacing using intense pulsed light: a preliminary study. Dermatol Surg. 2002; 28 (8):651–655

[112] Goldberg DJ, Cutler KB. Nonablative treatment of rhytids with intense pulsed light. Lasers Surg Med. 2000; 26(2):196–200

[113] Weiss RA, Goldman MP, Weiss MA. Treatment of poikiloderma of Civatte with an intense pulsed light source. Dermatol Surg. 2000; 26 (9):823–827, discussion 828

[114] Weiss RA, Weiss MA, Marwaha S, Harrington AC. Hair removal with a non-coherent filtered flashlamp intense pulsed light source. Lasers Surg Med. 1999; 24(2):128–132

[115] Gold MH, Bell MW, Foster TD, Street S. Long-term epilation using the EpiLight broad band, intense pulsed light hair removal system. Dermatol Surg. 1997; 23(10):909–913

8 Keg to Six Pack: Fat and Cellulite Treatments

Deanne Mraz Robinson and Daniel P. Friedmann

Summary

The male demand for cosmetic procedures targeting localized deposits of subcutaneous adipose tissue has grown rapidly over the past decade. Current therapeutic options are less invasive, decreasing downtime and adverse events, while providing a more natural aesthetic appearance. This chapter highlights the numerous available modalities for subcutaneous fat reduction in male patients.

Keywords: noninvasive fat reduction, tumescent liposuction, cryolipolysis, cryoadipolysis, high-intensity focused ultrasound, sodium deoxycholate

8.1 Background

Body contouring procedures are extremely popular, with up to 86% of people surveyed by the American Society for Dermatologic Surgery reporting being bothered by excess weight and 57% of them seeking body sculpting treatments.[1] Although men may face less social pressure to seek cosmetic enhancement, they are often motivated by the same desires as women, such as looking as good as possible for their age.[2] The male demand for cosmetic procedures targeting subcutaneous adipose tissue has expanded rapidly over the past decade, in part from the growth of less invasive therapeutic options for localized fat reduction with marginal downtime, limited adverse events, and a more natural appearance.[3] Between 2012 and 2017, noninvasive body contouring procedures in male patients increased by 60.64%, whereas liposuction decreased by 25.51%.[4,5]

8.2 Anatomy

Fat distribution is a sexually dimorphic phenomenon, with excess adiposity in men accumulating in the midline (e.g., abdominal and chest), whereas in premenopausal women it collects below the waist (e.g., gluteal, hips, thighs, knees, and calves).[6–8] The sex steroid hormone testosterone, analogous to estrogen in premenopausal women, may exert permissive effects on regional fat deposits by regulating the balance between lipid accumulation and mobilization, stimulating the latter in visceral tissue.[9,10] Age-related dysregulation of adipocyte lipid metabolism and decreased endogenous testosterone in men in turn leads to progressive abdominal fat deposition viscerally and decreased abdominal fat subcutaneously.[11,12] Women also develop central and upper body fat deposits at a later age than men, typically in the postmenopausal period due to a decrease in endogenous estrogen.[13] While visceral fat volume in men is 2.6 times that of premenopausal women, it is equivalent to that of postmenopausal women.[12]

The ideal male abdomen is square shaped with less natural sloping from the midline to lateral aspects and a lower waistline, slightly below the umbilicus, than its female counterpart (▶ Fig. 8.1).[14] The male upper body also displays a V-shaped taper from broad shoulders to a narrowed waist. Subcutaneous adipose tissue deposits in the waist and flanks increase waist circumference and decrease this V-shaped tapering.[15] Enlargement of the male breast, gynecomastia, either from excess subareolar and lateral pectoral fat—pseudogynecomastia, or subareolar glandular tissue and fat—is cosmetically unpleasant and psychologically distressing.[16] On the other hand, fat deposition in the anterior pectoral region, overlying the pectoralis major, can increase chest convexity and give a more masculine appearance.[15,17] Excess submental and submandibular fat deposits obscure the strong masculine jawline and leads to a decrease in cervicomental angle.[14] Evaluation and marking of any area undergoing treatment should be performed with the patient upright in anatomic position.

The architecture of the subcutaneous adipose tissue fibrous septa is markedly different between men and women, contributing to the more "firm" or "fibrous"

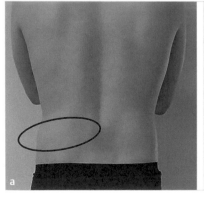 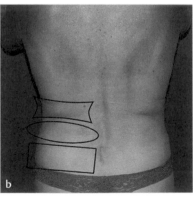

Fig. 8.1 (a) Bilateral male flanks marked by an ellipse. (b) Female hips (*rectangle*), waist (*ellipse*), and flanks (*polygon*). Note the lower waistline in the male patient, with the female waist equivalent to the male flank in anatomic position.

clinical presentation of subcutaneous fat in men.[18] Women have a higher percentage of fibrous septa that are perpendicular to the skin surface, while those of men are much more likely to be diagonal or parallel to the skin surface.[19]

8.3 Approach

Submental, chest, abdominal, and flank subcutaneous adipose tissue deposits are the most common areas of concern for male patients seeking body contouring procedures.[20] Available therapeutic options rely on the destruction by cooling, heating, or adipocyte disruption or dissolution, or physical removal by lipoaspiration, of subcutaneous adipocytes.[21] While the former techniques lead to subtle results with minimal downtime, the latter is a better option for patients wanting a more dramatic single-treatment result at the expense of a significant period of posttreatment recovery.

Prospective patients with significant visceral fat deposits should be excluded from abdominal body contouring, given that these treatments treat only subcutaneous adipose tissue. Patients with a history of progressive or cyclical weight gain are relatively contraindicated, given their propensity for postprocedure weight gain with suboptimal results. Men with emotional or psychological instability, eating disorders, body dysmorphic disorder, or unrealistic expectations (e.g., seeking immediate results, substantial weight loss, or perfection) are all more likely to be dissatisfied with treatment outcomes and should also be excluded.[22]

Substantial preexisting laxity of the overlying skin or underlying muscle due to prior rapid weight loss or advanced age may become exaggerated postprocedure. A thorough past medical, surgical, medication, and allergy history must be taken as patients with uncontrolled chronic medical conditions or who are at risk of perioperative bleeding (e.g., due to medically necessary long-term anticoagulation) are best treated with noninvasive body contouring devices. Patients taking medications that inhibit hepatic cytochrome P450 1A2 and 3A4, which interfere with lidocaine metabolism and may lead to toxic elevations in plasma lidocaine concentration, should either be treated noninvasively or stop the implicated medication(s) 1 week prior to tumescent liposuction.[23] The most common classes of these medications include antidepressants, antifungals, antivirals, and antibiotics.

8.4 Procedure

8.4.1 Cryoadipolysis

Cryoadipolysis, often incorrectly referred to as cryolipolysis,[24] is a procedure cleared by the Food and Drug Administration (FDA) for reducing the appearance of fat bulges in the abdomen, flank, and submental area, among other locations, in nonobese patients. Since adipocytes are preferentially sensitive to cold injury, prolonged cutaneous cooling induces adipocyte apoptosis, triggering a selective, delayed lobular panniculitis and subsequent targeted reduction in superficial subcutaneous fat, without clinical or histologic damage to overlying skin.[25,26] Transient pain, erythema, edema, bruising, and numbness are common complaints posttreatment, but alterations in serum lipid levels or liver function tests have not been reported.[27,28] Infrequently, intense neuropathic pain may develop several days posttreatment and may respond well to gabapentin or oral analgesics.[29] Fortunately, long-term peripheral nerve dysfunction has not been demonstrated.[30] Although these concerns have been reported equally among male and female patients, paradoxical adipose hyperplasia—a delayed increase in subcutaneous fat in the treated area that typically begins several months posttreatment—may be more common in men and patients of Hispanic background.[31] Hyperplasia or hypertrophy of disorganized adipocytes, perilobular septal thickening/fibrosis, and vascularity are seen on histology. Its etiology remains unclear, but local tissue hypoxia or reduced sympathetic innervation may be inciting metabolic activation of preexisting adipocytes or adipocyte progenitor cells.[32]

Currently available noninvasive technology utilizes a vacuum to elevate and compress a targeted fold of tissue into a cup-shaped plate for 35 minutes.[33] Prior treatment applicators, however, compressed fat within two opposing plates for 45 to 60 minutes at a higher temperature. A 75-minute nonvacuum conformable-surface applicator, with FDA clearance for treatment of thighs, has also been shown to be effective in areas where suction may be limited by anatomy or firmness of tissue, such as the periumbilical abdomen.[34] With subjects lying supine, a protective gel pad is draped over the treatment area immediately prior to applicator placement on the abdomen, while the flanks can be targeted with the patient on their side or prone. The applicator may then be secured in place with straps for the entirety of treatment, if needed. Submental cryoadipolysis can also be performed using a smaller applicator and protective liquid gel, with the subject sitting upright and similar straps supporting the device against the submentum.[35] At the conclusion of the treatment cycle, the cryoadipolysis applicator is immediately removed, and a manual massage of the treated area is performed. Posttreatment massage has been shown to produce significantly greater reductions in fat thickness due to reperfusion injury.[36] Combining cryoadipolysis with radial pulse (shockwave) therapy may also improve results.[37]

Treatment results are usually modest, with a single application to the flank having been shown to cause a 39.6-mL mean volume loss relative to the contralateral control in a clinical study.[38] Double-stacking or overlapping of applicators in the same session may lead to enhanced efficacy without an increase in adverse events.[39] A study of two overlapping applicator treatments in the same session for male pseudogynecomastia demonstrated significant improvement in 95% of subjects.[16]

8.4.2 High-Intensity Focused Ultrasound

High-intensity focused ultrasound (HIFU) uses high-frequency acoustic energy (2 MHz, > 1,000 W/cm^2) to rapidly raise adipose temperature above 55 to 58 °C, producing focal coagulative necrosis, while also disrupting adipocyte membranes secondary to mechanical effects (acoustic cavitation).[40,41] HIFU devices currently cleared by the FDA are indicated for noninvasive waist circumference reduction and target subcutaneous tissue at a focal depth of 1.3 cm; however, severe periprocedural pain and posttreatment ecchymosis have limited the use of this technology.[42]

8.4.3 Nonthermal Focused Ultrasound

Nonthermal focused ultrasound (NFU) varies significantly from HIFU by relying solely on adipocyte destruction via low-frequency (200 kHz, 17.5 W/cm^2) mechanical disruption.[43] NFU is FDA approved for noninvasive reduction of abdominal circumference at a depth of 1.5 cm. This nonthermal approach means dramatically less procedural pain and no downtime posttreatment, but requires multiple sequential treatment sessions for optimal, albeit subtle, results.[14] Localized posttreatment adverse events, including pain, erythema, and purpura, are transient and typically minimal.[44]

8.4.4 High-Intensity Focused Electromagnetic Field Therapy

High-intensity focused electromagnetic (HIFEM) technology has recently been shown to produce muscle fiber hypertrophy and hyperplasia, as well as induce local adipocyte apoptosis, leading to subcutaneous fat metabolism and a local increase in free fatty acids.[45–47] A flat applicator is fixed to the abdomen with a belt and each treatment is performed for 30 minutes, with the intensity slowly increased from 0% (ideally to 100%) based on patient tolerance. Four treatments over a 2-week period have been shown to reduce abdominal fat thickness by 19 and 23.3% after 1 and 3 months, respectively.[48] Other clinical trials have confirmed reductions in subcutaneous tissue thickness of 18.6% by magnetic resonance imaging (MRI) 2 months after four sessions[49] and 17.5% by computed tomography (CT) 1 month after eight sessions, the latter also noting a 14.8% hypertrophy of the rectus abdominis muscle.[50] One-year follow-up of subjects treated with HIFEM has demonstrated statistically significant long-term improvement in fat reduction (–14.63%), muscle thickness (19.05%), and diastasis recti reduction (–10.46%).[51]

8.4.5 Radiofrequency

Radiofrequency (RF) devices create an oscillating electrical field that generates heat from movement and collision of water molecules.[52] Since fat has a high electrical impedance and low thermal conductivity relative to overlying dermal tissue, an electrical field directed perpendicular to the skin surface and skin–subcutaneous interface is highly selective for subcutaneous tissue, leading to chromophore-independent thermal damage.[53] Purported mechanisms of fat reduction following RF include thermal stimulation of adipocyte metabolism via lipase-mediated enzymatic degradation of triglycerides and adipocyte apoptosis and rupture.[54,55]

Monopolar, or unipolar, and multipolar mechanisms of RF delivery are currently available for fat reduction, with the latter utilizing high-frequency electromagnetic radiation instead of an electric current to produce heat.[56] Trials of monopolar/unipolar RF (with a single electrode) or multipolar RF (three or more electrodes) for fat reduction in male patients, however, are lacking. Nevertheless, volumetric heating of subcutaneous tissue up to 20 mm in depth can be achieved, with optimal results requiring multiple weekly treatment sessions. Newer devices have built-in impedance and temperature monitoring to improve efficacy, safety, and operator dependency.

High-frequency, multipolar field RF has also been shown to produce significant abdominal fat reduction using an operator-independent device. An open-label trial showed a mean circumferential reduction of 4.93 cm in 35 patients after four weekly treatments, although 3 patients did not respond to therapy.[57] The body mass index (BMI) was effectively unchanged during the study period, and the best results were associated with subjects who had a higher initial BMI. Approximately 90% of subjects reported no pain with treatment.

Adverse events with RF devices most commonly include treatment-related pain and transient erythema. Posttreatment edema, purpura, postinflammatory hyperpigmentation, subcutaneous erythematous papules, blisters, and superficial burns—although relatively rare—are possible.[56]

8.4.6 Low-Level Laser Therapy

Although low-level laser therapy (LLLT) has been suggested to disrupt adipocyte cell membranes,[58] in vivo[59,60] and in vitro[21] studies have failed to corroborate this claim. Other purported effects on adipocyte apoptosis via complement activation or lipid metabolism via upregulated mitochondrial cytochrome C oxidase activity remain unvalidated.[61] The fact that the majority of photons from 635- or 850-nm LLLT light fail to penetrate into subcutaneous tissue does little to boost claims of subdermal efficacy.[21,62] Studies demonstrating improvement in abdominal circumference are compromised by lack of clinical controls, absent weight monitoring, short-term follow-up, or concomitant use of metabolic supplements.[63,64,65,66]

Nevertheless, LLLT devices are currently FDA approved for circumference reduction of the waist. Treatments are performed two to three times per week, requiring numerous sessions. Devices with light-emitting diode (LED) panels at a preset distance from the skin typically have nearly absent side effect profiles. A study of an LLLT device with LED panels directly approximating the skin in a controlled split-abdomen study showed no significant improvement in ultrasound-measured subcutaneous tissue thickness, but did report two cases of cutaneous ulceration.[67]

8.4.7 Infrared Diode Laser

A contact-cooled 1,060-nm diode laser device has been shown to produce controlled adipocyte injury by maintaining subcutaneous hyperthermia (42–47 °C), leading to a mean reduction of 18% in caliper-measured targeted fat thickness and 24% reduction in volume by MRI.[68] Treatment is performed with up to four rectangular applicators simultaneously for 25 minutes. Studies have shown significant improvement in subcutaneous fat deposits of the abdomen and flanks after a single treatment.[69,70] Posttreatment adverse events include tenderness, induration, and erythema.[71]

8.4.8 Injection Adipolysis

Sodium deoxycholate, or deoxycholic acid (DC), is an animal-derived secondary bile salt and biologic detergent that degrades adipocyte cell membranes.[72] Subcutaneous injection of DC produces concentration-dependent local adipolysis and mixed septal and lobular subcutaneous panniculitis composed of inflammatory cells recruited to clear cellular debris and free lipids.[73] Fat lobule atrophy and septal thickening/fibrosis are the end result, with the inflammatory cascade characteristically resolving within 1 month postinjection.[72,73] Data subanalysis from the two phase 3 pivotal trials in the United States and Canada (Reduced Frequency Immune [REFINE]-1 and -2) demonstrates that 77% of men treated with DC (ATX-101) achieved a clinically significant reduction in submental fat; 79% of men were also satisfied with the posttreatment appearance of their face/chin.[74]

The submental area is marked, taking care to avoid injecting into the immediate submandibular area, where there is risk of temporary demyelination of the marginal mandibular nerve. Injection points are performed approximately 1 cm apart using a 1-mL syringe and 30-gauge needle, with 0.2 mL of product injected at each point with the needle perpendicular to the skin surface. Using a greater amount of product (three to four vials, 6–8 mL) in the first session may lead to better results early on and encourage patients to complete the treatment series.[74] It is expected that less product will therefore be

needed with subsequent monthly treatments. Transient injection site pain, edema, numbness, ecchymosis, erythema, and induration/fibrosis are commonly observed postprocedure. Alopecia has been reported from submental injections, but often resolves spontaneously following the end of therapy within several months.[75] Intra-arterial DC injection with resulting sludge embolus formation and tissue necrosis is another rare potential complication.[76]

The effects, and side effect profile, of DC can, however, be tempered with the addition of phosphatidylcholine (PC). PC acts as a physiologic buffer, serving as a vehicle for DC diffusion beyond the injection site via liposome formation, and mitigating the rate of immediate loss of cell viability. Whereas injection of DC leads to immediate cell membrane lysis, the onset of lysis with PC/DC is delayed until 2 weeks postinjection.[77] Retrospective studies have confirmed the efficacy and safety of PC/DC in targeting focal areas of abdominal subcutaneous fat after multiple sessions.[78]

8.4.9 Tumescent Liposuction

Despite the increasing popularity of noninvasive body sculpting devices and injectables, traditional tumescent liposuction remains the gold standard for subcutaneous lipoplasty with unmatched single-session results.[79] Predicated on Klein's tumescent technique, this procedure uses microcannulas to contour subcutaneous adipose tissue comfortably under local anesthesia alone, with minimal postoperative downtime and nominal risk to underlying structures or overlying skin.[80,81]

Direct percutaneous large-volume infiltration of dilute lidocaine with epinephrine in buffered physiologic saline produces complete, prolonged local anesthesia and hemostasis of cutaneous and subcutaneous tissues, eliminating the need for general anesthesia (▶ Table 8.1).[80] The physical compressive effects of interstitial tumescent fluid on subcutaneous capillaries and the vasoconstriction produced by epinephrine combine to slow the systemic absorption of lidocaine, preventing third spacing and virtually eliminating blood loss with lipoaspiration.[82] Tumescent lidocaine dosages of 45 mg/kg are exceptionally safe, yielding peak plasma concentrations below levels associated with mild toxicity, regardless of the speed of infiltration.[83]

The planned treatment areas are first marked with a blue surgical pen, creating a topographic map. Intradermal blebs of anesthetic solution (6-mL syringe, 30-gauge needle,) are injected, through which tumescent fluid infiltration is then started. A variable-rate peristaltic pump is used to rapidly infiltrate subcutaneous tissue by means of a 21-gauge (neck) or 18- to 20-gauge (body) spinal needle. Microcannula entry sites, known as adits, may be either 2-mm incisions (no. 11 blade) or 1.5- to 2-mm-diameter round openings (biopsy punch) placed in the periphery, often in natural skin folds.

Longitudinal movement of a microcannula (12–14 gauge) in a pistonlike in-and-out motion will cause small fat fragments sucked into its aperture(s) to be rasped away from their fibrous stroma and immediately aspirated, creating tunnels within the subcutaneous layer.[84] "Pretunneling" with a microcannula not under suction or an Nd:YAG (neodymium:yttrium aluminum garnet) or diode laser device (920–1440 nm) helps break up fibrous subcutaneous connective tissue, which allows for greater and more rapid fat removal. Avoiding large cannulas (or larger microcannulas without pretunneling) also mitigates the risk of subcutaneous irregularities. Removal of repeated small volumes from multiple adits in an overlapping, fanning pattern also optimizes outcomes, especially in more fibrous areas like the abdomen and flanks. A uniform pinch test in the treated area denotes the end of treatment.

Absorbent pads are applied over open entry sites to collect drainage, and the patient is dressed in compression garments to promote drainage, speeding the resolution of subcutaneous edema and induration.[85] A high degree of uniform compression should be maintained until 24 hours after drainage has ceased.[86] Surgical area pain and tenderness are expected and controlled with a short course of low-dose narcotics followed by over-the-counter oral analgesics. Ecchymosis is generally mild and dependent in nature, often migrating inferiorly. Suctioning of deep fat near the mandibular ramus is avoided in order to decrease the risk of marginal mandibular nerve injury. Adits heal by secondary intention, with perilesional erythema and mild ecchymosis expected in the short term. Bleeding or hematoma formation is only a factor following liposuction of the male breast, albeit rare with high-grade compression.[86]

Postoperative photos are not taken until 3 to 4 months posttreatment. Whereas liposuctioned areas will resist weight gain, fatty deposits may subsequently accumulate viscerally or in other areas of the body.[87]

8.5 Before and After Examples

8.5.1 Case 1: Tumescent Liposuction of the Male Chest

The patient is a 38-year-old Caucasian male with pronounced fat deposits of the chest due to weight gain over the last several years, consistent with pseudogynecomastia (▶ Fig. 8.2a). Laser-assisted tumescent liposuction was performed, using 0.1% lidocaine with 1:1,000,000 epinephrine tumescent solution. Approximately 750 mL of subcutaneous fat was aspirated bilaterally with a 12-gauge cannula. A 600-µm laser fiber emitting 1,440-nm (15 W, 50 Hz) energy was utilized prior to suctioning to help emulsify fat. Marked reduction in chest fat deposits is evident at the 3-month follow-up (▶ Fig. 8.2b; the image has been altered to hide the patient's upper chest tattoo).

8.5.2 Case 2: Tumescent Liposuction of the Male Abdomen, Waist, and Flanks

The patient is a 55-year-old Caucasian male with subcutaneous fat deposits of the upper/lower abdomen, waist, and flanks, resistant to diet and exercise (▶ Fig. 8.3a). Laser-assisted tumescent liposuction was performed, using 0.1% lidocaine with 1:1,000,000 epinephrine tumescent solution. Approximately 1,000 mL of subcutaneous fat was aspirated bilaterally with a 12- and 14-gauge cannula. A 600-µm laser fiber emitting 1,440-nm (15 W, 50 Hz) energy was utilized prior to suctioning to help emulsify fat. A significant reduction in fat deposits is evident at the 4-month follow-up (▶ Fig. 8.3b).

8.5.3 Case 3: Cryoadipolysis of Male Flanks

The patient is a 35-year-old Caucasian male with subcutaneous fat deposits isolated to the flanks, resistant to

Table 8.1 Tumescent anesthetic formulation

Ingredients	Dose (volume)
0.9% sodium chloride	1 L
1% lidocaine hydrochloride	500 mg (50 mL) for 0.05% 1,000 mg (100 mL) for 0.1%
1:1,000 epinephrine	0.65 mg (0.65 mL) for 1:1,500,000 1.0 mg (1.0 mL) for 1:1,000,000
8.4% sodium bicarbonate	10 mEq (10 mL)

Note: The recommended concentration of lidocaine and epinephrine required per liter for effective tumescent anesthesia varies by body area. The upper and medial abdomen, and chest typically require higher concentrations (1,000–1,250 mg/L lidocaine, 1.0 mg/L epinephrine) than the waist/flanks (750–1,000 mg/L, 0.65–1.0 mg/L) and the lateral abdomen (500–750 mg/L, 0.65 mg/L).

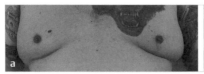
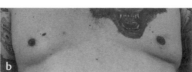

Fig. 8.2 (a) Before and (b) 3 months following laser-assisted tumescent liposuction of pseudogynecomastia.

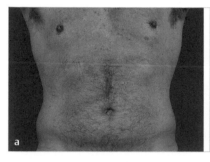
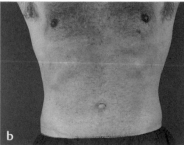

Fig. 8.3 **(a)** Before and **(b)** 4 months following laser-assisted tumescent liposuction of the upper and lower abdomen, waist, and flanks.

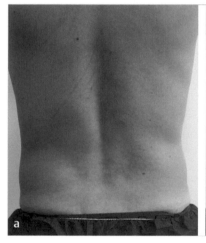
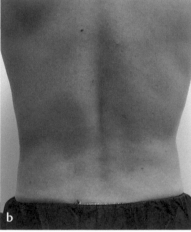

Fig. 8.4 **(a)** Before and **(b)** 3 months after a single session of cryoadipolysis for noninvasive fat reduction of the flanks. One suction applicator was used on each side. (Courtesy of Catherine DiGiorgio, MD.)

diet and exercise (▶ Fig. 8.4a). Noninvasive fat reduction was performed using a cryoadipolysis device with a curved suction applicator. One applicator cycle was used on each side in a single treatment session. A significant reduction in flank fat is evident at the 3-month follow-up (▶ Fig. 8.4b).

8.5.4 Case 4: High-Intensity Focused Electromagnetic Therapy of Upper Abdomen

The patient is a 41-year-old Caucasian male with upper abdominal fat deposits and muscle laxity (▶ Fig. 8.5a). Noninvasive muscle toning and subcutaneous fat reduction was performed with HIFEM therapy. Six treatments were performed over a 3-week period. Significant improvement in subcutaneous fat and muscle tone of the upper abdomen was seen at the 3-month follow-up (▶ Fig. 8.5b).

8.5.5 Case 5: Cryoadipolysis of Male Outer Thighs

The patient is a 28-year-old Caucasian male with outer thigh fat lipodystrophy (▶ Fig. 8.6a) secondary to tumescent liposuction of the upper/lower abdomen. Noninvasive fat reduction was performed with a nonvacuum

conformable-surface applicator for targeted cryoadipolysis. A significant reduction in subcutaneous fat of the outer thighs was seen 4 months after a single treatment session (▶ Fig. 8.6b).

8.6 Conclusion

Body contouring procedures for fat reduction in men have increased considerably as therapeutic options continue to trend toward less invasive, with decreased downtime and better side effect profiles. That said, tumescent liposuction remains the gold standard with unmatched single session results. Regardless of the choice of treatment, it is important to have not only a fundamental understanding of the male anatomy, specifically the distribution and location of the adipose tissue, but also the desired appearance or outcome. Current non and minimally invasive treatments include cryoadipolysis, light, laser and energy modalities such as infrared diode laser, radiofrequency, ultrasound, high intensity focused electromagnetic therapy; and injection adipolysis. Each have unique risks, benefits, and expected outcomes, and it is important to obtain a thorough history and examination as well as have a complete discussion of options when contemplating the best approach for your patient's goals. Although well-designed studies are limited, combination treatment may produce superior, more rapid results.

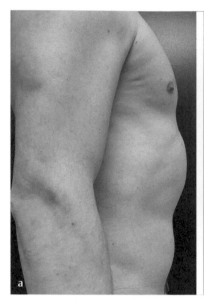
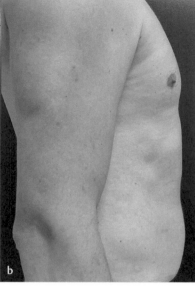

Fig. 8.5 (a) Before and (b) 3 months after 6 sessions of high-intensity focused electromagnetic therapy for upper abdominal muscle toning and subcutaneous fat reduction.

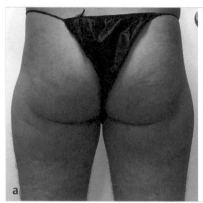
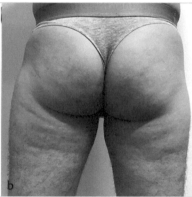

Fig. 8.6 (a) Before and (b) 4 months after a single treatment session with a nonvacuum conformable-surface applicator for cryoadipolysis of the outer thighs.

8.7 Pearls

- Excess adiposity accumulates in the midline (chest, abdomen) in men compared to below the waist in women, and these areas—along with the flanks, and submentum—are the most common areas of concern in male patients seeking treatment.
- The ideal male abdomen is square shaped with less sloping of flanks with a lower waistline than female counterparts, while excess submental and submandibular fat can obscure a strong masculine jawline.
- Exclude patients with significant visceral fat and appropriately counsel patients with substantial preexisting laxity of overlying skin regarding potential for exaggeration post procedure.
- Despite increased popularity of non-invasive and minimally invasive body sculpting procedures, liposuction remains the gold standard with unparalleled single session results.

References

[1] American Society for Dermatologic Surgery. 2018 ASDS Consumer Survey on Cosmetic Dermatologic Procedures. 2019. Available at: https://www.asds.net/Portals/0/PDF/consumer-survey-2018-infographic.pdf/. 2019. Accessed April 8, 2019

[2] Cox SE. Commentary on male body contouring. Dermatol Surg. 2017; 43 Suppl 2:S194–S195

[3] Sadick NS. The pathophysiology of the male aging face and body. Dermatol Clin. 2018; 36(1):1–4

[4] The American Society for Aesthetic Plastic Surgery. 2012 Cosmetic Surgery National Data Bank Statistics. 2013. Available at: https://www.surgery.org/sites/default/files/ASAPS-2012-Stats.pdf/. Accessed April 8, 2019

[5] The American Society for Aesthetic Plastic Surgery. 2017 Cosmetic Surgery National Data Bank Statistics. 2018 Available at: https://www.surgery.org/sites/default/files/ASAPS-Stats2017.pdf/. Accessed April 8, 2019

[6] Pulit SL, Karaderi T, Lindgren CM. Sexual dimorphisms in genetic loci linked to body fat distribution. Biosci Rep. 2017; 37(1): BSR20160184

[7] Ley CJ, Lees B, Stevenson JC. Sex- and menopause-associated changes in body-fat distribution. Am J Clin Nutr. 1992; 55(5):950–954

[8] Björntorp P. The regulation of adipose tissue distribution in humans. Int J Obes Relat Metab Disord. 1996; 20(4):291–302

[9] Björntorp P. Adipose tissue distribution and function. Int J Obes. 1991; 15 Suppl 2:67–81

[10] Björntorp P. Hormonal control of regional fat distribution. Hum Reprod. 1997; 12 Suppl 1:21–25

[11] Zamboni M, Rossi AP, Fantin F, et al. Adipose tissue, diet and aging. Mech Ageing Dev. 2014; 136–137:129–137

[12] Kotani K, Tokunaga K, Fujioka S, et al. Sexual dimorphism of age-related changes in whole-body fat distribution in the obese. Int J Obes Relat Metab Disord. 1994; 18(4):207–2

[13] Shimokata H, Tobin JD, Muller DC, Elahi D, Coon PJ, Andres R. Studies in the distribution of body fat: I. Effects of age, sex, and obesity. J Gerontol. 1989; 44(2):M66–M73

[14] Coleman KM, Lawrence N. Male body contouring. Dermatol Surg. 2017; 43 Suppl 2:S188–S193

[15] Singh B, Keaney T, Rossi AM. Male body contouring. J Drugs Dermatol. 2015; 14(9):1052–1059

[16] Munavalli GS, Panchaprateep R. Cryolipolysis for targeted fat reduction and improved appearance of the enlarged male breast. Dermatol Surg. 2015; 41(9):1043–1051

[17] Pilanci O, Basaran K, Aydin HU, Cortuk O, Kuvat SV. Autologous fat injection into the pectoralis major as an adjunct to surgical correction of gynecomastia. Aesthet Surg J. 2015; 35(3):NP54–NP61

[18] Keaney TC, Naga LI. Men at risk for paradoxical adipose hyperplasia after cryolipolysis. J Cosmet Dermatol. 2016; 15(4):575–577

[19] Querleux B, Cornillon C, Jolivet O, Bittoun J. Anatomy and physiology of subcutaneous adipose tissue by in vivo magnetic resonance imaging and spectroscopy: relationships with sex and presence of cellulite. Skin Res Technol. 2002; 8(2):118–124

[20] Wat H, Wu DC, Goldman MP. Noninvasive body contouring: a male perspective. Dermatol Clin. 2018; 36(1):49–55

[21] Brown SA, Rohrich RJ, Kenkel J, Young VL, Hoopman J, Coimbra M. Effect of low-level laser therapy on abdominal adipocytes before lipoplasty procedures. Plast Reconstr Surg. 2004; 113(6):1796–1804, discussion 1805–1806

[22] Svedman KJ, Coldiron B, Coleman WP, III, et al. ASDS guidelines of care for tumescent liposuction. Dermatol Surg. 2006; 32(5):709–716

[23] Klein JA. Cytochrome P450 3A4 and lidocaine metabolism. In: Klein JA, ed. Tumescent Technique: Tumescent Anesthesia and Microcannular Liposuction. St. Louis, MO: Mosby, Inc.; 2000:131–141

[24] Friedmann DP, Mishra V. Cryolipolysis and laser lipolysis: misnomers in cosmetic dermatology. Dermatol Surg. 2015; 41(11):1327–1328

[25] Manstein D, Laubach H, Watanabe K, Farinelli W, Zurakowski D, Anderson RR. Selective cryolysis: a novel method of non-invasive fat removal. Lasers Surg Med. 2008; 40(9):595–604

[26] Zelickson B, Egbert BM, Preciado J, et al. Cryolipolysis for noninvasive fat cell destruction: initial results from a pig model. Dermatol Surg. 2009; 35(10):1462–1470

[27] Stevens WG, Pietrzak LK, Spring MA. Broad overview of a clinical and commercial experience with CoolSculpting. Aesthet Surg J. 2013; 33(6):835–846

[28] Klein KB, Zelickson B, Riopelle JG, et al. Non-invasive cryolipolysis for subcutaneous fat reduction does not affect serum lipid levels or liver function tests. Lasers Surg Med. 2009; 41(10):785–790

[29] Keaney TC, Gudas AT, Alster TS. Delayed onset pain associated with cryolipolysis treatment: a retrospective study with treatment recommendations. Dermatol Surg. 2015; 41(11):1296–1299

[30] Coleman SR, Sachdeva K, Egbert BM, Preciado J, Allison J. Clinical efficacy of noninvasive cryolipolysis and its effects on peripheral nerves. Aesthetic Plast Surg. 2009; 33(4):482–488

[31] Jalian JM, Guddea ENG, Beutrour SC, Caliano RD, Friedman PM, Paradoxical adipose hyperplasia secondary to cryolipolysis: an under-reported entity? Lasers Surg Med. 2015; 47(6):476–478

[32] Jalian HR, Avram MM, Garibyan L, Mihm MC, Anderson RR. Paradoxical adipose hyperplasia after cryolipolysis. JAMA Dermatol. 2014; 150(3):317–319

[33] Kilmer SL. Prototype CoolCup cryolipolysis applicator with over 40% reduced treatment time demonstrates equivalent safety and efficacy with greater patient preference. Lasers Surg Med. 2017; 49(1):63–68

[34] Friedmann DP. Cryolipolysis for noninvasive contouring of the periumbilical abdomen with a nonvacuum conformable-surface applicator. Dermatol Surg. 2019; 45(9):1185–1190

[35] Leal Silva H, Carmona Hernandez E, Grijalva Vazquez M, Leal Delgado S, Perez Blanco A. Noninvasive submental fat reduction using colder cryolipolysis. J Cosmet Dermatol. 2017; 16(4):460–465

[36] Boey GE, Wasilenchuk JL. Enhanced clinical outcome with manual massage following cryolipolysis treatment: a 4-month study of safety and efficacy. Lasers Surg Med. 2014; 46(1):20–26

[37] Hunt JA. Cryolipolysis and radial pulse therapy. Prime N Am. 2013; 1:74–75

[38] Garibyan L, Sipprell WH, III, Jalian HR, Sakamoto FH, Avram M, Anderson RR. Three-dimensional volumetric quantification of fat loss following cryolipolysis. Lasers Surg Med. 2014; 46(2):75–80

[39] Suh DH, Park JH, Kim BY, Lee SJ, Moon JH, Ryu HJ. Double stacking cryolipolysis treatment of the abdominal fat with use of a novel contoured applicator. J Cosmet Laser Ther. 2019; 21(4):238–242

[40] Fatemi A. High-intensity focused ultrasound effectively reduces adipose tissue. Semin Cutan Med Surg. 2009; 28(4):257–262

[41] Haar GT, Coussios C. High intensity focused ultrasound: physical principles and devices. Int J Hyperthermia. 2007; 23(2):89–104

[42] Shalom A, Wiser I, Brawer S, Azhari H. Safety and tolerability of a focused ultrasound device for treatment of adipose tissue in subjects undergoing abdominoplasty: a placebo-control pilot study. Dermatol Surg. 2013; 39(5):744–751

[43] Brown SA, Greenbaum L, Shtukmaster S, Zadok Y, Ben-Ezra S, Kushkuley L. Characterization of nonthermal focused ultrasound for noninvasive selective fat cell disruption (lysis): technical and preclinical assessment. Plast Reconstr Surg. 2009; 124(1):92–101

[44] Teitelbaum SA, Burns JL, Kubota J, et al. Noninvasive body contouring by focused ultrasound: safety and efficacy of the contour I device in a multicenter, controlled, clinical study. Plast Reconstr Surg. 2007; 120(3):779–789

[45] Weiss RA, Bernardy J. Induction of fat apoptosis by a non-thermal device: mechanism of action of non-invasive high-intensity electromagnetic technology in a porcine model. Lasers Surg Med. 2019; 51(1):47–53

[46] Duncan D, Dinev I. Noninvasive induction of muscle fiber hypertrophy and hyperplasia: effects of high-intensity focused electromagnetic field evaluated in an in-vivo porcine model—a pilot study. Aesthet Surg J. 2020; 40(5):568–574

[47] Halaas Y, Bernardy J. Mechanism of nonthermal induction of apoptosis by high-intensity focused electromagnetic procedure: biochemical investigation in a porcine model. J Cosmet Dermatol. 2020; 19(3):605–611

[48] Katz B, Bard R, Goldfarb R, Shiloh A, Kenolova D. Ultrasound assessment of subcutaneous abdominal fat thickness after treatments with a high-intensity focused electromagnetic field device: a multicenter study. Dermatol Surg. 2019; 45(12):1542–1548

[49] Kinney BM, Lozanova P. High intensity focused electromagnetic therapy evaluated by magnetic resonance imaging: safety and efficacy study of a dual tissue effect based non-invasive abdominal body shaping. Lasers Surg Med. 2019; 51(1):40–46

[50] Kent DE, Jacob CI. Simultaneous changes in abdominal adipose and muscle tissues following treatments by high-intensity focused electromagnetic (HIFEM) technology-based device: computed tomography evaluation. J Drugs Dermatol. 2019; 18(11):1098–1102

[51] Kinney BM, Kent DE. MRI and CT assessment of abdominal tissue composition in patients after high-intensity focused electromagnetic therapy treatments: one-year follow-up. Aesthet Surg J. 2020; 40(12):NP686–NP693

[52] Franco W, Kothare A, Goldberg DJ. Controlled volumetric heating of subcutaneous adipose tissue using a novel radiofrequency technology. Lasers Surg Med. 2009; 41(10):745–750

[53] de Felipe I, Redondo P. Animal model to explain fat atrophy using nonablative radiofrequency. Dermatol Surg. 2007; 33(2):141–145

[54] Franco W, Kothare A, Ronan SJ, Grekin RC, McCalmont TH. Hyperthermic injury to adipocyte cells by selective heating of subcutaneous fat with a novel radiofrequency device: feasibility studies. Lasers Surg Med. 2010; 42(5):361–370

[55] Kaplan H, Gat A. Clinical and histopathological results following TriPollar radiofrequency skin treatments. J Cosmet Laser Ther. 2009; 11(2):78–84

[56] Lolis MS, Goldberg DJ. Radiofrequency in cosmetic dermatology: a review. Dermatol Surg. 2012; 38(11):1765–1776

[57] Fajkošová K, Machovcová A, Onder M, Fritz K. Selective radiofrequency therapy as a non-invasive approach for contactless body contouring and circumferential reduction. J Drugs Dermatol. 2014; 13(3):291–296

[58] Neira R, Arroyave J, Ramirez H, et al. Fat liquefaction: effect of low-level laser energy on adipose tissue. Plast Reconstr Surg. 2002; 110 (3):912–922, discussion 923–925

[59] Medrado AP, Trindade E, Reis SRA, Andrade ZA. Action of low-level laser therapy on living fatty tissue of rats. Lasers Med Sci. 2006; 21 (1):19–23

[60] Caruso-Davis MK, Guillot TS, Podichetty VK, et al. Efficacy of low-level laser therapy for body contouring and spot fat reduction. Obes Surg. 2011; 21(6):722–729

[61] Avci P, Nyame TT, Gupta GK, Sadasivam M, Hamblin MR. Low-level laser therapy for fat layer reduction: a comprehensive review. Lasers Surg Med. 2013; 45(6):349–357

[62] Esnouf A, Wright PA, Moore JC, Ahmed S. Depth of penetration of an 850 nm wavelength low level laser in human skin. Acupunct Electrother Res. 2007; 32(1–2):81–86

[63] Jackson RF, Stern FA, Neira R, Ortiz-Neira CL, Maloney J. Application of low-level laser therapy for noninvasive body contouring. Lasers Surg Med. 2012; 44(3):211–217

[64] Jackson RF, Dedo DD, Roche GC, Turok DI, Maloney RJ. Low-level laser therapy as a non-invasive approach for body contouring: a randomized, controlled study. Lasers Surg Med. 2009; 41(10):799–809

[65] McRae E, Boris J. Independent evaluation of low-level laser therapy at 635 nm for non-invasive body contouring of the waist, hips, and thighs. Lasers Surg Med. 2013; 45(1):1–7

[66] Savoia A, Landi S, Vannini F, Baldi A. Low-level laser therapy and vibration therapy for the treatment of localized adiposity and fibrous cellulite. Dermatol Ther (Heidelb). 2013; 3(1):41–52

[67] Jankowski M, Gawrych M, Adamska U, Ciescinski J, Serafin Z, Czajkowski R. Low-level laser therapy (LLLT) does not reduce subcutaneous adipose tissue by local adipocyte injury but rather by modulation of systemic lipid metabolism. Lasers Med Sci. 2017; 32(2):475–479

[68] Decorato JW, Chen B, Sierra R. Subcutaneous adipose tissue response to a non-invasive hyperthermic treatment using a 1,060 nm laser. Lasers Surg Med. 2017; 49(5):480–489

[69] Bass LS, Doherty ST. Safety and efficacy of a non-invasive 1060 nm diode laser for fat reduction of the abdomen. J Drugs Dermatol. 2018; 17(1):106–112

[70] Sweeney DL, Wang EB, Austin E, Jagdeo J. Combined hyperthermic 1060 nm diode laser lipolysis with topical skin tightening treatment: case series. J Drugs Dermatol. 2018; 17(7):780–785

[71] Schilling L, Saedi N, Weiss R.. 1060 nm diode hyperthermic laser lipolysis: the latest in non-invasive body contouring. J Drugs Dermatol. 2017; 16:48–52

[72] Rotunda AM. Injectable treatments for adipose tissue: terminology, mechanism, and tissue interaction. Lasers Surg Med. 2009; 41(10): 714–720

[73] Walker PS, Lee DR, Toth BA, Bowen B. Histological analysis of the effect of ATX-101 (deoxycholic acid injection) on subcutaneous fat: results from a phase 1 open-label study. Dermatol Surg. 2020; 46(1):70–77

[74] Shridharani SM, Behr KL. ATX-101 (deoxycholic acid injection) treatment in men: insights from our clinical experience. Dermatol Surg. 2017; 43 Suppl 2:S225–S230

[75] Grady B, Porphirio F, Rokhsar C. Submental alopecia at deoxycholic acid injection site. Dermatol Surg. 2017; 43(8):1105–1108

[76] Lindgren AL, Welsh KM. Inadvertent intra-arterial injection of deoxycholic acid: a case report and proposed protocol for treatment. J Cosmet Dermatol. 2020; 19(7):1614–1618

[77] Duncan D. Commentary on: Metabolic and structural effects of phosphatidylcholine and deoxycholate injections on subcutaneous fat: a randomized, controlled trial. Aesthet Surg J. 2013; 33(3):411–413

[78] Duncan DI, Hasengschwandtner F. Lipodissolve for subcutaneous fat reduction and skin retraction. Aesthet Surg J. 2005; 25(5):530–543

[79] Friedmann DP. A review of the aesthetic treatment of abdominal subcutaneous adipose tissue: background, implications, and therapeutic options. Dermatol Surg. 2015; 41(1):18–34

[80] Klein JA. The tumescent technique for liposuction surgery. Am J Cosmet Surg. 1987; 4:263–267

[81] Tierney EP, Kouba DJ, Hanke CW. Safety of tumescent and laser-assisted liposuction: review of the literature. J Drugs Dermatol. 2011; 10(12):1363–1369

[82] Klein JA. Tumescent technique for local anesthesia improves safety in large-volume liposuction. Plast Reconstr Surg. 1993; 92(6):1085–1098, discussion 1099–1100

[83] Klein JA, Jeske DR. Estimated maximal safe dosages of tumescent lidocaine. Anesth Analg. 2016; 122(5):1350–1359

[84] Klein JA. Surgical technique: microcannular tumescent liposuction. In: Klein JA, ed. Tumescent Technique: Tumescent Anesthesia and Microcannular Liposuction. St. Louis, MO: Mosby, Inc.; 2000:248–270

[85] Klein JA. Post-tumescent liposuction care. Open drainage and bimodal compression. Dermatol Clin. 1999; 17(4):881–889, viii

[86] Klein JA. Postliposuction care: open drainage and bimodal compression. In: Klein JA, ed. Tumescent Technique: Tumescent Anesthesia and Microcannular Liposuction. St. Louis, MO: Mosby, Inc.; 2000:281–293

[87] Hernandez TL, Kittelson JM, Law CK, et al. Fat redistribution following suction lipectomy: defense of body fat and patterns of restoration. Obesity (Silver Spring). 2011; 19(7):1388–1395

9 Not too Tight: Skin Tightening Procedures

Jordan V. Wang, Nazanin Saedi, and Girish S. Munavalli

Summary

In recent years, the popularity of cosmetic procedures has continued to rise, including those that serve to treat fine lines and wrinkles and skin laxity. Traditionally, women have comprised the vast majority of patients. However, men now represent a growing portion of patients. Due to several important differences in anatomy, perspectives, and preferences, the treatment approach to skin tightening should be tailored to men when treating this particular group. Practitioners should be knowledgeable about the various types of treatment that are available and understand the unique approach in order to continue to deliver effective, tailored, and high-quality care.

Keywords: aesthetics, skin tightening, lasers, ultrasound therapy, radiofrequency microneedling, wrinkles

9.1 Background

Over the past decade, the field of aesthetics has witnessed remarkable growth. What had originally started as a small subspecialty built around injectable neuromodulators and soft-tissue fillers has now grown to encompass numerous lasers and medical devices utilizing various technologies. According to the American Society for Dermatologic Surgery (ASDS), members performed more than 12.5 million procedures in 2018 alone, which was 7.8 million in 2012.[1] The top procedures were skin cancer treatments, injectable neuromodulators and soft-tissue fillers, and laser-, light-, or energy-based procedures. In the past 7 years, there was a 78% increase in soft-tissue filler treatments, a 74% increase in laser-, light-, or energy-based procedures, and a nearly 400% increase in body contouring procedures.[1] The numbers continue to grow each year as new devices and technologies are brought to the aesthetic market. The reasons why people are turning to cosmetics to enhance their appearance is well apparent in the ASDS survey data (▶ Fig. 9.1).

While part of this growth is due to the more recent expansion of technology coupled with the innovation of newer medical devices, consumer-driven growth has continued to play an ever-expanding role. With the rise of social media platforms, networking websites, and mobile applications, consumers and patients are more connected to each other than ever before. The trend to take and easily transmit mobile phone camera photographs of one's self has fostered a social "sharing" of images centered on one's physical attributes. Especially with many mobile and computer applications that can "filter" or alter one's appearance in either subtle or substantial ways, the new reality is that the current technology has significantly changed the perception of beauty worldwide.[2,3,4]

Whereas the population of patients seeking cosmetic treatments has traditionally been predominately female, a growing number of men are now looking to have aesthetic procedures done. Due to the rapidly expanding market of male aesthetics, it is important for clinicians to understand the available treatment options, including skin tightening procedures (▶ Fig. 9.2). Despite more men doing aesthetic procedures, there still continues to be barriers in place for men. There tends to be a lack of acceptance or stigma of doing cosmetic procedures among peers, more so for men than women. Also, there tends to be a general lack of knowledge of what can be done for men that will not make them look unnatural or feminine. Due to anatomical differences, specifically increased skin thickness and collagen density, facial aging in general is

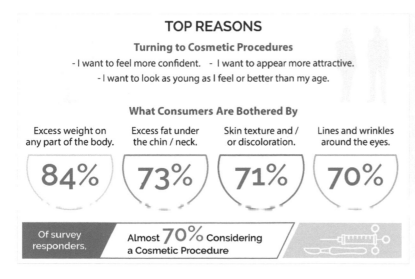

TOP REASONS

Turning to Cosmetic Procedures

- I want to feel more confident.   - I want to appear more attractive.
- I want to look as young as I feel or better than my age.

What Consumers Are Bothered By

Excess weight on any part of the body.	Excess fat under the chin / neck.	Skin texture and / or discoloration.	Lines and wrinkles around the eyes.
84%	73%	71%	70%

Of survey responders, Almost 70% Considering a Cosmetic Procedure

Fig. 9.1 Key factors behind the increase in cosmetic procedures. (Reproduced with permission from the American Society for Dermatologic Surgery: 2019 Annual Consumer Survey on Dermatologic Procedures.)

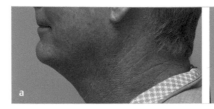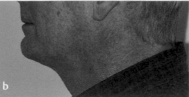

Fig. 9.2 (a) Before and (b) five months after single session of ThermiTight(R). (Courtesy of Jason D. Bloom, MD, FACS [Facial Plastic Surgeon].)

often less noticeable in men than in women.[5–7] However, males begin to experience decreases in skin thickness earlier on in their 20 s. Furthermore, a greater degree of muscle movement with facial expressions compared to women has been thought to contribute to deeper wrinkles.[8,9] Due to the rapidly expanding market of male aesthetics, it is important for clinicians to understand the available treatment options, including skin tightening procedures as a noninvasive option for men.

Cutaneous aging and skin laxity can be quite striking in both genders. Along with intrinsic aging, facial skin is particularly vulnerable to environmental stressors that patients are exposed to on a regular basis, such as ultraviolet radiation, smoke, and pollution. It has also been demonstrated that severe solar elastosis of the head and neck region was more common in men than in women.[10] These environmental insults can each lead to cellular stress and subsequent injury, where repetitive exposures can cause an accumulation of damage that can be harmful to cellular function, protein maturation, and normal skin physiology.[11,12,13,14] The skin's natural elasticity and firmness can be lost due to the resultant breakdown of collagen and elastin in addition to a reduction in fibroblast activity. Collagen types I and III represent approximately 75% of the dry weight of the dermis and 20 to 30% of its volume.[15] Fibroblasts generate new collagen, whereas matrix metalloproteinases (MMPs) degrade it, typically maintaining a balance. Ultraviolet radiation and other intrinsic and extrinsic sources of reactive oxygen species upregulate the production of MMPs, resulting in accelerated skin aging.[16] Elastin comprises 4% of the dry weight of the dermis and gives the skin its mechanical strength and ability to resist deformation, or elasticity.[17] Intrinsic aging causes atrophy of elastin fibers, whereas extrinsic aging, such as ultraviolet light exposure, causes a disorganization in the elastic fiber network resulting in solar elastosis.[18] The vital role of elastin in maintaining the structure of the extracellular matrix is well established; even the slightest decrease in the number of elastin fibers results in significant changes in skin elasticity and strength.

Clinically, these cellular and chemical effects can cause the familiar signs of cutaneous aging that people are accustomed to seeing, such as fine lines and wrinkles, thinning, roughness, dyspigmentation, coarseness, and decreased elasticity. Since skin laxity is a common cosmetic complaint of those seeking consultations, physicians should be familiar with recognizing and treating this condition.

9.2 Indications

The gold standard for correcting skin laxity and achieving tightening is surgical correction, such as rhytidectomy. Although consistently and uniformly effective, surgical procedures can be invasive, risky, costly, and inappropriate for some patients. As such, the demand for less invasive treatment modalities has increased. Minimally invasive skin tightening devices, when utilized correctly, can be effective in treating skin laxity. An individual modality may be more fitting to a specific patient depending on the clinical grade, depth, and degree of the laxity in addition to the preference for concurrent resurfacing and desired outcomes. An individualized treatment plan is always recommended in order to achieve ideal clinical outcomes as opposed to a one-size-fits-all approach in aesthetics.

9.3 Patient Selection

The importance of patient selection cannot be emphasized enough, especially since it represents a critical part for determining adequate clinical outcomes and patient satisfaction. When selecting patients for treatments of skin laxity using minimally invasive methods, it is best for patients to have mild to moderate skin laxity. Too significant or severe skin laxity may be more suitable for an invasive or surgical approach, such as a rhytidectomy (facelift), which may offer better outcomes.

In addition to proper patient selection, the management of expectations is equally as important. Minimally invasive modalities can be effective, but only in the right clinical scenario. It is crucial to advise patients of the limitations of skin tightening procedures that utilize medical devices, especially when compared to surgical options in patients with significant skin laxity. Less than ideal outcomes would be the rule rather than the exception in some scenarios involving severe laxity, and postprocedural results may not adequately satisfy the patient. Sufficiently addressing patient expectations is vital to ensure a high level of patient satisfaction and subsequent patient retention. Men are often less inclined to undergo large surgical operations from plastic surgeons and may prefer decreased postprocedural downtime often due to work commitments.

Prior to any procedures and ideally during the visit for aesthetic consultation, multiple photographs should be taken. Photographs from various angles using appropriate, standardized lighting are recommended. These photographs can help demonstrate the level of skin laxity to patients prior to any treatments being completed and can also be used to grade treatment effects for comparison. Although clinical scales for skin laxity have been developed, they are neither universally used nor specific for male patients.[19,20] Occasionally, patients may believe that treatments have not resulted in clinical improvements, in which case, these photographs can be of immense benefit to the practitioner.

Before treatment, patients should completely clean the treatment area of natural skin oils and impurities, as well as topical products or cosmetic makeup using a gentle wash and cleanser. In men, strong cleansers are often not required due to a lack of significant cosmetic makeup, including waterproof products. Topical, tumescent, or intradermal anesthesia can be used, such as combination of topical benzocaine, lidocaine, and tetracaine or topical lidocaine alone, as examples. Breathing of a gas mixture of nitrous oxide and oxygen can also be utilized in-office, either as a standalone or as an adjunct to other pain management modalities. If topical numbing products are used, they should be wiped off completely, and the area should be recleaned with either alcohol, chlorhexidine, hypochlorous acid, or another similar agent prior to initiating treatment.

9.4 Treatment Options

9.4.1 Microneedling

Microneedling, known as percutaneous collagen induction (PCI) therapy, has been utilized to treat a variety of cutaneous conditions, including skin laxity.[21,22] Extremely small needles are used to pierce the epidermis and dermal layers to create columns of physical injury. The depth of penetration can be selected depending on the condition and site, which can also be layered to create larger areas of controlled injury. After the damaged collagen is removed, new synthesis and remodeling subsequently occur, which are supported by the stimulation of various growth factors and fibroblasts.[23] A recent study showed significant improvements in global wrinkle score, skin laxity, and skin texture at 150 days following a series of four microneedling treatments in 48 subjects.[24] Although the results from microneedling can be modest, it represents an inexpensive modality that can concurrently treat the epidermis. Whereas these devices are primarily used for improving skin texture, treating minimal skin laxity may also be possible. The depths of needle penetration may offer improved results when increased for males with thicker skin, especially on the cheeks.

Whereas traditional devices initially came in the form of manual rollers, newer automated devices such as pens are now more commonly utilized.[25] The newer pens allow for rapid adjustments of depth and frequency in addition to the hygienic use of disposable, single-use tips. A thin layer of gliding solution is recommended at faster speeds to allow for easy movement without "catching" of the skin. Automated pens should be held perpendicular, and multiple passes in different directions are recommended. For microneedling, the treatment endpoint is typically transient pinpoint bleeding.

Ablative and Nonablative Lasers

Ablative resurfacing lasers represent the traditional gold standard for the treatment of facial rejuvenation and skin laxity. By targeting water in the skin for vaporization, lax skin can be selectively targeted for removal. Due to complete epithelial destruction, new collagen formation occurs after the prolonged downtime that is required for full re-epithelialization. Treatments are associated with increased risks of adverse events, such as dyspigmentation and scarring. Compared to newer modalities, treatments are limited to superficial depths.

The introduction of nonablative lasers was met with both greater acceptance and increased demand due to its decreased postprocedural downtime when compared to their ablative counterparts. Adverse events are also more limited. The thermal energy can reach and bulk heat the dermis to induce physiologic changes as described earlier, while sparing the overlying epidermis with concurrent superficial cooling. Although better tolerated than the ablative lasers, clinical outcomes are more modest due to less thermal injury being delivered.

In 2004, fractional photothermolysis was introduced, which resulted in a paradigm shift in aesthetic treatment options.[26] In contrast to treating the entire skin, only portions are treated by using thermal injury to create small columns, termed microscopic treatment zones (MTZs). Their density, width, and depth can be controlled by the practitioner. Male patients may tolerate greater densities if required. Since these damaged columns are surrounded by untreated and unaffected skin, the duration of postprocedural downtime is significantly decreased because these act as healing reservoirs. Ablative fractional resurfacing may also be superior to its traditional counterpart for treating skin laxity, since it has the ability to penetrate deeper into the dermis.[27] As with nonfractionated devices, ablative modalities still offer improved clinical outcomes compared to nonablative devices. Confluent and fractionally ablative modalities can also be combined safely to offer effective results.[28] Due to limited depths, ablative and nonablative lasers are more suited to treat mild skin laxity or if other epidermal skin conditions are simultaneously being treated.

9.4.2 Radiofrequency

Radiofrequency (RF) has been used as a method to cause controlled dermal heating for purposes of skin tightening since 2001.[29] Instead of harnessing the power of light, RF uses an electric current to deliver energy to the dermis for thermal collagen remodeling.[30] Heat is generated from the tissue resistance to the movement of electrons within the RF field to typically heat the area between 43 and 45 °C, whereas the epidermis is cooled. The depth of penetration is inversely proportional to the frequency. The mechanisms by which RF devices produce skin tightening are volumetric heating of the dermal structures, such as collagen and fascia, and induction of a wound healing response. An earlier study in 2003 demonstrated the safety and efficacy of a single RF treatment for periorbital skin laxity in 86 patients, which included several objective and subjective measures.[31] In addition to clinical improvements, electron microscopy has also evidenced thicker collagen fibers associated with treatments.[32]

Numerous devices deliver RF energy in various modes, including unipolar, monopolar, bipolar, and multipolar. Unipolar RF is difficult to control with greater chance to cause deeper tissue damage, whereas multipolar RF can deliver more uniform wavelength penetration.[33] Monopolar RF typically utilizes a grounding plate, where the energy is driven deeper down through the skin's layers and structures. Monopolar energy can be delivered in a stamped mode, gliding movement, or subcutaneous fiber, and recent analyses have demonstrated monopolar RF's seemingly effective and safe treatments.[34,35] In comparison, bipolar and multipolar RFs deliver the energy between the poles of the handpiece, and the depth of penetration is controlled by the distance between them. Bipolar and multipolar devices do not deliver RF energy as deep, since the current has a controlled distribution that is limited to the volume between the electrodes.[36] For this reason, they have been suggested to be more helpful for either younger patients who desire prevention or those with mild laxity.[37] Newer devices are equipped with subdermal probes and real-time monitoring to increase patient safety and reduce the potential for overheating, which can cause unintended burns, local damage, blistering, necrosis, and scarring. RF devices can typically cause deeper effects than the previously mentioned modalities. Male patients with greater laxity may benefit from monopolar RF due to deeper penetration.

9.4.3 Radiofrequency Microneedling

The concept of fractionation has classically been applied to lasers, particularly resurfacing lasers, such as the carbon dioxide laser. However, fractionation has also been applied to RF as well. In recent years, RF has been combined with traditional microneedling, termed "RF microneedling." This is by definition, a fractional treatment. The device utilizes a small needle array to penetrate the epidermal and dermal layers and deliver RF energy through the needles to the dermis.[25,38] Physicians can choose to use either insulated or noninsulated needles. Insulated needles deliver energy focused at the tips of the needles, whereas noninsulated needles deliver RF energy from a larger focus to cause more thermal injury. Tips can

also be used in monopolar and bipolar modes, which control the flow of the RF energy. Noninsulated tips and monopolar modes are thought to deliver increased and deeper injury, but also with an increased risk of adverse events. Multiple delivery systems differ in needle length, needle coating, needle sharpness, and method of needle insertion. A recent study showed improvements in wrinkle reduction, skin tightening, and lifting of the mid to lower face using a noninsulated RF microneedling system in 49 patients undergoing 3 monthly treatments.[39] Skin laxity, particularly of the lower face and neck, is an excellent indication for RF microneedling treatment.

The addition of RF energy can increase the amount and depth of controlled injury to the dermis compared to traditional microneedling. Treatments can be layered to create additional injury at various depths, which supports enhanced neocollagenesis and remodeling, above and beyond the trauma induced by microneedling alone. In contrast to traditional microneedling, no gliding solution is needed and pinpoint bleeding is not necessarily expected depending on the treatment parameters. The needles penetrate and retract instead of oscillating, so it is important to allow for full retraction before moving sites in order to prevent dragging and unintended thermal damage to the skin (▶ Fig. 9.3).

Again, patient selection is critical. Thinner skin seems to respond better than thicker, sebaceous skin, which may make some male patients not great candidates for RF microneedling or male patients might not get as much improvement. Mild to moderate skin laxity is also more responsive than severe skin laxity. Laxity and rhytids of the lower face (perioral, mid-cheeks, jawline, neck) have been documented to respond given their more "volume-depleted" nature. This is in contrast to the upper face (periocular, forehead), where dynamic muscle movement is more responsible as the etiology of the rhytides.

9.4.4 Ultrasound

Devices have more recently harnessed ultrasound energy for skin tightening procedures. A distinct advantage of ultrasound is the ability to directly visualize the dermis and subcutaneous structures before initiating treatment, so that practitioners can ensure that energy is being delivered where it is wanted and needed. Focused ultrasound waves induce a vibration of the molecules in the dermis, which in turn generates friction and thermoviscous losses that create heating.[30] Unlike other energy modalities, ultrasound energy can safely penetrate deeper into the tissue to briefly raise temperatures above 60 °C to produce small thermal coagulation points without heating superficial skin structures, which can allow for greater temperatures and controlled injury.[40] Thus, selective targeting of key facial anatomic structures, such as

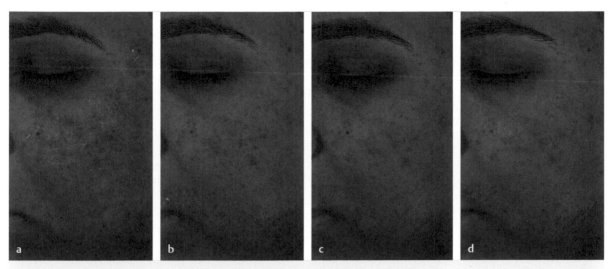

Fig. 9.3 Male patient following radiofrequency microneedling at (a) immediate post, (b) 2 days post, (c) 4 days post, and (d) 7 days post treatment demonstrating post-procedural downtime and healing. (Courtesy of Jordan V Wang, MD, MBE, MBA and Roy Geronemus, MD.)

the superficial musculoaponeurotic system (SMAS), at 4 to 5 mm of depth is possible. Microfocused ultrasound causes collagen fibers in the mid to deep reticular layer of the dermis and subdermis to become denatured and stimulate new collagen formation.[41] It has safely and effectively been used for skin tightening and lifting with little downtime and risk for complications since its introduction in 2009.[42] An early study published in 2010 demonstrated in a Food and Drug Administration (FDA) pivotal fashion, the safe and effective use of ultrasound to tighten facial and neck skin in 36 patients. This included a brow elevation of 1.7 mm at 90 days following the single treatment.[43]

Ultrasound devices can cause dramatic skin tightening responses for significant skin laxity due to its deeper penetration compared to other available modalities. Treatments have been proven to be relatively safe and well tolerated by patients of all skin types, including skin of darker color.[44,45] Men who have more laxity will not experience as much improvement as women. Newer technology has led to more recent refinements of the available medical devices, which should continue to improve clinical outcomes in the near future (▶ Fig. 9.4).

More recently, a new ultrasound device has become available that uses utilize a Synchronous Ultrasound Parallel Beam Technology (SUPERB™) (Sofwave, Yoqneam, Israel) (▶ Fig. 9.4). This particular device uses 7 parallel transducers that are in direct contact with the skin, which supports the incorporation of feedback-controlled skin cooling. The high-intensity, high-frequency, parallel beams allow most of the thermal injury to remain localized at depths of 0.5-2 mm, with the treatment centered at 1.5 mm. At this depth, there can be improvement of fine lines and wrinkles, which can translate to clinical skin tightening.

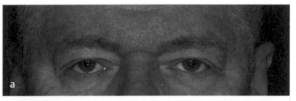
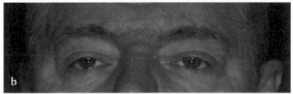

Fig. 9.4 (a) Male patient at baseline and (b) 3 month follow-up after single treatment with synchronous ultrasound parallel beam technology (Sofwave, Yoqneam, Israel). (Courtesy of Jordan V Wang, MD, MBE, MBA and Roy G Geronemus, MD.)

9.5 Postprocedural Expectations

Proper patient education regarding postprocedural expectations is vital to patient care. Discussion should be tailored to the particular procedure that was completed and should include both short- and long-term expectations, especially regarding healing time. For example, patients may experience mild inflammation and swelling from most treatments, which are expected and typically subside within hours. For mild discomfort, patients can be instructed to take acetaminophen. Any significant bleeding, bruising, swelling, and pain that is not typical should prompt the patient to contact the practitioner. Instructions should be provided both orally and in writing.

Patients should be reminded that it may take time to see clinical improvement and multiple treatments are often necessary. Although some improvements may be seen shortly within several weeks following treatment, neocollagenesis and collagen remodeling occur over a period of several months. The expectation is that it can take at least 6 months to witness maximal clinical improvements.

In order to reduce downtime and optimize treatment outcomes, topical products that contain hyaluronic acid or similar collagen-stimulating peptides can be applied regularly by patients. Many formulations have been designed and are widely available to be used in conjunction with minimally invasive procedures. However, caution is warranted when treatments involve epidermal injury, since the applied products should be designed for dermal application. For example, various cases have reported facial granulomas associated with the periprocedural use of topical products containing vitamin C in conjunction with microneedling.[46] Periprocedural products may work to sensitize the local immune system. Whereas the medical literature is limited, recent focus has also examined the use of platelet-rich plasma (PRP) for cutaneous rejuvenation.[47] However, studies have been small and were not standardized for the collection and administration of PRP. PRP continues to hold promise, since it contains a supratherapeutic level of numerous growth factors and cytokines that can stimulate cellular proliferation, differentiation, and regeneration.

9.6 Adverse Events

Depending on the utilized treatment modality, various postprocedural complications are possible. Following treatment with most aesthetic medical devices, the most commonly experienced events include mild temporary pain, swelling, bruising, and occasionally bleeding if the epidermis is treated. These typically improve within minutes to hours and then resolve within several hours. Postprocedural dyspigmentation can also occur, especially when the epidermis is treated, such as with microneedling or ablative lasers. Most cases are temporary in nature, such as postinflammatory hypo- and hyperpigmentation. This can take several weeks to months to resolve, and the use of postprocedural topical steroids or hydroquinone may be helpful in severe or refractory cases. The risks for dyspigmentation are greater in patients with darker skin tones, such as African American or Asian patients. Extra care must be taken when treating skin of color, and these patients should always be reminded of this possible adverse event in order to offer full disclosure of potential risks and expected outcomes.

More serious and severe complications can certainly occur, including scarring, local damage to nerves and vascular structures, and infection. Modalities that are meant to offer treatment of greater depths can variably increase the risk for deeper damage to local structures, including the injury to larger nerves. In rare cases, transient palsies can occur from either the treatment itself or inflammation of the area, which can take several days to weeks for normal function to return. Patients should be counseled on the nature of this adverse event and the need for continued monitoring. In contrast, scarring represents a more permanent and disfiguring adverse event. Patients should be informed of this unfortunate outcome and be reassured that they will be closely managed to limit and ameliorate any permanent effects, which can include additional laser treatments, especially after allowing for the scar to first settle for adequate evaluation.

Any patients who complain of increasing pain, swelling, or other associated effects should be triaged appropriately. Clinical staff should be adequately trained on how to recognize serious adverse events, especially via the telephone. They should have a low threshold to recommend that patients return to clinic for full evaluation by the performing practitioner.

In all instances of patient complications, adequate support and counseling coupled with close observation are necessary. Patients should be reminded that these were risks that were thoroughly discussed prior to the procedure and assured that they will be managed closely and appropriately moving forward. Bringing patients back for frequent visits not only may help alleviate their concerns but can also prevent them from seeking additional care from outside providers, who may not be as familiar or well suited to caring for these particular complications. Practitioners should also remain available to these patients in order to maintain patient satisfaction and repair patient trust if needed. It is extremely important to establish and build a strong patient–practitioner relationship, especially in these circumstances.

9.7 Conclusion

Cutaneous aging and skin laxity represent common aesthetic complaints for patients. Whereas treatments have traditionally focused on women, men are increasingly seeking cosmetic treatments. It has been suggested that aesthetic procedures in men favor small modifications that produce conservative and subtle changes.[8] With the various treatment modalities and the numerous medical devices that are available, physicians should become familiar with the potential treatment options and be able to tailor individualized treatment approaches. Sufficient knowledge, in addition to adequate training, is necessary for the delivery of high-quality patient-centered care.

9.8 Pearls

- During consultations for skin tightening procedures, patient education remains the foundation, and accurately conveying the expectations of any treatment is key to preserving both patient satisfaction and retention.

- When performing radiofrequency microneedling, it is important to make sure the skin is stretched taut to allow for proper insertion of the needles and delivery of energy.
- Newer treatment modalities and devices are seemingly released every year, so it is important for practitioners to review the data behind each of them and obtain first-hand experiences before making any recommendations.
- When performing radiofrequency microneedling, make sure that the needles are fully retracted from the skin before moving to the next location in order to prevent dragging and unintended damage to the skin.
- The scheduling of patient calls and follow-up appointments should be based on the downtime of the treatment performed in order to offer adequate oversight.

References

[1] American Society for Dermatologic Surgery. 2018 ASDS survey on dermatologic procedures. 2018. Available at: https://www.asds.net/portals/0/PDF/procedures-survey-results-presentation-2018.pdf
[2] Ramphul K, Mejias SG. Is "Snapchat dysmorphia" a real issue? Cureus. 2018; 10(3):e2263
[3] Rajanala S, Maymone MBC, Vashi NA. Selfies-living in the era of filtered photographs. JAMA Facial Plast Surg. 2018; 20(6):443–444
[4] Wang JV, Rieder EA, Schoenberg E, Zachary CB, Saedi N. Patient perception of beauty on social media: professional and bioethical obligations in esthetics. J Cosmet Dermatol. 2020; 19(5):1129–1130
[5] Farhadian JA, Bloom BS, Brauer JA. Male aesthetics: a review of facial anatomy and pertinent clinical implications. J Drugs Dermatol. 2015; 14(9):1029–1034
[6] Shuster S, Black MM, McVitie E. The influence of age and sex on skin thickness, skin collagen and density. Br J Dermatol. 1975; 93(6):639–643
[7] Lee Y, Hwang K. Skin thickness of Korean adults. Surg Radiol Anat. 2002; 24(3–4):183–189
[8] Sedgh J. The aesthetics of the upper face and brow: male and female differences. Facial Plast Surg. 2018; 34(2):114–118
[9] Weeden JC, Trotman CA, Faraway JJ. Three dimensional analysis of facial movement in normal adults: influence of sex and facial shape. Angle Orthod. 2001; 71(2):132–140
[10] Karagas MR, Zens MS, Nelson HH, et al. Measures of cumulative exposure from a standardized sun exposure history questionnaire: a comparison with histologic assessment of solar skin damage. Am J Epidemiol. 2007; 165(6):719–726
[11] Tobin DJ. Introduction to skin aging. J Tissue Viability. 2017; 26(1):37–46
[12] Nkengne A, Bertin C. Aging and facial changes: documenting clinical signs, part 1—clinical changes of the aging face. Skinmed. 2013; 11(5):281–286
[13] Mokos ZB, Ćurković D, Kostović K, Čeović R. Facial changes in the mature patient. Clin Dermatol. 2018; 36(2):152–158
[14] Cui H, Kong Y, Zhang H. Oxidative stress, mitochondrial dysfunction, and aging. J Signal Transduct. 2012; 2012:646354
[15] Bolognia J, Jorizzo JL, Schaffer JV. Dermatology. 3rd ed. Philadelphia, PA: Elsevier Saunders; 2012.G
[16] Kammeyer A, Luiten RM. Oxidation events and skin aging. Ageing Res Rev. 2015; 21:16–29
[17] Naouri M, Atlan M, Perrodeau E, et al. Skin tightening induced by fractional CO(2) laser treatment: quantified assessment of variations in mechanical properties of the skin. J Cosmet Dermatol. 2012; 11(3):201–206
[18] Heinz A, Huertas AC, Schräder CU, Pankau R, Gosch A, Schmelzer CE. Elastins from patients with Williams-Beuren syndrome and healthy individuals differ on the molecular level. Am J Med Genet A. 2016; 170(7):1832–1842
[19] Leal Silva HG. Facial laxity rating scale validation study. Dermatol Surg. 2016; 42(12):1370–1379
[20] Alexiades-Armenakas M, Rosenberg D, Renton B, Dover J, Arndt K. Blinded, randomized, quantitative grading comparison of minimally invasive, fractional radiofrequency and surgical face-lift to treat skin laxity. Arch Dermatol. 2010; 146(4):396–405
[21] Ramaut L, Hoeksema H, Pirayesh A, Stillaert F, Monstrey S. Microneedling: Where do we stand now? A systematic review of the literature. J Plast Reconstr Aesthet Surg. 2018; 71(1):1–14
[22] Hou A, Cohen B, Haimovic A, Elbuluk N. Microneedling: a comprehensive review. Dermatol Surg. 2017; 43(3):321–339
[23] Alster TS, Graham PM. Microneedling: a review and practical guide. Dermatol Surg. 2018; 44(3):397–404
[24] Ablon G. Safety and effectiveness of an automated microneedling device in improving the signs of aging skin. J Clin Aesthet Dermatol. 2018; 11(8):29–34
[25] Puiu T, Mohammad TF, Ozog DM, Rambhatla PV. A comparative analysis of electric and radiofrequency microneedling devices on the market. J Drugs Dermatol. 2018; 17(9):1010–1013
[26] Manstein D, Herron GS, Sink RK, Tanner H, Anderson RR. Fractional photothermolysis: a new concept for cutaneous remodeling using microscopic patterns of thermal injury. Lasers Surg Med. 2004; 34(5):426–438
[27] Ortiz AE, Goldman MP, Fitzpatrick RE. Ablative CO2 lasers for skin tightening: traditional versus fractional. Dermatol Surg. 2014; 40 Suppl 12:S147–S151
[28] Munavalli GS, Turley A, Silapunt S, Biesman B. Combining confluent and fractionally ablative modalities of a novel 2790 nm YSGG laser for facial resurfacing. Lasers Surg Med. 2011; 43(4):273–282
[29] Gold MH. Noninvasive skin tightening treatment. J Clin Aesthet Dermatol. 2015; 8(6):14–18
[30] Greene RM, Green JB. Skin tightening technologies. Facial Plast Surg. 2014; 30(1):62–67
[31] Fitzpatrick R, Geronemus R, Goldberg D, Kaminer M, Kilmer S, Ruiz-Esparza J. Multicenter study of noninvasive radiofrequency for periorbital tissue tightening. Lasers Surg Med. 2003; 33(4):232–242
[32] Kist D, Burns AJ, Sanner R, Counters J, Zelickson B. Ultrastructural evaluation of multiple pass low energy versus single pass high energy radiofrequency treatment. Lasers Surg Med. 2006; 38(2):150–154
[33] Mazzoni D, Lin MJ, Dubin DP, Khorasani H. Review of non-invasive body contouring devices for fat reduction, skin tightening and muscle definition. Australas J Dermatol. 2019; 60(4):278–283
[34] Carruthers J, Fabi S, Weiss R. Monopolar radiofrequency for skin tightening: our experience and a review of the literature. Dermatol Surg. 2014; 40 Suppl 12:S168–S173
[35] Weiss RA, Weiss MA, Munavalli G, Beasley KL. Monopolar radiofrequency facial tightening: a retrospective analysis of efficacy and safety in over 600 treatments. J Drugs Dermatol. 2006; 5(8):707–712
[36] Krueger N, Sadick NS. New-generation radiofrequency technology. Cutis. 2013; 91(1):39–46
[37] Gentile RD, Kinney BM, Sadick NS. Radiofrequency technology in face and neck rejuvenation. Facial Plast Surg Clin North Am. 2018; 26(2):123–134
[38] Weiner SF. Radiofrequency microneedling: overview of technology, advantages, differences in devices, studies, and indications. Facial Plast Surg Clin North Am. 2019; 27(3):291–303
[39] Gold M, Taylor M, Rothaus K, Tanaka Y. Non-insulated smooth motion, micro-needles RF fractional treatment for wrinkle reduction and lifting of the lower face: International study. Lasers Surg Med. 2016; 48(8):727–733
[40] Gutowski KA. Microneedling with radiofrequency for skin tightening. Clin Plast Surg. 2016; 43(3):577–582
[41] Fabi SG. Noninvasive skin tightening: focus on new ultrasound techniques. Clin Cosmet Investig Dermatol. 2015; 8:47–52

[42] MacGregor JL, Tanzi EL. Microfocused ultrasound for skin tightening. Semin Cutan Med Surg. 2013; 32(1):18–25

[43] Alam M, White LE, Martin N, Witherspoon J, Yoo S, West DP. Ultrasound tightening of facial and neck skin: a rater-blinded prospective cohort study. J Am Acad Dermatol. 2010; 62(2):262–269

[44] Minkis K, Alam M. Ultrasound skin tightening. Dermatol Clin. 2014; 32(1):71–77

[45] Juhász M, Korta D, Mesinkovska NA. A review of the use of ultrasound for skin tightening, body contouring, and cellulite reduction in dermatology. Dermatol Surg. 2018; 44(7):949–963

[46] Soltani-Arabshahi R, Wong JW, Duffy KL, Powell DL. Facial allergic granulomatous reaction and systemic hypersensitivity associated with microneedle therapy for skin rejuvenation. JAMA Dermatol. 2014; 150(1):68–72

[47] Schoenberg E, Hattier G, Wang JV, Saedi N. Platelet-rich plasma (PRP) for facial rejuvenation: an early examination. Clin Dermatol. 2020; 38 (2):251–253

10 Aesthetic Concerns in Skin of Color Patients

Andrew Alexis and Michelle Henry

Summary

Men of color represent a diverse segment of the male patient population with specific aesthetic concerns and unique considerations. This cohort includes, but is not limited to, individuals of African, Asian (East and South), Hispanic/Latin American, and Middle Eastern ancestry who are more likely to have Fitzpatrick skin phototypes IV to VI. Despite the considerable size and projected growth of this population, there is a paucity of published literature or research studies addressing aesthetic concerns in men with skin of color. Understanding the needs of ethnic skin is critical to obtaining good patient outcomes in the field of aesthetic dermatology. Although there is an appreciation for the fundamental differences between different Fitzpatrick skin types, there is a distinct lack of research and management guidelines specifying differences in ethnic skin. This chapter will serve as an introduction and guide to evaluating, assessing, and treating the unique and diverse aesthetic concern in men of color.

Keywords: aesthetics, men, skin of color, procedures, follicular disorders

10.1 Background

10.1.1 Anatomy and Physiology of Ethnic Skin

Differences in the skin structure and physiology of ethnic skin require differences in safety considerations and potential efficacy. The care and management of aesthetic skin concerns in men of color necessitates an understanding of the physiologic differences of ethnic skin, and the resultant treatment modifications required to ensure the appropriate settings for energy-based devices, techniques for injectable fillers, and dosages for prescription medications. In the field of aesthetics in particular, according to the latest data by the American Society for Aesthetic Plastic Surgery, ethnic minorities (Hispanics, African Americans, Asians) are the quickest growing fraction of the aesthetic procedure market.[1] From 2017 to 2018, the number of ethnic patients seeking minimally invasive cosmetic procedures increased three times more than the number of Caucasians at a global level. Reasons for this exponential growth include increased exposure and access to procedures, targeted advertising, and socioeconomic advancement of certain cohorts in these popula- tions. Ethnic patients have unique natural features and cosmetic concerns that require a thorough understanding by the dermatologists and cosmetic surgeons who will treat these patients.[2] Further, ethnic populations have unique cultural beliefs and ideologies that need to be taken into consideration, and physicians trained to practice only on white patients will be ill equipped to offer optimal clinical care to patients of color. All of this underscores that it is critical for physicians treating aesthetic concerns in ethnic men to anticipate potential differences in skin response, recognize therapeutic limitations, and appreciate patient concerns.

The amount of epidermal melanin is the most apparent difference in individuals of color (► Table 10.1). Whereas skin of all races and ethnicities contains the same number and distribution of melanocytes, individuals with darker skin have melanocytes that produce larger melanosomes that are more singly dispersed and contain greater quantities of melanin. Moreover, the melanin contained in the melanosomes of darker skinned individuals undergoes a slower rate of degradation.[3] However, melanocytes in those with darker complexions often show a labile, exaggerated response to cutaneous injury.[4–7]

Several regulatory factors are involved in these differences; notably neuregulin 1 (NRG1) that accelerates the production and pigmentation of melanocytes has been shown to be expressed and secreted in higher levels by fibroblasts and keratinocytes of darker skin types compared to lighter skin types.[8] Moreover, the RAB27A melanosome transport molecule has been shown to be expressed in higher levels in darker skinned individuals.[9] As melanin provides photoprotection from damaging ultraviolet (UV)

Table 10.1 Common Aesthetic Concerns in Men with Skin of Color

Postinflammatory hyperpigmentation
Melasma
Other dyschromia
Dermatosis papulose nigra
Textural irregularities (e.g., enlarged pores, roughness)
Oily skin
Acne scars
Hypertrophic scars/keloids
Pseudofolliculitis barba
Acne keloidalis nuchae
Rhytides
Hair loss

light, darker skin is less susceptible to photoaging, which allows the epidermis and dermis of those individuals to retain their original structure throughout the aging process to a greater extent compared to lighter skinned individuals. Transmission of UVA light through the epidermis is 17.5% in pigmented skin and 55.5% in Caucasians, whereas the transmission of UVB through the epidermis is 5.7% for pigmented skin compared to 29.4% for Caucasians.[10]

Aside from pigmentation, the structure and function of the epidermis and dermis are different between the various ethnicities. The stratum corneum of black skin contains a greater number of corneocyte layers, with each layer presenting increased intracellular cohesion and compactness compared to white skin. Moreover, the content of lipids in the stratum corneum was shown to differ between ethnicities, with the cholesterol-to-ceramide ratio being the highest in Asians, intermediate in Caucasians, and lowest in African Americans.[11,12] Corneocyte size does not differ between skin of different ethnicities, but higher levels of desquamation have been noted in black skin compared to white skin (▶ Table 10.1).[13]

Transepidermal water loss (TEWL), which refers to the total amount of water vapor lost through the skin and related appendages under nonsweating conditions, has been shown in some studies to differ between racial/ethnic populations, with Asians having the highest amount of TEWL after tape stripping. Differences in the skin hydration and pH of different ethnicities have yet to be determined due to lack of consistent parameters and results across various clinical studies.[14-16]

Hair structure and biology also differ between various ethnic groups. Asian, Caucasian, and African hairs exhibit distinct characteristics in density, diameter, shape, mechanical properties, and composition. Hair of African origin is spiral, with frequent twists that have random reversals in direction, pronounced flattening, and irregular diameter.[17] African hair also exhibits increased dryness, lower moisture content, less total sebum, and increased fragility due to decreased tensile strength compared to Caucasian hair.[3] Asian hair has the greatest diameter with circular geometry, and hair follicles that are more metabolically active than other ethnicities. Caucasian hair is intermediate in diameter and shape and presents the greatest tensile strength among the ethnic groups. In terms of content, keratin and other proteins are similar across the various ethnic groups (▶ Table 10.1).[18]

Due to the interplay between structural, functional, and cultural factors, the frequency of dermatologic and aesthetic concerns varies by racial/ethnic population.[1,20,21,22] Aesthetic concerns that disproportionately affect men with skin of color include disorders of hyperpigmentation, aesthetic sequelae of follicular disorders, dermatosis papulosa nigra, and keloids or hypertrophic scars.[22,23] In addition to these, there are concerns that are prevalent across all populations but may have unique considerations in men of color. A comprehensive list of the range

Table 10.2 Common Aesthetic Procedures in Men with Skin of Color

Chemical peels
Laser hair removal
Electrodessication
Nonablative laser resurfacing/photorejuvenation
Botulinum toxin
Soft tissue fillers
Hair restoration (e.g., transplantation, platelet-rich plasma)

of common aesthetic concerns in men with skin of color is presented in ▶ Table 10.1.

Minimally invasive treatments are essential tools in the management of leading aesthetic concerns in men of color. The most common minimally invasive procedures used to address aesthetic concerns in male patients with skin of color are listed in ▶ Table 10.2. As a result of structural and functional characteristics, performing aesthetic procedures in this patient population is associated with a higher risk of complications, most notably postinflammatory pigment alteration and hypertrophic scarring or keloid formation. However, with careful selection of device or peeling agent, use of conservative treatment parameters, and judicious pre- and posttreatment precautions, minimally invasive procedures can be performed safely and effectively in men of color.

10.2 Managing Hyperpigmentation

Hyperpigmentation is among the leading aesthetic concerns in men of color. It is frequently seen as a sequela of inflammatory disorders (e.g., acne, atopic dermatitis, psoriasis, etc.), a primary pigmentary disorder (e.g., melasma, lentigines, photo-induced hyperpigmentation, maturational hyperpigmentation, etc.), or as a complication of dermatologic procedures and treatments. Minimally invasive procedures including chemical peels,[24-29] fractional lasers,[30,31,32,33,34] Q-switched lasers,[35,36,37,38,39,40,41,42,43,44,45,46,47,48,49] picosecond lasers,[50,51,52,53,54,55,56,57,58] and microneedling[59,60,61,62,63,64,65]—typically in conjunction with topical skin lightening agents—have been used successfully on patients with higher skin phototypes and are a mainstay in the overall management of hyperpigmentation. Minimally invasive procedures contribute to the treatment of hyperpigmentation either by increasing penetration of topical skin lightening agents (e.g., chemical peels, fractional lasers, and microneedling) or by removing excess pigment (e.g., fractional lasers, Q-switched lasers, picosecond lasers, and chemical peels). Combining multiple modalities is often necessary to achieve the most efficacious results, but must be done with caution as excessive epidermal and dermal injury associated with the above procedures can result in iatrogenic dyspigmentation.

Although Q-switched lasers have been widely used in East Asian skin types (up to skin phototype III), their safety in more darkly pigmented individuals (e.g., skin phototypes IV–VI) is limited due to a higher rate of dyspigmentation—including irreversible guttate hypopigmentation. In a Thai study of men with melasma, five weekly 30% glycolic acid peels combined with weekly low-fluence Q-switched (LFQS) neodymium:yttrium aluminum garnet (Nd:YAG) laser demonstrated greater improvement in melasma than weekly glycolic acid peels alone. However, relapse rates were high and dyspigmentation associated with LFQS laser was observed. In a U.S. study involving melasma patients with skin phototypes II to V, monthly LFQS Nd:YAG lasers in combination with microdermabrasion and topical skin lightening agents resulted in significant improvement without treatment-associated dyspigmentation.[66] As such, careful patient selection (favor lighter/intermediate skin types), lower frequency of treatments (monthly vs. weekly), lower fluences (e.g., 2 laser passes at 1.6–2.0 J/cm^2),[67] and combination of skin lightening agents are advised when considering LFQS in the treatment of melasma.

Low-energy 1,927-nm nonablative fractional laser has emerged as a safe and effective modality for treating hyperpigmentation in skin phototypes IV to VI. Two studies have included patients with higher Fitzpatrick skin phototypes (up to VI) with favorable results.[30,68] This technology has the advantage of being able to extrude dermal pigmentation and enhance penetration of topical skin lightening agents while maintaining a very low risk safety profile.

10.2.1 Chemical Peels

Chemical peeling is a versatile minimally invasive procedure that plays a key role in the management of a broad range of aesthetic concerns in men of color (▶ Table 10.3). They are particularly useful as an adjunct in the treatment of hyperpigmentation (in combination with topical skin lightening agents) and for the improvement of textural irregularities such as the appearance of enlarged follicular openings. They are also an effective approach to overall skin rejuvenation in the context of photoaging or for the purpose of skin care maintenance—enhancing radiance, reducing dyschromia, and improving texture.

Superficial peeling agents are preferred for safety reasons—given the higher risk of dyspigmentation and scarring from medium and deep peels in patients with skin of color. Salicylic acid and glycolic acid peels are the most widely utilized, but other suitable peeling agents include mandelic acid, Jessner's peel, and low-concentration trichloroacetic acid (e.g., 15% TCA). In a recent retrospective study, the overall complication rate of superficial chemical

Table 10.3 Best practices for performing laser/light based procedures in men of color (modified from Alexis AF, British Journal of Dermatology, 2013;169(3): 91–97)[1]

- Laser Wavelength—consider chromophore (especially risk of absorption by epidermal melanin); longer wavelengths associated with less epidermal absorption and therefore greater safety in patients with higher skin phototype

- Laser treatment parameters—employ settings that minimize extent of epidermal and dermal injury (typically more conservative than in SPT I–III, often requiring a greater number of sessions), e.g., lower fluences and longer pulse durations for laser hair removal; lower treatment densities (microthermal zones cm2) for fractional laser resurfacing

- Pre- and post-treatment sun protection (sun-protective behaviors, broad-spectrum sunscreen SPF ≥ 30)

- Consider pre- (≥ 2 weeks prior) and post treatment bleaching agents (e.g., hydroquinone 4% cream)

- Judicious epidermal cooling, e.g., slower treatment speeds when using lasers with contact cooling; pausing between passes of resurfacing lasers to reduce bulk heating; ice packs post-procedure

- Consider topical corticosteroids post-treatment (to reduce inflammation), especially when significant post-procedure erythema or edema noted

[1]Alexis AF. Lasers and light-based therapies in ethnic skin: treatment options and recommendations for Fitzpatrick skin types V and VI. The British journal of dermatology, 2013;169 (3):91–97.

peels in skin phototypes III to VI was 3.8%.[69] Key strategies to improving outcomes when performing chemical peels in male patients with skin of color are summarized in ▶ Table 10.4. Avoidance of over-application or, in the case of peels requiring neutralization, prolonged time of application is important for minimizing the risk of complications. As such, judicious application and close observation for impending signs or symptoms of irritation are of paramount importance.

10.2.2 Laser Treatments

Nonablative fractional lasers can be used for a broad range of aesthetic indications in men with skin of color.[70,71] The 1,550-nm erbium-doped fractional laser has been used extensively in patients of color[72,73,74,75] and is particularly useful in the treatment of acne scarring, textural irregularities, and features of photoaging (▶ Fig. 10.1). Postinflammatory hyperpigmentation (PIH) is a significant risk but can be managed by conservative treatment parameters—most notably, a lower range of treatment densities, pre- and posttreatment hydroquinone, as well as strict sun protection.

Other resurfacing technologies with broad applications in men of color include the microsecond pulsed Nd:YAG

1,064-nm laser[71,76,77] and picosecond lasers.[51,52,78] Submillisecond (300- to 650-microsecond) pulsed Nd:YAG can be used for the treatment of acne scars, keloids/hypertrophic scars, acne, dyschromia, and photoaging in patients of color. This approach has the advantage of being safe on all skin types and not requiring pretreatment anesthetic. However, multiple treatments are generally required to achieve clinically meaningful results. The 755-nm picosecond laser with the diffractive lens array (DLA) has been studied in the treatment of unwanted scars, pigmented lesions, and striae in patients with skin of color (Fitzpatrick skin phototypes IV–VI). Self-limited erythema and hyperpigmentation were the most common adverse events.[51]

Resurfacing with fractional radiofrequency (RF) has recently been demonstrated in a study involving 35 subjects with skin type VI who received three sessions of facial treatments, 4 weeks apart using a fractional RF device with 24-pin coated tip.[79] Safety and efficacy in the treatment of wrinkles, acne scars, and overall appearance were observed.

Table 10.4 Best practices for performing chemical peels in men of color

- Utilize superficial peeling agents (e.g. glycolic acid 20-50%, salicylic acid 20-30%, mandelic acid 40%, trichloroacetic acid 15%)

- Discontinue topical retinoids or exfoliate skin care procedures (e.g., exfoliating masks, mechanical brush cleansing, etc.) at least 7 days prior to chemical peel

- Monitor patient closely during chemical peel

- Customize number of layers applied and duration of application according to individual patient tolerability

- Utilize portable fan and cool compresses to reduce stinging/burning

- Neutralize or abort peel in areas demonstrating signs or symptoms of irritation during peel

- Consider pre- and post-treatment topical skin lightening agents (for reduced risk of iatrogenic hyperpigmentation and enhanced efficacy in the management of hyperpigmentation)

10.3 Laser Hair Removal

Long-wavelength lasers in the near-infrared spectrum (especially the 800- to 810-nm diode and 1,064-nm Nd:YAG laser) have revolutionized the treatment of follicular disorders with aesthetic sequelae in men of color such as pseudofolliculitis barbae[80,81,82,83,84,85,86,87,88,89,90,91] and acne keloidalis nuchae.[92,93,94,95,96] Laser hair removal has also been shown to be effective as an alternative therapy for dissecting cellulitis of the scalp[97,98] and hidradenitis suppuritiva.[99] Whereas the 755-nm alexandrite laser has been used on lighter complexioned individuals with Fitzpatrick skin phototypes III to V,[82,94,100] the 800- to 810-nm and 1,064-nm Nd:YAG laser is preferred for intermediately pigmented phototypes IV to V and richly pigmented phototypes V to VI, respectively, based on their risk-to-benefit ratio. In a study comparing Er:YAG laser resurfacing to long-pulsed Nd:YAG laser for the treatment of acne keloidalis nuchae in Egyptian men, both groups experienced a significant reduction in papules and plaque size, whereas a significant decrease in plaque count was only seen in the Er:YAG group.[93] When using laser hair removal in men of color, utilizing lower fluences, longer wavelengths, and efficient epidermal cooling are key to maximizing safety. For millisecond pulsed lasers, the use of longer pulse durations are recommended for higher phototypes with richly pigmented skin in order to facilitate epidermal cooling and thereby minimize risk of pigmentary complications.

10.4 Injectable Fillers and Neuromodulators

10.4.1 Approach

The restoration of a youthful male face to combat the age-related loss of skeletal, muscle, and fat compartment volume is increasingly achieved with noninvasive procedures such as fillers and neuromodulators. The overarching goal for all patients, regardless of their gender or ethnicity, is to achieve harmonization in facial topography and rejuvenation. The aging process, however, affects different ethnicities distinctly, and different ethnicities have distinct structural characteristics that affect facial treatment planning. For example, individuals

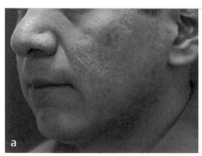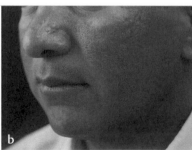

Fig. 10.1 A Hispanic man with acne scarring before (**a**) and after (**b**) laser resurfacing with 1550-nm erbium-doped fractional laser.

of African American origin, aside from having relative intrinsic protection against photoaging, have a thicker dermis and do not experience sagging, rhytids, and facial tissue ptosis to the same degree as their Caucasian counterparts. Signs of aging in these patients are more evident in the periorbital, perioral, and midface region and less on the upper third of the face. Patients of Asian origin present with a wide bitemporal, bizygomatic width, shorter face, and low projection of the midface. They have flatter, broader foreheads, retrognathia, and microgenia, and the aging process typically results in disharmonies in the lower third of the face. Aside from structural facial differences, ethnic patients are also susceptible to discoloration and scarring; thus, when treating them with injectable agents such as soft-tissue fillers and neuromodulators, the technique needs to be modified to minimize risk of these complications.

10.4.2 Procedure

Several types of fillers, notably hyaluronic acid (HA), calcium hydroxyapatite (CaHa), and poly-L-lactic acid (PLLA), have been used safely and effectively in individuals of diverse ethnic backgrounds.[101–103] Strategies to minimize the risk for hyperpigmentation (PIH) after soft-tissue filler injection include longer, slower injection times and avoidance of a multiple puncture technique. In a clinical trial of 150 patients (skin types IV–VI) evaluating the safety and efficacy of hyaluronic fillers, 13% of multiple puncture techniques resulted in hyperpigmentation compared with 2% of linear threading.[102] Moreover, due to the presence of larger, multinucleated fibroblasts, ethnic skin is 3 to 18 times more prone to the development of keloid formation; physicians should be cautious in treating patients with a history of hypertrophic scarring or keloid formation[3]. Nevertheless, in the study of Taylor et al,[102] none of the 150 patients developed a keloid.

The most important aspect of facial volumization in male patients of color is intimate knowledge of the structural differences between them and Caucasians and honoring the aesthetic ideals that they are aspiring toward.

Most often than not, individuals of ethnic backgrounds are not seeking a "Westernized" version but rather a "rejuvenated" version of themselves (▶ Fig. 10.2). For example, African American women usually experience fine lines, and loss of volume below the vermillion border, of the upper lip, and thus seek augmentation of the upper lip area.[104] This is achieved by superiorly rolling the lip using low-viscosity HA fillers such as Belotero (Merz Aesthetics, Raleigh, North Caroline, United States) or Restylane silk (Galderma, Fort Worth, Texas, United States). Moreover, the collagen content and collagen-production capacity of African Americans is higher than that of Caucasians, thus treating with soft-tissue fillers that have biostimulatory properties such as PLLA (Galderma) and CaHa (Radiesse; Merz Aesthetics) can be more effective in this population, and as a result they will require fewer treatments than their white counterparts.

Patients of Indian descent tend to have a smaller skeletal framework, which results in a more pronounced appearance of fat pad descent, and concentration of the bulk of the volume in the inner face.[105,106] In these patients, restoring volume to the facial frame (forehead, temples, and chin) can provide a more balanced, symmetric global appearance.

Early signs of aging, such as volume loss in the infraorbital area, are more pronounced in Asian patients due to the skeletal differences. In contrast to Caucasians, these patients typically prefer high cheekbones, seeking augmentation of the zygoma and lateral maxilla, and want to avoid further widening of the midface. Therefore, restoring the anterior projection of the infraorbital area and adding central projection while restoring volume to the forehead, chin, and nose is commonly sought to harmonize the Asian male face.[107] Lip enhancement is generally not indicated in Asians as the lip fullness is typical more than that of Caucasians. Asian individuals seek to embrace and optimize their Eastern facial features, with a general preference for an oval facial shape—full in the upper half and tapered from the cheek to chin.[108]

The use of neuromodulators is widespread among ethnic patients, particularly in combination with fillers, as

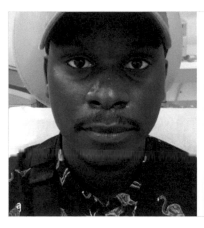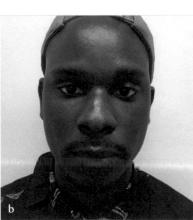

Fig. 10.2 A 37-year-old African American man before **(a)** and two weeks after **(b)** volumization with 2-mL hyaluronic acid filler in the midface.

the two treatments enhance the global clinical outcome. The most common area of application is the glabella, and results from clinical studies have shown that compared to Caucasian patients, the longevity and treatment response of neuromodulator may be greater in patients of color.[109] No population-specific adverse events or side effects have been noted with this treatment in this population.

10.5 Hair Restoration

10.5.1 Approach

Hair loss and scalp disorders affect men of color, and their treatment can be a challenge, as causative factors may be related to cultural hair practices. For example, hair practices such as dreadlocks, scarves, and tight braiding can weaken hair, especially in individuals of African origin who already have hair with decreased density and tensile strength.[110] The use of heat and chemical relaxers in hair straightening is widespread in this population, and in addition to hair loss, can aggravate or lead to scalp disorders and contact dermatitis.[111] Basic hair care has also been shown to be different, especially in the African American population who, due to a propensity for dryness and breakage, often shampoo their hair only once every week or once in 2 weeks. Whereas cultural practices predispose these individuals to traction alopecia, this population is also commonly affected by other forms of hair loss such as central centrifugal cicatricial alopecia (CCCA) and frontal fibrosing alopecia.

10.5.2 Traction Alopecia

Traction alopecia is a type of nonscarring hair loss that occurs by repetitive, prolonged tension to the hair. It is most commonly seen in individuals of African and Hispanic origin and is directly related to the hair grooming practices of these populations.[112,113] Cardinal signs of traction alopecia include perifollicular edema and peripilar casts, followed by evident hair loss, particularly in the frontal and temporal scalp[114,115]. Although the condition is nonscarring, persistence of hair grooming practices and lack of treatment can ultimately lead to destruction of the hair follicle and permanent hair loss. In cases of patients of color who present with signs of traction alopecia but who do not engage in hair practices that would result in such a phenotype, the differential diagnosis of frontal fibrosing alopecia, androgenetic alopecia, telogen effluvium, trichotillomania, and CCCA should be considered.[116] Treatment options for traction alopecia start with lifestyle changes as they relate to hair, which means styling the hair in a loose manner, and avoiding heat, and chemical relaxers.[117] In circumstances where the disease has progressed, treatments to suppress follicular inflammation, such as antibiotics or intralesional corticosteroid injections at the periphery of hair loss, can be used. In advanced conditions, where there is extensive destruction

of the hair follicle, surgical options such as hair transplantation need to be considered.[118]

10.5.3 Central Centrifugal Cicatricial Alopecia

CCCA, a term coined by the North American Hair Research Society (NAHRS), is an inflammatory condition that is almost unique to patients with skin of color and can be seen in men. A combination of genetics, hair structure, and hair care habits has been shown to be implicated in the pathophysiology of this condition. In CCCA, hair loss is common in the midscalp and vertex, which, together with loss of follicular openings, leads to a shiny appearance of the scalp.[119] Other signs and symptoms include frequent hair breakage, papules, pustules, and pruritus of the scalp. Dermoscopic evaluation can reveal presence of peripilar white halos that correspond to fibrosis surrounding the outer root sheath.[120] When treatment is sought in the early stages of disease, it is possible to prevent scarring and permanent hair loss. Strategies employed include antibiotics with anti-inflammatory properties such as doxycycline, topical or intralesional corticosteroids, and antimalarials such as hydroxychloroquine.[120] Hair transplantation is also an option when permanent hair loss has occurred; however, patients should be clear from inflammation as this can compromise the quality of graft survival.[121]

10.5.4 Lichen Planopilaris

Lichen planopilaris (LPP) is another type of scarring alopecia that often occurs in skin of color, particularly in individuals of Asian descent.[1] Characteristics of this condition include follicular erythema, hyperkeratosis, and scarring of the frontotemporal hairline. Other anatomic areas such as the eyebrows, eyelashes, and occipital scalp may be affected.[122,123] Unfortunately, to date, there is no successful treatment for LPP. Therapeutic strategies such as topical or intralesional corticosteroids, calcineurin inhibitors, hydroxychloroquine, mycophenolate mofetil, and oral 5-alpha reductase inhibitors (5aRi) have been shown to have relative efficacy in some patients.[124] Whereas regrowth of hair is rare in these patients, the main clinical goal is to slow down or stop progression of hair loss.

10.5.5 Hair Transplantation

With the development of modern methodologies, such as follicular unit extraction (FUE) and robotic hair transplantation, surgical hair restoration offers superior cosmetic outcomes. Whereas hair transplantation has universal guidelines regardless of the patient's ethnicities, surgeons should appreciate the differences in hair structure of their ethnic patients compared to their white patients, as it applies to hairline design, selection of donor site, and grafting.[125] For example, most Caucasian patients exhibit frontotemporal recession, whereas many Asians may have round, broad foreheads with the hairline following this pattern. Patients of African descent, on the other hand, have a straight hairline that follows almost a right angle at the frontotemporal junction. The hairline of Hispanics is varied, but physicians need to make note of the origin pattern when designing the new hairline.[126,127] Other considerations when performing hair transplantation in patients of skin of color include hair density, which is decreased in African patients compared to Asians and Caucasians, and the risk of hair transection, given the curlier nature of the hair shaft. No further modifications in technique are required regarding graft dissection and placement.

10.6 Conclusion

Men of color represent a diverse and rapidly growing segment of the aesthetic patient population. Structural and functional differences such as pigment lability and increased prevalence of keloid and hypertrophic scarring, as well as variations in features of photoaging, dictate special considerations and unique approaches to the aesthetic treatment of this population. In addition to more typical indications such as photoaging, aesthetic procedures can offer great benefit to the treatment of challenging follicular disorders that disproportionately affect men of color as well as pigmentary disorders and acne scarring. Careful selection of treatment modality and individualized consideration of optimal parameters are key to achieving successful outcomes in this diverse patient population with unique aesthetic concerns and dermatologic characteristics.

10.7 Pearls

- The gold standard for correcting skin laxity and achieving tightening is surgical correction, such as rhytidectomy. Although consistently and uniformly effective, surgical procedures can be invasive, risky, costly, and inappropriate for some patients. As such, the demand for less invasive treatment modalities has increased.
- It is crucial to inform patients of the limitations of skin tightening procedures that utilize medical devices, especially when compared to surgical options in patients with significant skin laxity.
- Ablative resurfacing lasers represent the traditional gold standard for the treatment of facial rejuvenation and skin laxity.
- Unlike other energy modalities, ultrasound energy can safely penetrate deeper into the tissue to briefly raise temperatures above 60 degrees Celsius to produce small thermal coagulation points without heating superficial skin structures, which can allow for greater temperatures and controlled injury.

References

[1] Lawson CN, Hollinger J, Sethi S, et al. Updates in the understanding and treatments of skin & hair disorders in women of color. Int J Womens Dermatol. 2017; 3(1) Suppl:S21–S37

[2] Henry M, Sadick N. Aesthetic considerations in female skin of color: what you need to know. Semin Cutan Med Surg. 2018; 37(4):210–216

[3] Taylor SC. Skin of color: biology, structure, function, and implications for dermatologic disease. J Am Acad Dermatol. 2002; 46(2) Suppl Understanding:S41–S62

[4] Andersen KE, Maibach HI. Black and white human skin differences. J Am Acad Dermatol. 1979; 1(3):276–282

[5] Berardesca E, Maibach H. Racial differences in skin pathophysiology. J Am Acad Dermatol. 1996; 34(4):667–672

[6] Montagna W, Carlisle K. The architecture of black and white facial skin. J Am Acad Dermatol. 1991; 24(6, Pt 1):929–937

[7] Weigand DA, Haygood C, Gaylor JR. Cell layers and density of Negro and Caucasian stratum corneum. J Invest Dermatol. 1974; 62(6): 563–568

[8] Choi W, Kolbe L, Hearing VJ. Characterization of the bioactive motif of neuregulin-1, a fibroblast-derived paracrine factor that regulates the constitutive color and the function of melanocytes in human skin. Pigment Cell Melanoma Res. 2012; 25(4):477–481

[9] Yoshida-Amano Y, Hachiya A, Ohuchi A, et al. Essential role of RA-B27A in determining constitutive human skin color. PLoS One. 2012; 7(7):e41160

[10] Lawson CN, Hollinger J, Sethi S, et al. Updates in the understanding and treatments of skin & hair disorders in women of color. Int J Womens Dermatol. 2015; 1(2):59–75

[11] Gambichler T, Matip R, Moussa G, Altmeyer P, Hoffmann K. In vivo data of epidermal thickness evaluated by optical coherence tomography: effects of age, gender, skin type, and anatomic site. J Dermatol Sci. 2006; 44(3):145–152

[12] Thomson ML. Relative efficiency of pigment and horny layer thickness in protecting the skin of Europeans and Africans against solar ultraviolet radiation. J Physiol. 1955; 127(2):236–246

[13] Corcuff P, Lotte C, Rougier A, Maibach HI. Racial differences in corneocytes. A comparison between black, white and oriental skin. Acta Derm Venereol. 1991; 71(2):146–148

[14] Primavera G, Berardesca E. Clinical and instrumental evaluation of a food supplement in improving skin hydration. Int J Cosmet Sci. 2005; 27(4):199–204

[15] Fluhr JW, Dickel H, Kuss O, Weyher I, Diepgen TL, Berardesca E. Impact of anatomical location on barrier recovery, surface pH and stratum corneum hydration after acute barrier disruption. Br J Dermatol. 2002; 146(5):770–776

[16] Berardesca E, Maibach HI. Transepidermal water loss and skin surface hydration in the non invasive assessment of stratum corneum function. Derm Beruf Umwelt. 1990; 38(2):50–53

[17] Ji JH, Park TS, Lee HJ, et al. The ethnic differences of the damage of hair and integral hair lipid after ultra violet radiation. Ann Dermatol. 2013; 25(1):54–60

[18] Laatsch CN, Durbin-Johnson BP, Rocke DM, et al. Human hair shaft proteomic profiling: individual differences, site specificity and cuticle analysis. PeerJ. 2014; 2:e506

[19] American Society for Aesthetic Plastic Surgery. Cosmetic Surgery National Data Bank: Statistics. Arlington Heights, IL: American Society for Aesthetic Plastic Surgery; 2018

[20] Alexis AF, Few J, Callender VD, et al. Myths and knowledge gaps in the aesthetic treatment of patients with skin of color. J Drugs Dermatol. 2019; 18(7):616–622

[21] Rossi A, Alexis AF. Cosmetic procedures in skin of color. G Ital Dermatol Venereol. 2011; 146(4):265–272

[22] Awosika O, Burgess CM, Grimes PE. Considerations when treating cosmetic concerns in men of color. Dermatol Surg. 2017; 43 Suppl 2: S140–S150

[23] Callender VD. Commentary on considerations when treating cosmetic concerns in men of color. Dermatol Surg. 2017; 43 Suppl 2: S151–S152

[24] Downie J, Schneider K, Goberdhan L, Makino ET, Mehta RC. Combination of in-office chemical peels with a topical comprehensive pigmentation control product in skin of color subjects with facial hyperpigmentation. J Drugs Dermatol. 2017; 16(4):301–306

[25] Sarkar R, Parmar NV, Kapoor S. Treatment of postinflammatory hyperpigmentation with a combination of glycolic acid peels and a topical regimen in dark-skinned patients: a comparative study. Dermatol Surg. 2017; 43(4):566–573

[26] Godse K, Sakhia J. Triple combination and glycolic peels in post-acne hyperpigmentation. J Cutan Aesthet Surg. 2012; 5(1):60–61

[27] Joshi SS, Boone SL, Alam M, et al. Effectiveness, safety, and effect on quality of life of topical salicylic acid peels for treatment of post-inflammatory hyperpigmentation in dark skin. Dermatol Surg. 2009; 35(4):638–644, discussion 644

[28] Garg VK, Sinha S, Sarkar R. Glycolic acid peels versus salicylic-mandelic acid peels in active acne vulgaris and post-acne scarring and hyperpigmentation: a comparative study. Dermatol Surg. 2009; 35(1):59–65

[29] Burns RL, Prevost-Blank PL, Lawry MA, Lawry TB, Faria DT, Fivenson DP. Glycolic acid peels for postinflammatory hyperpigmentation in black patients. A comparative study. Dermatol Surg. 1997; 23(3): 171–174, discussion 175

[30] Bae YC, et al. Treatment of post-inflammatory hyperpigmentation in patients with darker skin types using a low energy 1,927 nm non-ablative fractional laser: a retrospective photographic review analysis. Lasers Surg Med. 2020; 52(1):7–12

[31] Kaufman-Janette J, Cazzaniga A, Ballin A, Swanson-Garcell R. Effectiveness of a nutraceutical during non-ablative 1927 nm fractional laser on patients with facial hyperpigmentation and photoaging. J Drugs Dermatol. 2017; 16(5):501–506

[32] Lee SJ, Chung WS, Lee JD, Kim HS. A patient with cupping-related post-inflammatory hyperpigmentation successfully treated with a 1,927 nm thulium fiber fractional laser. J Cosmet Laser Ther. 2014; 16 (2):66–68

[33] Oram Y, Akkaya AD. Refractory postinflammatory hyperpigmentation treated fractional CO$_2$ laser. J Clin Aesthet Dermatol. 2014; 7(3):42–44

[34] Rokhsar CK, Ciocon DH. Fractional photothermolysis for the treatment of postinflammatory hyperpigmentation after carbon dioxide laser resurfacing. Dermatol Surg. 2009; 35(3):535–537

[35] Munavalli G. A split-face assessment of the synergistic potential of sequential Q-switched Nd:YAG laser and 1565 nm fractional non-ablative laser treatment for facial rejuvenation in Fitzpatrick skin type II-V patients. J Drugs Dermatol. 2016; 15(11):1335–1342

[36] Brown AS, Hussain M, Goldberg DJ. Treatment of melasma with low fluence, large spot size, 1064-nm Q-switched neodymium-doped yttrium aluminum garnet (Nd:YAG) laser for the treatment of melasma in Fitzpatrick skin types II-IV. J Cosmet Laser Ther. 2011; 13(6):280–282

[37] Moody MN, Landau JM, Vergilis-Kalner IJ, Goldberg LH, Marquez D, Friedman PM. 1,064-nm Q-switched neodymium-doped yttrium aluminum garnet laser and 1,550-nm fractionated erbium-doped fiber laser for the treatment of nevus of Ota in Fitzpatrick skin type IV. Dermatol Surg. 2011; 37(8):1163–1167

[38] Saedi N, Metelitsa A. Commentary on Q-switched 660-nm versus 532-nm Nd: YAG laser for the treatment for facial lentigines in Asian patients. Dermatol Surg. 2015; 41(12):1396–1397

[39] Noh TK, Chung BY, Yeo UC, Chang S, Lee MW, Chang SE. Q-switched 660-nm versus 532-nm Nd: YAG laser for the treatment for facial lentigines in Asian patients: a prospective, randomized, double-blinded, split-face comparison pilot study. Dermatol Surg. 2015; 41 (12):1389–1395

[40] Kim HS, Kim EK, Jung KE, Park YM, Kim HO, Lee JY. A split-face comparison of low-fluence Q-switched Nd: YAG laser plus 1550 nm fractional

[41] Saedi N, Chan HH, Dover JS. Treating lentigines in Asian patients with the Q-switched Alexandrite laser. J Drugs Dermatol. 2011; 10(12) Suppl:s14–s15

[42] Kim S, Cho KH. Treatment of procedure-related postinflammatory hyperpigmentation using 1064-nm Q-switched Nd:YAG laser with low fluence in Asian patients: report of five cases. J Cosmet Dermatol. 2010; 9(4):302–306

[43] Kim S, Cho KH. Treatment of facial postinflammatory hyperpigmentation with facial acne in Asian patients using a Q-switched neodymium-doped yttrium aluminum garnet laser. Dermatol Surg. 2010; 36(9):1374–1380

[44] Metelitsa AI. Commentary: treatment of facial postinflammatory hyperpigmentation with facial acne in Asian patients using a novel Q-switched neodymium-doped yttrium aluminum garnet laser. Dermatol Surg. 2010; 36(9):1381

[45] Park JM, Tsao H, Tsao S. Combined use of intense pulsed light and Q-switched ruby laser for complex dyspigmentation among Asian patients. Lasers Surg Med. 2008; 40(2):128–133

[46] Wang CC, Sue YM, Yang CH, Chen CK. A comparison of Q-switched alexandrite laser and intense pulsed light for the treatment of freckles and lentigines in Asian persons: a randomized, physician-blinded, split-face comparative trial. J Am Acad Dermatol. 2006; 54 (5):804–810

[47] Jang KA, Chung EC, Choi JH, Sung KJ, Moon KC, Koh JK. Successful removal of freckles in Asian skin with a Q-switched alexandrite laser. Dermatol Surg. 2000; 26(3):231–234

[48] Zhou X, Gold MH, Lu Z, Li Y. Efficacy and safety of Q-switched 1,064-nm neodymium-doped yttrium aluminum garnet laser treatment of melasma. Dermatol Surg. 2011; 37(7):962–970

[49] Vachiramon V, Sahawatwong S, Sirithanabadeekul P. Treatment of melasma in men with low-fluence Q-switched neodymium-doped yttrium-aluminum-garnet laser versus combined laser and glycolic acid peeling. Dermatol Surg. 2015; 41(4):457–465

[50] Lee MC, Lin YF, Hu S, et al. A split-face study: comparison of pico-second alexandrite laser and Q-switched Nd:YAG laser in the treatment of melasma in Asians. Lasers Med Sci. 2018; 33(8): 1733–1738

[51] Haimovic A, Brauer JA, Cindy Bae YS, Geronemus RG. Safety of a pico-second laser with diffractive lens array (DLA) in the treatment of Fitzpatrick skin types IV to VI: a retrospective review. J Am Acad Dermatol. 2016; 74(5):931–936

[52] Levin MK, Ng E, Bae YS, Brauer JA, Geronemus RG. Treatment of pigmentary disorders in patients with skin of color with a novel 755 nm picosecond, Q-switched ruby, and Q-switched Nd:YAG nanosecond lasers: a retrospective photographic review. Lasers Surg Med. 2016; 48(2):181–187

[53] Wang YJ, et al. Prospective randomized controlled trial comparing treatment efficacy and tolerance of picosecond alexandrite laser with a diffractive lens array and triple combination cream in female Asian patients with melasma. J Eur Acad Dermatol Venereol. 2020; 34(3): 624–63

[54] Chen YT, Lin ET, Chang CC, et al. Efficacy and safety evaluation of picosecond alexandrite laser with a diffractive lens array for treatment of melasma in Asian patients by VISIA imaging system. Photobiomodul Photomed Laser Surg. 2019; 37(9):559–566

[55] Jo DJ, Kang IH, Baek JH, Gwak MJ, Lee SJ, Shin MK. Using reflectance confocal microscopy to observe in vivo melanolysis after treatment with the picosecond alexandrite laser and Q-switched Nd:YAG laser in melasma. Lasers Surg Med. 2018

[56] Lee YJ, Shin HJ, Noh TK, Choi KH, Chang SE. Treatment of melasma and post-inflammatory hyperpigmentation by a picosecond 755-nm alexandrite laser in Asian patients. Ann Dermatol. 2017; 29(6):779–781

[57] Chalermchai T, Rummaneethorn P. Effects of a fractional picosecond 1,064 nm laser for the treatment of dermal and mixed type melasma. J Cosmet Laser Ther. 2018; 20(3):134–139

[58] Choi YJ, Nam JH, Kim JY, et al. Efficacy and safety of a novel picosecond laser using combination of 1 064 and 595 nm on patients

with melasma: a prospective, randomized, multicenter, split-face, 2% hydroquinone cream-controlled clinical trial. Lasers Surg Med. 2017; 49(10):899–907

[59] Cassiano DP, Espósito ACC, Hassun KM, Lima EVA, Bagatin E, Miot HA. Early clinical and histological changes induced by microneedling in facial melasma: a pilot study. Indian J Dermatol Venereol Leprol. 2019; 85(6):638–641

[60] Ismail ESA, Patsatsi A, Abd El-Maged WM, Nada EEAE. Efficacy of microneedling with topical vitamin C in the treatment of melasma. J Cosmet Dermatol. 2019

[61] Lima EVA, Lima MMDA, Paixão MP, Miot HA. Assessment of the effects of skin microneedling as adjuvant therapy for facial melasma: a pilot study. BMC Dermatol. 2017; 17(1):14

[62] Ustuner P, Balevi A, Ozdemir M. A split-face, investigator-blinded comparative study on the efficacy and safety of Q-switched Nd:YAG laser plus microneedling with vitamin C versus Q-switched Nd:YAG laser for the treatment of recalcitrant melasma. J Cosmet Laser Ther. 2017; 19(7):383–390

[63] Lima EdeA. Microneedling in facial recalcitrant melasma: report of a series of 22 cases. An Bras Dermatol. 2015; 90(6):919–921

[64] Budamakuntla L, Loganathan E, Suresh DH, et al. A randomised, open-label, comparative study of tranexamic acid microinjections and tranexamic acid with microneedling in patients with melasma. J Cutan Aesthet Surg. 2013; 6(3):139–143

[65] Kwon HH, Choi SC, Jung JY, Park GH. Combined treatment of melasma involving low-fluence Q-switched Nd:YAG laser and fractional microneedling radiofrequency. J Dermatolog Treat. 2019; 30 (4):352–356

[66] Kauvar AN. Successful treatment of melasma using a combination of microdermabrasion and Q-switched Nd:YAG lasers. Lasers Surg Med. 2012; 44(2):117–124

[67] Kauvar ANB. Commentary on the clinical and histological effect of a low-fluence Q-switched 1,064-nm neodymium: yttrium-aluminum-garnet laser for the treatment of melasma and solar lentigenes in Asians. Dermatol Surg. 2017; 43(9):1134–1136

[68] Brauer JA, Alabdulrazzaq H, Bae YS, Geronemus RG. Evaluation of a low energy, low density, non-ablative fractional 1927 nm wavelength laser for facial skin resurfacing. J Drugs Dermatol. 2015; 14(11): 1262–1267

[69] Vemula S, Maymone MBC, Secemsky EA, et al. Assessing the safety of superficial chemical peels in darker skin: a retrospective study. J Am Acad Dermatol. 2018; 79(3):508–513.e2

[70] Alexis AF. Lasers and light-based therapies in ethnic skin: treatment options and recommendations for Fitzpatrick skin types V and VI. Br J Dermatol. 2013; 169 Suppl 3:91–97

[71] Roberts WE, Henry M, Burgess C, Saedi N, Chilukuri S, Campbell-Chambers DA. Laser treatment of skin of color for medical and aesthetic uses with a new 650-microsecond Nd:YAG 1064 nm laser. J Drugs Dermatol. 2019; 18(4):s135–s137

[72] Kaushik SB, Alexis AF. Nonablative fractional laser resurfacing in skin of color: evidence-based review. J Clin Aesthet Dermatol. 2017; 10 (6):51–67

[73] Alexis AF, Coley MK, Nijhawan RI, et al. Nonablative fractional laser resurfacing for acne scarring in patients with Fitzpatrick skin phototypes IV-VI. Dermatol Surg. 2016; 42(3):392–402

[74] Clark CM, Silverberg JI, Alexis AF. A retrospective chart review to assess the safety of nonablative fractional laser resurfacing in Fitzpatrick skin types IV to VI. J Drugs Dermatol. 2013; 12(4):428–431

[75] Alexis AF. Fractional laser resurfacing of acne scarring in patients with Fitzpatrick skin types IV-VI. J Drugs Dermatol. 2011; 10(12) Suppl:s6–s7

[76] Lipper GM, Perez M. Nonablative acne scar reduction after a series of treatments with a short-pulsed 1,064-nm neodymium:YAG laser. Dermatol Surg. 2006; 32(8):998–1006

[77] Badawi A, Tome MA, Attoya A, Sami N, Morsy IA. Retrospective analysis of non-ablative scar treatment in dark skin types using the submillisecond Nd:YAG 1,064 nm laser. Lasers Surg Med. 2011; 43(2): 130–136

[78] Brauer JA, Kazlouskaya V, Alabdulrazzaq H, et al. Use of a picosecond pulse duration laser with specialized optic for treatment of facial acne scarring. JAMA Dermatol. 2015; 151(3):278–284

[79] Battle F, Battle S. Clinical evaluation of safety and efficacy of fractional radiofrequency facial treatment of skin type VI patients. J Drugs Dermatol. 2018; 17(11):1169–1172

[80] Emer JJ. Best practices and evidenced-based use of the 800 nm diode laser for the treatment of pseudofolliculitis barbae in skin of color. J Drugs Dermatol. 2011; 10(12) Suppl:s20–s22

[81] Kauvar AN. Treatment of pseudofolliculitis with a pulsed infrared laser. Arch Dermatol. 2000; 136(11):1343–1346

[82] Leheta TM. Comparative evaluation of long pulse alexandrite laser and intense pulsed light systems for pseudofolliculitis barbae treatment with one year of follow up. Indian J Dermatol. 2009; 54(4): 364–368

[83] Rogers CJ, Glaser DA. Treatment of pseudofolliculitis barbae using the Q-switched Nd:YAG laser with topical carbon suspension. Dermatol Surg. 2000; 26(8):737–742

[84] Ross EV, Cooke LM, Overstreet KA, Buttolph GD, Blair MA. Treatment of pseudofolliculitis barbae in very dark skin with a long pulse Nd:YAG laser. J Natl Med Assoc. 2002; 94(10):888–893

[85] Ross EV, Cooke LM, Timko AL, Overstreet KA, Graham BS, Barnette DJ. Treatment of pseudofolliculitis barbae in skin types IV, V, and VI with a long-pulsed neodymium:yttrium aluminum garnet laser. J Am Acad Dermatol. 2002; 47(2):263–270

[86] Schulze R, Meehan KJ, Lopez A, et al. Low-fluence 1,064-nm laser hair reduction for pseudofolliculitis barbae in skin types IV, V, and VI. Dermatol Surg. 2009; 35(1):98–107

[87] Smith EP, Winstanley D, Ross EV. Modified superlong pulse 810 nm diode laser in the treatment of pseudofolliculitis barbae in skin types V and VI. Dermatol Surg. 2005; 31(3):297–301

[88] Valeriant M, Terracina FS, Mezzana P. Pseudofolliculitis of the neck and the shoulder: a new effective treatment with alexandrite laser. Plast Reconstr Surg. 2002; 110(4):1195–1196

[89] Weaver SM , III, Sagaral EC. Treatment of pseudofolliculitis barbae using the long-pulse Nd:YAG laser on skin types V and VI. Dermatol Surg. 2003; 29(12):1187–1191

[90] Xia Y, Cho S, Howard RS, Maggio KL. Topical eflornithine hydrochloride improves the effectiveness of standard laser hair removal for treating pseudofolliculitis barbae: a randomized, double-blinded, placebo-controlled trial. J Am Acad Dermatol. 2012; 67(4):694–699

[91] Yamauchi PS, Kelly AP, Lask GP. Treatment of pseudofolliculitis barbae with the diode laser. J Cutan Laser Ther. 1999; 1(2):109–111

[92] Esmat SM, Abdel Hay RM, Abu Zeid OM, Hosni HN. The efficacy of laser-assisted hair removal in the treatment of acne keloidalis nuchae; a pilot study. Eur J Dermatol. 2012; 22(5):645–650

[93] Gamil HD, Khater EM, Khattab FM, Khalil MA. Successful treatment of acne keloidalis nuchae with erbium:YAG laser: a comparative study. J Cosmet Laser Ther. 2018; 20(7–8):419–423

[94] Tawfik A, Osman MA, Rashwan I. A novel treatment of acne keloidalis nuchae by long-pulsed alexandrite laser. Dermatol Surg. 2018; 44(3): 413–420

[95] Umar S. Selection criteria and techniques for improved cosmesis and predictable outcomes in laser hair removal treatment of acne keloidalis nuchae. JAAD Case Rep. 2019; 5(6):529–534

[96] Woo DK, Treyger G, Henderson M, Huggins RH, Jackson-Richards D, Hamzavi I. Prospective controlled trial for the treatment of acne keloidalis nuchae with a long-pulsed neodymium-doped yttrium-aluminum-garnet laser. J Cutan Med Surg. 2018; 22(2):236–238

[97] Krasner BD, Hamzavi FH, Murakawa GJ, Hamzavi IH. Dissecting cellulitis treated with the long-pulsed Nd:YAG laser. Dermatol Surg. 2006; 32(8):1039–1044

[98] Boyd AS, Binhlam JQ. Use of an 800-nm pulsed-diode laser in the treatment of recalcitrant dissecting cellulitis of the scalp. Arch Dermatol. 2002; 138(10):1291–1293

[99] Hamzavi IH, Griffith JL, Riyaz F, Hessam S, Bechara FG. Laser and light-based treatment options for hidradenitis suppurativa. J Am Acad Dermatol. 2015; 73(5) Suppl 1:S78–S81

[100] Badawi A, Kashmar M. Treatment of trichostasis spinulosa with 0.5-millisecond pulsed 755-nm alexandrite laser. Lasers Med Sci. 2011; 26(6):825–829

[101] Alexis AF, Alam M. Racial and ethnic differences in skin aging: implications for treatment with soft tissue fillers. J Drugs Dermatol. 2012; 11(8):s30–s32, discussion s32

[102] Taylor SC, Burgess CM, Callender VD. Safety of nonanimal stabilized hyaluronic acid dermal fillers in patients with skin of color: a randomized, evaluator-blinded comparative trial. Dermatol Surg. 2009; 35 Suppl 2:1653–1660

[103] Taylor SC, Downie JB, Shamban A, et al. Lip and perioral enhancement with hyaluronic acid dermal fillers in individuals with skin of color. Dermatol Surg. 2019; 45(7):959–967

[104] Burgess C, Awosika O. Ethnic and gender considerations in the use of facial injectables: African-American patients. Plast Reconstr Surg. 2015; 136(5) Suppl:28S–31S

[105] Sundaram H, Signorini M, Liew S, et al. Global Aesthetics Consensus Group. Global aesthetics consensus: botulinum toxin type a—evidence-based review, emerging concepts, and consensus recommendations for aesthetic use, including updates on complications. Plast Reconstr Surg. 2016; 137(3):518e–529e

[106] Sundaram H, Flynn T, Cassuto D, Lorenc ZP. New and emerging concepts in soft tissue fillers: roundtable discussion. J Drugs Dermatol. 2012; 11(8):s12–s24, discussion s25

[107] Liew S. Ethnic and gender considerations in the use of facial injectables: Asian patients. Plast Reconstr Surg. 2015; 136(5) Suppl:22S–27S

[108] Le TT, Farkas LG, Ngim RC, Levin LS, Forrest CR. Proportionality in Asian and North American Caucasian faces using neoclassical facial canons as criteria. Aesthetic Plast Surg. 2002; 26(1):64–69

[109] Tamura BM, Odo MY, Chang B, Cucé LC, Flynn TC. Treatment of nasal wrinkles with botulinum toxin. Dermatol Surg. 2005; 31(3):271–275

[110] Grimes PE. Skin and hair cosmetic issues in women of color. Dermatol Clin. 2000; 18(4):659–665

[111] Swee W, Klontz KC, Lambert LA. A nationwide outbreak of alopecia associated with the use of a hair-relaxing formulation. Arch Dermatol. 2000; 136(9):1104–1108

[112] Mirmirani P, Khumalo NP. Traction alopecia: how to translate study data for public education: closing the KAP gap? Dermatol Clin. 2014; 32(2):153–161

[113] Khumalo NP, Gumedze F. Traction: risk factor or coincidence in central centrifugal cicatricial alopecia? Br J Dermatol. 2012; 167(5):1191–1193

[114] Samrao A, Price VH, Zedek D, Mirmirani P. The "Fringe Sign": a useful clinical finding in traction alopecia of the marginal hair line. Dermatol Online J. 2011; 17(11):1

[115] Samrao A, Chen C, Zedek D, Price VH. Traction alopecia in a ballerina: clinicopathologic features. Arch Dermatol. 2010; 146(8):930–931

[116] Heath CR, Taylor SC. Alopecia in an ophiasis pattern: traction alopecia versus alopecia areata. Cutis. 2012; 89(5):213–216

[117] James J, Saladi RN, Fox JL. Traction alopecia in Sikh male patients. J Am Board Fam Med. 2007; 20(5):497–498

[118] Ozçelik D. Extensive traction alopecia attributable to ponytail hairstyle and its treatment with hair transplantation. Aesthetic Plast Surg. 2005; 29(4):325–327

[119] Olsen EA, Callender V, McMichael A, et al. Central hair loss in African American women: incidence and potential risk factors. J Am Acad Dermatol. 2011; 64(2):245–252

[120] Miteva M, Tosti A. Dermoscopy guided scalp biopsy in cicatricial alopecia. J Eur Acad Dermatol Venereol. 2013; 27(10):1299–1303

[121] Callender VD, Lawson CN, Onwudiwe OC. Hair transplantation in the surgical treatment of central centrifugal cicatricial alopecia. Dermatol Surg. 2014; 40(10):1125–1131

[122] Miteva M, Whiting D, Harries M, Bernardes A, Tosti A. Frontal fibrosing alopecia in black patients. Br J Dermatol. 2012; 167(1):208–210

[123] Miteva M, Tosti A. The follicular triad: a pathological clue to the diagnosis of early frontal fibrosing alopecia. Br J Dermatol. 2012; 166(2):440–442

[124] Moreno-Ramírez D, Ferrándiz L, Camacho FM. Diagnostic and therapeutic assessment of frontal fibrosing alopecia. Actas Dermosifiliogr. 2007; 98(9):594–602

[125] Park JH, You SH, Kim N. Frontal hairline lowering with hair transplantation in Asian women with high foreheads. Int J Dermatol. 2019; 58(3):360–364

[126] Epstein J, Bared A, Kuka G. Ethnic considerations in hair restoration surgery. Facial Plast Surg Clin North Am. 2014; 22(3):427–437

[127] Lam SM, Karamanovski E. Hair restoration in the ethnic patient and review of hair transplant fundamentals. Facial Plast Surg Clin North Am. 2010; 18(1):35–42

11 Aesthetic Concerns in Transgender Patients

Yunyoung C. Chang and Jennifer L. MacGregor

Summary

Transgender and nonbinary gender patients are an important population of consideration in male aesthetic dermatology. Although the reported prevalence and visibility of the transgender population has risen over the past decade, those who transition continue to encounter obstacles when it comes to receiving medical and cosmetic care by trained providers. Barriers to access include limited outreach, unfamiliarity of the patient on available procedures, insufficient numbers of trained providers, lack of psychosocial and community support, high costs, and delays while undergoing psychological evaluations. Dermatologists may play a central role in the aesthetic care of the transgender patient, by improving outreach, increasing patient education, adopting more inclusive office procedures, allowing quicker access to transitioning procedures, and offering safe, minimally invasive, and less time-consuming aesthetic treatments. It is important to note that transgender aesthetic preferences may not follow the traditional binary ideals of beauty, including "masculine versus feminine," and should be tailored as per individual patients. Although the impact of minimally invasive dermatologic procedures may be more modest than surgical treatments, dermatologic enhancements can help align appearance with a patient's gender identity, improve self-confidence, and, ultimately, improve the quality of life in the transgender population. This chapter will review the process of gender transition, available minimally invasive procedures for the face and body, and illustrative case examples.

Keywords: transgender, nonbinary, gender affirmation, nonsurgical cosmetic procedures, minimally invasive cosmetic procedures, noninvasive cosmetic procedures, masculinization, feminization

11.1 Background

11.1.1 Epidemiology of the Transgender Population

The prevalence of the transgender population has shown an upward trend, with study estimates reporting double the prevalence rates compared to a decade ago.[1,2] One recent study reported about 0.6% of adults, approximately 1.4 million, and 0.7% of youth aged 13 to 17 years, or approximately 150,000 youth, identify as transgender in the United States.[1] With the growth in the transgender population, medical providers including dermatologists must strive to improve their overall understanding, awareness, and knowledge in the medical care for this population.

11.2 Gender Transitioning

11.2.1 Overview: Medications and Surgical Procedures for Gender Transition

Gender transitioning refers to a process of aligning one's gender presentation with one's internal gender identity. Gender transitioning can occur on multiple levels, including social transitions, medical treatments, and/or surgical transformations.[3] Social transitions involve using a preferred name and pronouns, and some may legally change their name.

The use of cross-sex hormone therapy for medical reassignment has become more commonplace in the transgender population.[4] Transgender males (biologically female transitioning to male) may choose to undergo hormonal therapy with exogenous testosterone,[4] which suppresses female secondary sex characteristics and masculinizes transgender men. The physical changes can begin within 3 months of initiating therapy, including medically induced menopause, changes in the distribution of fat on the face and body, enhanced muscle mass, and increased libido. Later changes include increased clitoral size, vaginal skin atrophy, and a deepened voice.[4] Skin changes that occur with testosterone therapy include increased facial and body hair, increased oil production and acne, and male pattern hair loss.[4] Nonbinary individuals may also choose to undergo medical therapy, by balancing hormones based on their personal goals.

For transgender females (biologically male transitioning to female), hormonal therapy includes hormonal supplementation with estrogen, with or without antiandrogen therapies like spironolactone or cyproterone acetate.[4] The goal of therapy is to induce female secondary sex characteristics, including breast formation, fat redistribution, muscle mass reduction, testicular size decrease, and female patterned hair growth.[4,5] The skin can become drier and thinner, with less oil production and smaller pore size. The rate at which these desired physical changes occur after hormonal therapy initiation varies, ranging from within a few months to 2 to 3 years.[5] This rate will also depend on other factors, like genetics and age at which you start therapy. Although medical therapy alone may lead to significant visible changes (▶ Fig. 11.1), some patients desire faster, more immediate, and more striking physical changes. Minimally invasive aesthetic treatments, which will be discussed in detail later, can be used to further enhance the desired feminine appearance by softening and balancing features, contouring the face and body, and providing

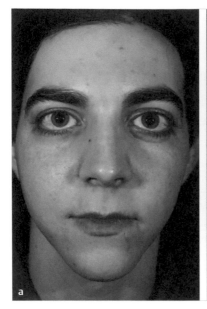 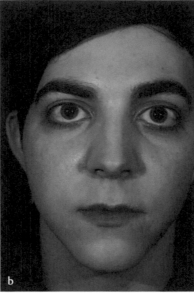

Fig. 11.1 (a) Before and (b) after hormonal therapy. Aesthetic changes include wider and more rounded convexities at temple and cheek. Also note the midface appears fuller with a softer and less angular contour through the mandible and chin.

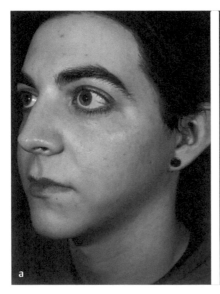 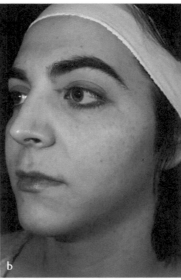

Fig. 11.2 (a) Before and (b) after facial fillers in the same patient resulted in additional widening at the temple, cheek, and tear trough with a softer and more rounded contour to the mandible and chin. The lips are subtly enhanced to reveal a more natural, feminine lip projection with elevated mouth corners.

more immediate results (▶ Fig. 11.2, ▶ Fig. 11.3, ▶ Fig. 11.4, ▶ Fig. 11.5, ▶ Fig. 11.6, ▶ Fig. 11.7).

Surgical gender reassignment procedures are also available for transgender patients in addition to medical therapy.[5] Based on guidelines set by the World Professional Association for Transgender Health (WPATH) and the Endocrine Society, transgender patients should have undergone 1 year of hormonal therapy and living as the desired gender prior to gender reassignment surgeries.[4] For transgender males, surgical options include oophorectomy, hysterectomy, scrotoplasty, phalloplasty, metoidioplasty, and chest masculinization surgery.[6] Procedures available for transgender females include removal of the testes (orchiectomy), creating a neovagina (vaginoplasty),

breast augmentation surgery, tracheal shave to soften the "Adam's apple" (chondrolaryngoplasty), and voice feminization surgery. Facial plastic surgery is commonly pursued to soften facial contours, including rhinoplasty, fat transfer, forehead and chin implants, brow lift and forehead lift surgery, and orthognathic surgery.[5] A population study published by Boston Medical Center between 2004 and 2015 reported 35% subjects had undergone at least one gender-affirming surgery, suggesting that the majority of transgender patients do not undergo any type of gender-affirmation surgery.[7] This low rate may be due to multiple reasons, including paucity of providers, high financial cost, lack of interest, or aversion to invasive procedures.

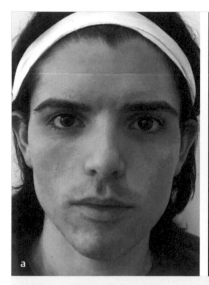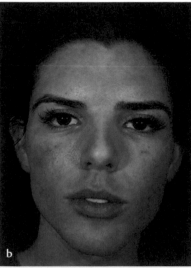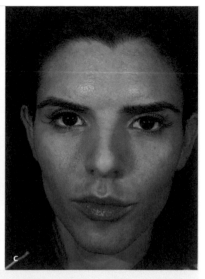

Fig. 11.3 **(a)** Before and **(b)** after laser hair removal to the lower face and neck, showing reduction in shadowing and softening of skin texture. This patient also received injectables to the upper face with botulinum toxin to smooth and gently arch the brow and facial fillers to the mid and lower face to enhance convexity of cheek, lips, and smooth contour of the mandible and chin. **(c)** After botulinum toxin injection to the masseter muscle, the face appears more heart shaped.

11.2.2 Quality of Life Relating to Gender Identity and Aesthetic Procedures

Research has shown that transgender individuals report a low quality of life (QOL) and high incidence of mental health issues. In effect, medical and surgical gender-affirming surgeries are associated with higher QOL and high patient satisfaction.[8,9] Despite this, even after transitioning, the transgender population continues to be at risk of lower QOL and mental health issues than the general population.[10] Cosmetic concerns are especially tied to the emotional well-being of transgender patients because, by definition, their perceived gender identity and desired aesthetic presentation to the world differ from their biological sex. Improving the cosmetic appearance of transgender individuals based on their individual aesthetics may, in turn, further improve their QOL.

11.2.3 Barriers to Care

In order to improve access to medical care, providers must consider the many barriers transgender individuals face as they navigate the transition process. Barriers to good medical care include patients' unfamiliarity with available procedures, paucity of trained providers in transgender health, delays while undergoing psychological evaluations, and high costs associated with required medications and surgical procedures. Additionally, distant location from metropolitan areas or large medical centers and lack of family or social support make access difficult for many patients. Medical providers may also become a barrier to good care. Physicians have the power to make themselves available or unavailable to transgender patients, provide transgender-friendly or transgender-unfriendly office environment, and to provide or delay prescriptions and cosmetic treatments at a pace that may not fit with the patient's desired timeline. Board-certified providers may charge more money for procedures, and lack of insurance coverage for cosmetic procedures may be cost prohibitive for those patients without available resources. Confronted with societal pressures to conform to a binary gender system and ideals of beauty while faced with these barriers to receiving treatment, transgender patients may experience worsening anxiety, depression, and despair. Given these barriers, some patients pursue medical and aesthetic care beyond traditional medical providers,[11] and may turn to illegal products, international internet prescriptions, or unlicensed or untrained providers. Unfortunately, cases of transgender patients resorting to "pumping," or using liquid silicone, or receiving care from secondary providers have been reported,[12,13] with associated complications. In contrast, it is optimal to receive aesthetic care from board-certified, trained medical physicians with experience in these procedures and dealing with the possible complications.

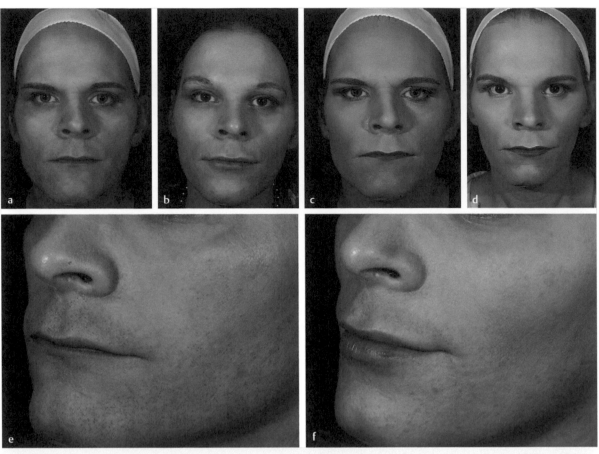

Fig. 11.4 (a) Before and (b) after injectable fillers to soften the temples, lift and smooth the depressed nasal root and reduce the prominent supraorbital brow ridges (with makeup removed). Additional lift to the brow was achieved after polydioxanone thread lifting, two treatments of microfocused ultrasound as well as botulinum toxin injection. (c) Before and (d) after with makeup showing the overall impact of upper face treatment as well as lower face. The lower face was treated with botulinum toxin injection to masseters to produce a more heart-shaped tapered jawline and fillers were used to enhance lip volume as well as lift the mouth corners and soften the chin/prejowl sulcus. Note that her lips will be treated in several sessions over time to gradually build volume while preserving a natural shape. (e) Before and (f) after oblique side angle showing the effect of lower face smoothing achieved with injectable facial filler, botulinum toxin, polydioxanone thread lifting, and laser hair removal.

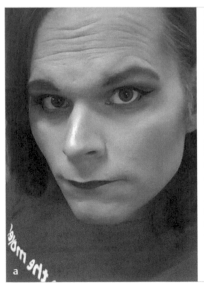

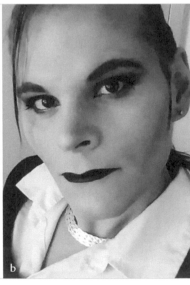

Fig. 11.5 (a,b) The patient's own "selfie" photos showing the before and after change achieved though minimally invasive aesthetic procedures including injectable fillers, botulinum toxin, microfocused ultrasound skin tightening, polydioxanone thread lifting, and laser hair removal.

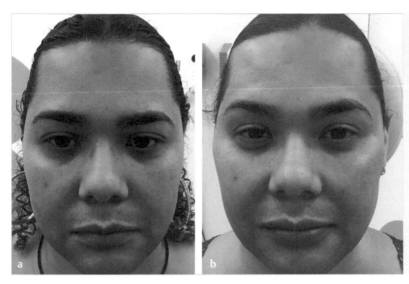

Fig. 11.6 (a) Before and **(b)** after single-session treatment with little to no downtime. This patient received botulinum toxin to the glabella and injectable filler to lift the tear trough and enhance convexities of the cheek and temple.

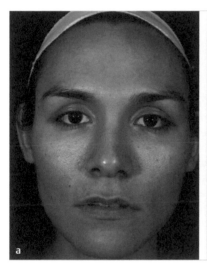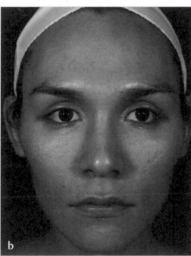

Fig. 11.7 (a) Before and **(b)** after injectable botulinum toxin to the upper face and masseters to create a brow lift and more heart-shaped face with tapering at the jawline. Injectable fillers were placed to widen the temples and cheeks as well as lift the mouth corners and plump body of the lip. Laser hair removal was also started for the upper lip and chin.

11.3 Improving Aesthetic Care through Minimally Invasive Aesthetic Procedures

11.3.1 Minimally Invasive Aesthetic Procedures

In addition to medical and surgical treatment options, all transgender patients may benefit from adjunct minimally invasive aesthetic procedures provided by dermatologists and other board-certified physicians. Minimally invasive aesthetic procedures may be more immediately available, provide results in a relatively short period of time with minimal downtime, and improve ultimate outcome during the transition process, thereby bridging the gap in receiving medical care and achieving desired aesthetic goals. Minimally invasive procedures are especially important for patients prior to and during the first year of hormonal/medical therapy while patients await physical changes and/or gender affirmation surgery. More immediately available procedures may help ease gender dysphoria, further increase self-esteem, and improve satisfaction with appearance and QOL.

Clinical Pearl: Never assume you know what your patient sees in the mirror or what procedure they might be seeking. Dermatologists should ask their transgender patients vague questions to assess their unique concerns. Consider asking "tell me what concerns you have" or simply looking in the mirror and saying "tell me what you see." Be sure to ask about what other treatments or procedures they are considering or have already planned so that you work within the framework of their overall transition with other physicians they might be working with (surgeons, psychiatrists, and endocrinologists).

Dermatologists can address specific cosmetic concerns including gender-affirming facial and body-contouring, hormone-related skin changes, and surgery-related scarring.[14,15] Injectables, like botulinum toxin injections and filler treatments, are performed in an outpatient medical setting with minimal risk and little downtime compared to surgical interventions. Facial injectables can be started immediately to enhance or diminish certain features and to masculinize or feminize features according to patients' aesthetic goals. Laser treatments and body-contouring devices are also available immediately and have high safety standards when performed by trained providers. With these noninvasive procedures, there is minimal need for psychologic vetting, medical pretreatment, or other delays that are routinely required prior to hormonal therapy and invasive surgery. They may also be more cost-effective for patients with more limited resources. In cisgender patients, minimally invasive aesthetic procedures have been shown to improve body image and QOL.[16]

Despite the growing medical literature regarding hormonal therapy and surgical procedures for gender transitioning, educational resources and published data regarding minimally invasive aesthetic procedures for transgender patients are sparse. Recently published reviews outline current dermatologic literature to instigate thought around this topic, but more detailed procedural outlines, case series, and larger studies on how dermatologists can contribute to the cosmetic transformation of the transgender patient would be helpful for the dermatologic community.[14,15,17,18,19] Studies are currently underway to assess QOL data in transgender individuals who have received minimally invasive aesthetic services. Growing literature may cultivate an increased number of providers qualified and comfortable in performing aesthetic treatments in this population, thereby increasing access and QOL, as well as aid in future counseling efforts. The remainder of this chapter will review the role of medical providers, detail available minimally invasive cosmetic procedures relating specifically to the transgender population, and exhibit with our case examples.

11.3.2 Role of Dermatologists and Other Medical Providers

Dermatologists and other medical care providers should keep an open mind when assessing transgender patients for aesthetic procedures, as goals may be to feminize, masculinize, both, or neither. Transgender individuals' aesthetic goals may diverge from the traditional gender paradigm of "masculine" or "feminine" ideals of beauty (▶ Table 11.1).[19,20,21] Accordingly, we advocate for a more flexible assessment of transgender patients. Practitioners should inquire about a patient's individual goals during the initial consultation and throughout follow-up visits, listen

Table 11.1 Traditionally "masculine" versus "feminine" facial features

Traditionally "masculine" features

- Higher, possibly receding hairline
- Wider more angular forehead
- Flat horizontal brow
- More prominent supraorbital brow ridges
- Wider mouth with thinner lips
- Longer, more square chin
- Wider more square lower face
- Beard hair or more coarse lower face skin texture
- Acute nasolabial angle

Traditionally "feminine" features

- Lower hairline
- Smooth, convex forehead
- Brows arch above softer orbital rim
- Eyes appear more open and/or wider set
- Convex, prominent cheek contour
- Heart-shaped, more tapered lower face
- Smaller lower face to upper face proportion
- Fuller vermillion contour and fuller lip body
- More obtuse nasolabial angle

to all patients, and discuss openly about their preferences, prior to proceeding with recommendations and treatments. As mentioned earlier, mental health issues remain a big issue in the transgender population. If any symptoms of mood changes or depression are detected, dermatologists should ensure that patients have a working relationship with a psychiatrist as well as strong social support.

As with all patients, the patient–physician relationship is important when dealing with transgender patients. Medical providers should avoid patronizing language regarding the patient's decisions, listen deliberately, and develop an individualized plan to help moving forward with the transition process. The office medical forms should be comprehensive of all gender orientations, and clinical staff should also be trained to inquire and address patients with their preferred pronouns and names. With supportive care and better outreach, dermatologists can bring more transgender patients into the care of board-certified and trained physicians.

11.3.3 Patient Preferences

A recent cross-sectional survey study of 327 people showed that a majority of transgender men reported prioritizing their face as the most essential body part to have changed, over the face or genitals.[14] These patients stated that they were mostly concerned about cosmetic procedures "looking good," more so than the risk of scars, complications, or other risks. In contrast, transgender women reported their face as the most essential body part to have changed. Of facial procedures, transgender women

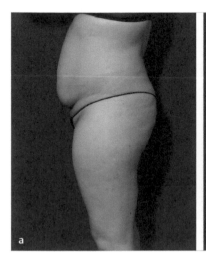
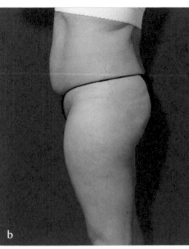

Fig. 11.8 (a) Before and (b) 2 months after abdominal cryolipolysis combined with three twice-monthly sessions of pulsed focused ultrasound in a transgender woman.

stated hair removal was the most preferred cosmetic treatment, followed by surgery and then injectables.[14] Transgender women reported seeking procedures mostly from plastic surgeons,[14] which may be due to patient preference, prior physician relationship, better outreach, or ease of access.

Clinical Pearl: Transgender men and women may have different priorities when it comes to cosmetic and aesthetic treatments, with a majority of transgender men focusing more on the chest and transgender women focusing more on the face based on one study. It is important to ask about individual patient preferences when performing initial consultations.

It would be helpful to have before and after treatment photos of transgender patients who have undergone available dermatologic procedures available to help with outreach and to allow for transgender patients to relate to the subjects, rather than relying on results from cisgender patient images. We postulate that minimally invasive aesthetic procedures performed by dermatologists may become more common and sought after in both transgender men and transgender women with better outreach as well as additional literature on the available procedures, patient preferences, and typical outcomes.

11.4 Available Procedures and Illustrative Examples

11.4.1 Transgender men (female to male transition)

Transgender men benefit from dermatologic care and minimally invasive aesthetic treatments, and more awareness on available procedures is needed in the general public. As stated previously, transgender men report that their primary aesthetic concern is their chest, rather than their face or genitals. In our experience, pseudogynecomastia (residual breast tissue) posthormonal therapy with exogenous testosterone does not respond well to minimally invasive treatments like cryolipolysis (▶ Fig. 11.8), and we routinely refer these patients for surgical correction. Noninvasive body contouring, like cryolipolysis and pulsed focused ultrasound, of other body areas, particularly in the abdomen, flanks, and submental regions, may be sought after and remains a good treatment option in transgender men.

Although possibly not a primary concern for transgender men, facial aesthetic treatments may be sought after by transgender men, and effective treatment options are available. Some transgender male patients report fluctuation in bone structure during testosterone injection cycles. We recommend baseline and follow-up photographs and evaluation at regular time points every few weeks to assess these changes and to achieve the desired outcome in transgender men. Facial contouring using injectable treatments has been used effectively in our practice to refine and enhance facial features. For the upper face, botulinum toxin injections are effective at flattening and strengthening the brow, with injection points in the forehead region. For the mid and lower face, injectable fillers can be used to create a more prominent and angular cheekbone and jawline (▶ Fig. 11.9). Of note, many transgender male patients in our experience prefer more medial cheek volumization as compared to lateral cheekbone heightening. On the face, facial hair growth preferences vary, with some transgender men electing to maintain new hair growth or shave, whereas others pursue laser hair removal after testosterone therapy. In transgender men, testosterone therapy may trigger or worsen increased oil production, acne, folliculitis, hyperpigmentation, and scarring.[22] Dermatologists can play a supportive role in controlling acne and folliculitis through medical therapy as well as giving skincare recommendations.[18] Scarring and

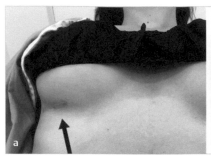
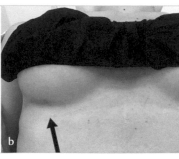

Fig. 11.9 (a) Before and (b) after two sessions of nonablative fractional laser resurfacing to blend breast augmentation scars in a transgender woman.

dyspigmentation from both acne and surgical procedures can be improved using topical retinoids, antioxidants, and peeling agents as well as multiple fractional laser resurfacing or microneedling with radiofrequency treatments. Some patients may develop male pattern or androgenetic alopecia during and after transitioning, in which approved therapies including topical minoxidil and follicular unit hair transplantation may be considered.

Clinical Pearl: In transgender men, testosterone therapy induces many changes in the skin and aesthetic contour of the face, including oily skin, acne, hair loss, and bone structure changes. Aesthetics may fluctuate during hormone injection cycles, so it is important to ask patients about this. Hormone therapy alone may not be sufficient to achieve a traditionally masculine jawline—these patients may benefit from injectable fillers.

11.4.2 Transgender Women (Male to Female Transition)

Transgender women report facial aesthetics is of primary importance to have changed when transitioning.[14] The face is less easily hidden from the outside world, as compared to the chest or genitals. Traditionally, "feminine" features include smooth facial outline, convex forehead with lower hairline, high, arched brows, open eyes, prominent cheek contour, fuller lips, and heart-shaped face structure (▶ Table 11.1). Medical therapy may help induce a more female appearance to the skin and face. Estrogen therapy reduces the thickness and growth rate of hair on the face as well as chest, back, and arms, but it rarely eliminates all the coarse, thick terminal hairs in the beard region. Laser hair removal in patients with dark hairs is an easy initial treatment for most transgender women[14] and can make a huge difference in patient satisfaction in our experience (▶ Fig. 11.3, ▶ Fig. 11.4, ▶ Fig. 11.7). Important to note, it often takes more than the average six to eight treatment sessions for optimal response in the authors' experience, and electrolysis remains an option for patients who are not candidates for laser hair removal. Other changes expected from estrogen therapy include mild softening and rounding of the forehead and filling in of the temple, cheek/midface and

mandible, resulting from shifts in and increase of the subcutaneous fat. These changes ultimately result in less angular facial features (▶ Fig. 11.1), but may take 2 or more years to fully develop.

Patients wishing for more rapid or additional enhancements may consider minimally invasive treatments, such as injectable botulinum toxin, soft-tissue fillers, thread lifting (with polydioxanone or Poly-L-lactic acid sutures), and energy-based tightening devices, which can all be used in combination for optimal results (▶ Fig. 11.3, ▶ Fig. 11.4, ▶ Fig. 11.5, ▶ Fig. 11.6, ▶ Fig. 11.7). Patients with prominent supraorbital brow ridges, low-set, flat, or heavy eyebrows, and depressed nasal root may benefit from upper face botulinum toxin, filler injectables, thread lifting, and skin tightening in combination. Specifically, transgender women tend to have more prominent facial muscles at baseline, including a stronger frontalis, heavier and more prominent glabella complex, and larger, hypertrophied masseter muscles. These muscles can be treated with botulinum toxin injections to relax, soften, and atrophy the muscles as needed (▶ Fig. 11.3, ▶ Fig. 11.4, ▶ Fig. 11.6, ▶ Fig. 11.7). In our experience, transgender women typically require higher dosages of botulinum toxin than their cisgender counterparts to achieve optimal response. Over years of treatment, shrinkage or thinning of these muscle groups can be seen, without the need for surgical intervention and may be an option in patients who are unwilling to undergo surgery. Flat or heavy eyebrows may be lifted chemically using botulinum toxin ("liquid brow lift"), resulting in an average of 1-mm lift and also opening up of the eyes (▶ Fig. 11.3, ▶ Fig. 11.4a, ▶ Fig. 11.6, ▶ Fig. 11.7). Strategically placed filler injections around the brow and in the temples may further lift the eyebrow (▶ Fig. 11.4a, ▶ Fig. 11.7). Thread lifts with barbs or cones can be placed in the forehead from the frontotemporal hairline to lift up, and microfocused ultrasound of the forehead stimulates collagen to produce a gradual brow lift (▶ Fig. 11.4a). Those with particularly heavy brows or prominent supraorbital brow ridges that are not adequately improved with minimally invasive techniques may elect for surgical treatment for more dramatic improvements. Patients with a flatter midface and cheek and hollow tear troughs may benefit from volumization and widening of the facial structures to enhance the convexities, soften the contours, and augment a heart-shaped face (▶ Fig. 11.2, ▶ Fig. 11.3, ▶ Fig. 11.6, ▶ Fig. 11.7). This can be obtained with filler injections to the lateral cheeks, temples, tear troughs, and forehead to enhance bone structure, as well as botulinum toxin injections at high doses to the masseter muscle to slim the jawline (▶ Fig. 11.2, ▶ Fig. 11.3, ▶ Fig. 11.4b, ▶ Fig. 11.7). Of note, patients of all gender identities or also based on ethnic preference may wish to maintain a stronger or angular jawline, and this should be asked of the patient.

For the lower face, the lips can be defined and shaped based on patient aesthetics by adding volume to the vermilion border (▶ Fig. 11.2) and/or volumized by adding filler to the body of the lip at the wet–dry border (▶ Fig. 11.3, ▶ Fig. 11.4b, ▶ Fig. 11.7). The angular and depressed areas of the perioral and chin area can also be softened with the use of filler injections to blend the contrasting facial regions and shadows (▶ Fig. 11.4b, c). The chin can be volumized to create a pointier and more tapered jawline, and botulinum toxin injections to the chin can be used to relax mentalis dimpling.

Some transgender female patients may present already pleased with their natural features, just wishing for a small, subtle enhancement of their beauty or to make small adjustments to specific areas. Individual aesthetics, personal preferences, and/or cultural influences may determine a patient's ultimate aesthetic goals. As a case illustration, the patient in ▶ Fig. 11.7 was happy with her overall appearance on initial presentation, and small changes made a significant improvement in her overall proportions and confidence. Our patient requested a higher, more arched brow and a more "feminine" jawline. A single session of injectable botulinum toxin to the glabellar complex and masseters, along with strategically placed droplets of hyaluronic acid (HA) filler to the temples, lateral cheeks, body of the lip, and perioral region, allowed us to open up her eyes and widen the upper face to achieve a more "heart-shaped face" (▶ Fig. 11.7). Improving facial proportions, by widening the upper face, lifting the nasolabial angle, or adding small volumes of filler to the nasal root or nasal dorsum (nonsurgical or "liquid" rhinoplasty) as well as the lips can make a larger nose appear less prominent and more lifted (▶ Fig. 11.4, ▶ Fig. 11.5, ▶ Fig. 11.7).

At the time of writing this chapter, there have been little data in the medical literature about transgender women's attitudes or preferences on body contouring. Based on the authors' experience, the primary areas of concern for body contouring tend to be the abdomen, flanks, inner thighs, and bra line adiposity, and these areas respond well to cryolipolysis, pulsed focused ultrasound, and radiofrequency fat reduction devices (▶ Fig. 11.10). Some patients request hip and buttock augmentation, which can be obtained through a series of filler injections with PLLA.[23] Prior to treatment, we must counsel that the volume of product required over multiple sessions for these

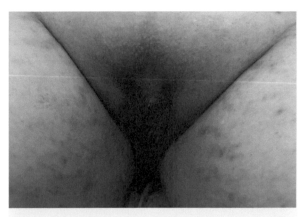

Fig. 11.10 Postoperative result of vaginoplasty in a transgender woman. Scars are not noticeable and require no treatment. She was recently treated for folliculitis and will first receive a topical regimen to fade resulting pigmentation.

areas is large and may be cost prohibitive.[11,13] Fat harvesting and transplantation may be another option for these patients.

It is also important to note potential negative dermatologic side effects from estrogen therapy that may present in transgender women during the transition process. Melasma is known to be triggered or worsened with exogenous estrogens and may present as a new aesthetic concern for transgender women. Melasma can occur anytime during and after transitioning, and it is unclear if it improves off of estrogen therapy. Melasma may respond partially to topical treatments, including sunscreens, hydroquinone, chemical peels, antioxidants, and retinoids. Laser treatments, like low-density, low-energy 1927-nm fractional resurfacing, and picosecond devices are also options to accelerate lightening of pigmentation and to maintain remission.[24] New angiomas or broken capillaries due to estrogen can also be treated with lasers, like the 532-nm potassium titanyl phosphate (KTP) laser or 595-nm pulsed dye laser (PDL). Similarly, new leg veins secondary to estrogen can be treated with vascular lasers or with sclerotherapy. New-onset cellulite from hormonal therapy can be temporarily smoothened with radiofrequency and infrared-based energy devices. New-onset striae can be treated with vascular lasers, nonablative fractional resurfacing, microneedling, biostimulatory fillers, or a combination. In patients with preexisting androgenetic alopecia or "male pattern hair loss," estrogen therapy typically does not improve a receding hairline or halt progression of disease. Topical minoxidil and platelet-rich plasma (PRP) are treatment options and may be continued in transgender females to prevent worsening of hairline recession. Transgender women may also be evaluated for follicular unit hair transplantation to restore a lower frontal hairline and to cover a thinning vertex, especially if longer hairstyles are desired. Importantly, maintenance treatments with topical minoxidil should be continued after hair transplantation. Following estrogen therapy, some of our patients have also reported loss of mandibular size and structure, resulting in skin laxity and submental adiposity. These patients may benefit from jawline and chin filler (HA, PLLA, calcium hydroxyapatite [CaHA]) to replace mandibular size, thread lifts to the lower face to support the skin, skin tightening with radiofrequency or microfocused ultrasound, and fat reduction with cryolipolysis or deoxycholate injections. In addition, surgical reassignment surgeries, including breast augmentation (top surgery), vaginoplasty (bottom surgery), and chondrolaryngoplasty (Adam's apple surgery"), yield scarring in most patients. If these scars are undesirable, vascular lasers, laser resurfacing, or microneedling with radiofrequency are available treatment options that have yielded good results in our patients (▸ Fig. 11.11, ▸ Fig. 11.12).

Clinical Pearl: A combination of aesthetic procedures is likely the best option for reaching desired aesthetic outcomes in transgender women, including facial contouring to produce softer lines, body contouring, and treatment of estrogen-related skin conditions like melasma. Be specific when discussing goals (e.g., do you think you might like a more arched or angled brow, fuller lower lip, etc.)

11.4.3 Nonbinary Gender Status

Although some transgender individuals identify as male or female, others may not identify with a specific preset gender. There has been an increased awareness of nonbinary or intersex gender status through media, art, film, and politics.[25-28] Individuals with nonbinary status may be due to ambiguous genitalia at birth, personal preference, or both. These individuals may choose to decide a gender identity in early adulthood or remain nonbinary gender status throughout adulthood. Many advocates recommend holding off on medical, surgical, and aesthetic treatment options until this decision is made after infancy or childhood. Medical professionals should ask what pronouns or names these patients prefer and all electronic or paper forms should be inclusive for all gender identities. Dermatologists should always have an open discussion about individual aesthetic preferences, without assuming a traditionally binary aesthetic system.

Clinical Pearl: Many transgender patients will not like to view their clinical photographs, so always ask if they want to see photos before showing them. Seeing an image where you look different than you hope or envision can be upsetting. Instead, ask open-ended questions, listen carefully to individual preferences, and

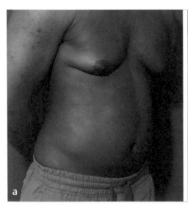
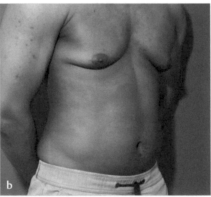

Fig. 11.11 A transgender man (a) before and (b) after coolsculpting to the chest. No change is seen and the patient ultimately sought surgical correction.

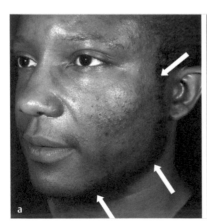
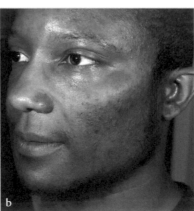

Fig. 11.12 (a) Before and (b) immediately after a single session of facial fillers to strengthen and contour the temple, zygoma, mandible, and chin with calcium hydroxylapatite. Testosterone-induced acne is also seen and the patient has started topical retinoids and a brightening/peeling regimen.

base treatment recommendations on this open dialogue. At each visit, ask what they like (or don't) and remain flexible about changing the plan according to interim results.

11.5 Conclusion

Dermatologists can play a critical role in the gender transition process for transgender and nonbinary gender status individuals, by aiding in general dermatologic skin conditions arising from hormonal treatments as well as offering minimally invasive aesthetic procedures. Although medical and surgical reassignment treatments may induce aesthetic transformations, barriers to access and anatomic changes may be slower and more subtle than desired. Some transgender patients may also be averse to surgical options and subsequent scarring. Minimally invasive aesthetic procedures can bridge the gap by allowing for immediate treatment options, serving as an adjunct to medical or surgical therapy, or as an alternative in patients who do not want to undergo surgery yet still desire aesthetic enhancements. We predict more patients will seek minimally invasive aesthetic treatments, especially with better outreach and awareness. Thus, more dermatologic literature is needed on the most effective, safest treatments we can provide to our patients. Importantly, we should not make assumptions about any patient's aesthetic preferences but should rather have an open discussion about these preferences throughout our evaluation procedure. Rather than being patronizing or clinging to one's own preconceptions of gender status, medical providers should listen to their patients and personalize treatments based on individual patient's needs. When we ask our transgender patients about suggestions they would give to their doctors, we repeatedly hear: "I feel that doctors should listen more than talk and try to understand where the patient is coming from rather than their own opinions. Everyone's journey is different." We hope this book chapter is the first of many steps to understand and provide the best care for our transgender and nonbinary patients.

11.6 Pearls

- Minimally invasive aesthetic procedures provide results in a relatively short period of time with minimal downtime, and improve ultimate outcome during the transition process, thus bridging the gap in receiving medical care and achieving desired aesthetic goals.
- A majority of transgender women reported their face as the most essential body part to have changed.
- In contrast, transgender men reported prioritizing their chest over the face or genitals.
- Pseudogynecomastia (residual breast tissue) post-hormonal therapy with exogenous testosterone does not respond well to minimally invasive treatments like cryolipolysis and such patients are routinely referred for surgical correction.
- In transgender men, testosterone therapy may trigger or worsen increased oil production, acne, folliculitis, hyperpigmentation, and scarring.
- Dermatologists can play a critical role in the gender transition process for transgender and non-binary gender status individuals, by aiding dermatologic skin conditions arising from hormonal treatments as well as offering minimally-invasive aesthetic procedures.

References

[1] The Williams Institute UCLA School of Law. Estimates of Transgender Populations in States with Legislation Impacting Transgender People (Update): How Many Adults Identify as Transgender in the United States? June 2016. Available at: http://williamsinstitute.law.ucla.edu/wp-content/uploads/How-Many-Adults-Identify-as-Transgender-in-the-United-States.pdf. Accessed Nov 11 2018

[2] The Williams Institute UCLA School of Law. Estimates of Transgender Populations in States with Legislation Impacting Transgender People (Update): Age of Individuals who Identify as Transgender in the United States, Jan 2017. Available at: https://williamsinstitute.law.ucla.edu/wp-content/uploads/TransAgeReport.pdf. Accessed Nov 11, 2018

[3] White Hughto JM, Reisner SL, Pachankis JE. Transgender stigma and health: a critical review of stigma determinants, mechanisms, and interventions. Soc Sci Med. 2015; 147:222–231

[4] Unger CA. Hormone therapy for transgender patients. Transl Androl Urol. 2016; 5(6):877–884

[5] Tangpricha V, den Heijer M. Oestrogen and anti-androgen therapy for transgender women. Lancet Diabetes Endocrinol. 2017; 5(4):291–300

[6] Irwig MS. Testosterone therapy for transgender men. Lancet Diabetes Endocrinol. 2017; 5(4):301–311

[7] Kailas M, Lu HMS, Rothman EF, Safer JD. Prevalence and types of gender-affirming surgery among a sample of transgender endocrinology patients prior to state expansion of insurance coverage. Endocr Pract. 2017; 23(7):780–786

[8] Gorin-Lazard A, Baumstarck K, Boyer L, et al. Is hormonal therapy associated with better quality of life in transsexuals? A cross-sectional study. J Sex Med. 2012; 9(2):531–541

[9] Wierckx K, Van Caenegem E, Elaut E, et al. Quality of life and sexual health after sex reassignment surgery in transsexual men. J Sex Med. 2011; 8(12):3379–3388

[10] Jellestad L, Jäggi T, Corbisiero S, et al. Quality of life in transitioned trans persons: a retrospective cross-sectional cohort study. BioMed Res Int. 2018; 2018:8684625

[11] Walker H.. Body of work: from DIY hormones to silicone injections, why some trans women choose to transition outside the medical industry. Out Magazine. 2019:75–78

[12] Murariu D, Holland MC, Gampper TJ, Campbell CA. Illegal silicone injections create unique reconstructive challenges in transgender patients. Plast Reconstr Surg. 2015; 135(5):932e–933e

[13] Pinto TP, Teixeira FDB, Barros CRDS, et al. Use of industrial liquid silicone to transform the body: prevalence and factors associated with its use among transvestites and transsexual women in São Paulo, Brazil. Cad Saude Publica. 2017; 33(7):e00113316

[14] Ginsberg BA, Calderon M, Seminara NM, Day D. A potential role for the dermatologist in the physical transformation of transgender people: a survey of attitudes and practices within the transgender community. J Am Acad Dermatol. 2016; 74(2):303–308

[15] Ginsberg BA. Dermatologic care of the transgender patient. Int J Womens Dermatol. 2016; 2(1):65–67

[16] Sobanko JF, Dai J, Gelfand JM, Sarwer DB, Percec I. Prospective cohort study investigating changes in body image, quality of life, and self-esteem following minimally invasive cosmetic procedures. Dermatol Surg. 2018; 44(8):1121–1128

[17] Marks DH, Awosika O, Rengifo-Pardo M, Ehrlich A. Dermatologic surgical care for transgender individuals. Dermatol Surg. 2019; 45(3): 446–457

[18] Boos MD, Ginsberg BA, Peebles JK. Prescribing isotretinoin for transgender youth: A pledge for more inclusive care. Pediatr Dermatol. 2019; 36(1):169–171

[19] Ascha M, Swanson MA, Massie JP, et al. Nonsurgical Management of Facial Masculinization and Feminization. Aesthet Surg J. 2019; 39(5): NP123–NP137

[20] Altman K. Facial feminization surgery: current state of the art. Int J Oral Maxillofac Surg. 2012; 41(8):885–894

[21] Carruthers JD, Glogau RG, Blitzer A, Facial Aesthetics Consensus Group Faculty. Advances in facial rejuvenation: botulinum type a, hyaluronic acid dermal fillers and combination therapies-consensus recommendations. Plast Reconstr Surg. 2008; 121(5) Suppl:5S–30S

[22] Wierckx K, Van de Peer F, Verhaeghe E, et al. Short- and long-term clinical skin effects of testosterone treatment in trans men. J Sex Med. 2014; 11(1):222–229

[23] Lin MJ, Dubin DP, Khorasani H. Poly-L-lactic acid for minimally invasive gluteal augmentation. Dermatol Surg. v

[24] Trivedi MK, Yang FC, Cho BK. A review of laser and light therapy in melasma. Int J Womens Dermatol. 2017; 3(1):11–20

[25] Cory Dawson, Hanne Gaby Odiele, Emily Quinn, Pidgeon Pagonis, Evaan Kheraj. These Activists Get REAL About Being Intersex. https://video.teenvogue.com/watch/these-activists-get-real-about-being-intersex. Released on June 27, 2017. Accessed April 10, 2019

[26] Hanne Gaby, Chase Strangio, Katrina Karkazis, LaLa Zannell, Maria Tridas, Lucy Diavolo, Wazi Maret. 5 Common Misconceptions About Sex and Gender. https://video.teenvogue.com/watch/5-common-misconceptions-about-sex-and-gender. Released on March 29, 2019. Accessed April 10, 2019

[27] https://www.rivergallo.com/about. Accessed April 10, 2019

[28] Susan Miller (USA Today). California becomes first state to condemn intersex surgeries on children. https://www.usatoday.com/story/news/nation/2018/08/28/intersex-surgeries-children-california-first-state-condemn/1126185002/. Published August 28, 2018. Accessed on April 10, 2019

12 Bringing it All Home: Conclusions and Future Considerations

Brian P. Hibler, Merrick A. Brodsky, Andrés M. Erlendsson, and Anthony M. Rossi

Summary

This chapter summarizes the fundamental approaches to the male cosmetic patient with regard to various aesthetic treatments. Increasingly, men are becoming more conscious about the health and appearance of their skin, and the demand for cosmetic procedures among male patients is steadily rising. Appreciating differences in anatomy, biochemical differences in skin, and different aesthetic ideals between male and female patients is critical for achieving the best outcome. Alterations in current aesthetic techniques and dosing, gender-specific uses of existing devices, and overall approaches need to be modified to obtain results suitable for the male patient. More than ever, tailoring minimally invasive cosmetic procedures to match an individual's gender (or gender identity) is becoming an important objective. Herein, we review the key take-home points and approaches to the male cosmetic patient.

Keywords: male, aesthetics, cosmetics, gender, sexual dimorphism, dermal fillers, neuromodulators, hair transplantation, lasers

12.1 Background

The demand for cosmetic procedures among male patients is steadily rising. Additionally, younger male patients are becoming more proactive by choosing preventative skin care treatments. Appreciating differences in anatomy, biochemical differences in skin, and different aesthetic ideals between male and female patients is critical for achieving the best outcome.[1,2] Alterations in current aesthetic techniques and dosing, gender-specific uses of existing devices, and overall approaches need to be modified to obtain results suitable for the male patient. Although once overlooked, tailoring minimally invasive cosmetic procedures to match an individual's gender (or gender identity) is becoming an important objective. In this chapter, we summarize the key take-home points and approaches to the male cosmetic patient.

12.2 Anatomy

Similar to women, men deal with signs of intrinsic and extrinsic aging, including issues such as photoaging, fat loss, and wrinkles. However, male skin—on both the face and the body—has several important differences to consider. Moreover, differences in key defining facial and body features produce what is considered a "male" or "female" physique, knowledge of which is paramount for physicians performing cosmetic procedures.

12.2.1 The Skin

There are a number of anatomical and biochemical differences between male and female skin. In general, male skin is thicker,[3–6] and androgens have been shown to play a major role in regulating dermal thickness.[7] As men age, the collagen content decreases at a steady rate; meanwhile, due to the effects of estrogen, female skin maintains its thickness until more abrupt thinning occurs after menopause. This later but more rapid decline leads to increased signs of aging relative to male counterparts in the late fifth to sixth decades of life.[8] Overall, men have greater skeletal muscle mass than women.[9] There are sex differences in facial muscle movement, with men having greater facial movement after adjusting for facial size[10]; when combined with their thicker skin, these factors can result in deeper facial furrows. Decreased adherence to photoprotection can also lead to increased signs of extrinsic photoaging in men, including dyspigmentation, rhytid formation, and solar elastosis. For example, the Favre–Racouchot disease is a cosmetic dermatosis induced by chronic sun exposure often seen in concert with other signs of photoaging (e.g., cutis rhomboidalis nuchae, periorbital rhytids), and is more common in fair-skinned male patients with history of significant ultraviolet (sun) exposure.[11]

Male facial skin typically has a greater sebum output than female skin, leading to more oily and acne-prone skin, though there can be variability between individuals.[12] Sebum production may be increased by androgens[13] and decreased by estrogens,[14,15] and the greatest gender differences in sebum production are observed after age 50.[12,13] On the other hand, the increased number of sebaceous glands translates to decreased risk of facial xerosis compared with females, and can result in having naturally shinier facial skin. Various hygiene practices can also lead to different skin concerns in men versus women, such as frequent shaving resulting in sensitive skin and local irritation or "razor burn."

12.2.2 Facial Features

A major concern among men considering facial cosmetic procedures is a worry about "looking done," or drastically changing their appearance. Although they may not be able to communicate the specific features differentiating a traditionally "male" versus "female" face, most men are subconsciously aware of factors that are considered more masculine or feminine (▶ Table 12.1).

The overall skeletal framework of the head is different between men and women, with women having a skull about four-fifths the size of the male skull.[16] Men and women have different craniofacial shapes; as such,

Table 12.1 Differences in key male and female facial/body characteristics

Facial features	
• Larger skull	• Smaller skull
• Strong brow ridge	• Soft brow ridge
• Straight eyebrows	• Arched, curved eyebrows
• Equally proportioned upper/lower facial features	• More prominent upper face features
• Angular shapes with prominent bones and muscles	• Heart-shaped face with fuller cheeks, smoother forms
• Broad nose	• Narrow nose
• Strong, chiseled jawline	• Narrower, softer jawline
• Square chin	• Smaller, pointed chin
• Thinner upper lip	• Fuller upper lip
Body contours	
• V-shaped torso	• Curvilinear torso
• Defined pectoralis and abdominal wall muscles	• Hourglass shape, widest point at hips

women seek to have a tapered, heart-shaped face with more prominent upper facial features, whereas men desire a more square, chiseled jawline with equally proportioned facial features between the upper and lower face.[17]

Assessment of the upper, mid, and lower face highlights key sexual dimorphic traits. Men prefer a more horizontal, lower-set eyebrow position than females, which is an important consideration when performing neuromodulation of the forehead. Additionally, the male forehead is flatter compared with a convex, feminine forehead. Tear troughs can be a cosmetic concern for both men and women, though men tend to develop more severe sagging of the lower eyelid at a later age.[18] The inferior orbital rim tends to recede laterally in females, whereas males have recession of the entire inferior orbital rim, which may contribute to the gender differences in periocular aging.[19] The development of malar mounds and festoons is likely multifactorial, including the natural aging process, genetics, sun exposure, and smoking. Of note, at the malar eminence, where there is maximal cheek projection, women have, on average, 3 mm thicker subcutaneous fat.[20] Men naturally have thinner upper lips than women, and although lip augmentation with fillers may not be as commonly requested, for the right patient it may be aesthetically appealing. Although thinning of the lips occurs with age in both sexes, restoring volume to produce a large upper lip should be done conservatively for a natural-appearing outcome. Male pattern baldness and treatment of facial and neck hair are other common cosmetic concerns. Treatment of male pattern baldness can produce a more youthful, masculine look. However, when it comes to hair reduction treatments for excess growth, overtreatment on the face and beard area may create a feminine appearance, necessitating appropriate skill and experience of the treating physician. The lower face, particularly a square jawline, is considered a defining male feature that is highly sought after. A strong jawline can be achieved through multiple avenues, which may include reduction of jowls, submental fat reduction, or enhancement of the jawline with dermal fillers.

12.2.3 Body Contouring

The ideal male body entails a trim, athletic build with a "V-shaped" torso, where the body's greatest width is at the shoulders and tapers to the narrowest point at the waist. As men age, however, they often develop areas of fat, which accumulate in the abdomen, flanks, breast, and the neck and chin. These are often targeted via either invasive, minimally invasive, or noninvasive body contouring techniques.

One of the first steps in achieving a "V-shaped" torso includes reduction of fat deposits at the flanks, or "love handles," and sculpting of the abdomen. Liposuction of the abdomen was the most common surgical cosmetic procedure for men as of 2018.[21] Along with contouring the abdomen, surgical breast reduction for gynecomastia and pseudogynecomastia is increasing in popularity and was the second most popular surgical cosmetic procedure for men in 2018. Male surgical breast reduction increased by nearly 50% between 2014 and 2018, and increased by almost 200% over the past 20 years.[21,22] Increasingly, less invasive treatments including cryolipolysis, radiofrequency (RF) treatments, and low-level laser therapy are being employed to target focal areas of excess fat. A temperature-controlled multifrequency monopolar RF device (truSculpt 3D, Cutera, Brisbane, California, United States) was shown to decrease abdominal fat by 24% at 12 weeks after a single treatment.[23] In a similar fashion, a monopolar RF device with targeted pressure energy (BTL Unison, BTL Industries, Boston, Massachusetts, United States) significantly improved gluteofemoral cellulite after four weekly treatments as measured by clinical and ultrasound assessment.[24]

For men who desire increased definition of a particular muscle group, implants, such as pectoral or calf implants, may be placed to create cosmetic fullness. Other strategies, including pectoral and abdominal wall "etching," can be performed to create the perception of increased tone. New devices utilizing high-intensity focused electromagnetic (HIFEM) technology (Emsculpt, BTL Industries) are showing promising results for abdominal body sculpting via abdominal muscle hypertrophy and simultaneous reduction in subcutaneous fat.[25] This approach is also being explored for noninvasive buttock lifting and toning of gluteal muscles.[26] Small applicators have been approved by the Food and Drug Administration (FDA) for use on the arms, calves, and thighs, though studies of their efficacy at this time are limited.[27]

12.3 Approach to Aesthetic Procedures in the Male Patient

There are many ways in which performing cosmetic procedures in male patients differs from that in female patients. This may include modifications in the cosmetic consultation or alterations in the technique of the procedure. Although the key aspects of various cosmetic procedures have already been reviewed in extensive detail in the earlier chapters, here we will summarize important points regarding the general approach to cosmetic procedures in male patients.

12.3.1 Cosmetic Consultation

One of the most important aspects of performing cosmetic procedures on any patient is the initial consultation. It is important to assess the patient's own perception of their body and what enhancements they would like to make. Men often seek cosmetic treatment to appear "good for their age," to appear more youthful, and improve their perceived competitiveness in the workplace.[28] In a study of male patients seeking elective cosmetic procedures, the crow's feet and tear troughs were rated most likely to be treated first, followed by forehead wrinkles.[28] Unlike females who are often more in tune to cosmetic trends, male patients are frequently unsure of their options for rejuvenation. Other times, male patients may present for consultation at the behest of their partner, and don't know what they want other than to look "refreshed" or "more youthful." As such, it is always important to have the patient look into the mirror and describe what features concern them and what they desire to change. At this point, depending on the desired outcome, they can be informed of their surgical and nonsurgical options,

The timing of specific cosmetic procedures may vary between men and women. Increasingly, younger males are looking for preventative rejuvenation to maintain their appearance. The cosmetic concerns of younger versus older patients may shift focus; younger males may be more concerned with body contouring and fat reduction, whereas older males may be concerned by deep static rhytids and loss of soft tissue in the face. When starting to perform cosmetic procedures in male patients, it is important to take a staged approach. Men often desire subtle augmentation, such that it is not readily apparent they had cosmetic work performed.

Concerns about body image are often assumed to relate predominantly to females, but are becoming increasingly prevalent among men. Although most bodily concerns are not pathological, 1 in 50 men meet the diagnostic criteria for body dysmorphic disorder (BDD).[29] Signs of BDD include mirror checking or avoidance, reassurance seeking, touching disliked areas, excessive exercise, comparing appearance with that of others, excessive tanning, and seeking cosmetic procedures.[30] Patients with BDD are prevalent in aesthetic practices, and it is important to be able to identify these individuals.

BDD typically starts during teenage years and without proper intervention continues throughout adulthood.[31] Individuals with BDD exhibit poor insight into the condition and will seek cosmetic or dermatological treatment to treat the perceived "defects" rather than confront the underlying dysmorphia. Patients with BDD are hard to satisfy, and cosmetic procedures rarely improve their bodily perception. Dissatisfied BDD patients are more likely to threaten with malpractice lawsuits than others, and thus, extensive documentation is especially important when consulting these patients.[32] Treating BDD patients cosmetically may also feed into their dysmorphia by acknowledging that there is a "defect" to treat and that can potentially make the condition worse. If concerns about BDD arise during a consultation, BDD screening instruments such as "Cosmetic Procedure Screening Questionnaire (COPS) for Body Dysmorphic Disorder" can be used to assess the patient.[33] Trying to reassure the patient that their body is "normal" is not advised. Instead, focusing on the time, distress, disability, cost, or lost opportunities triggered by the bodily obsession can help put the problem into context and support a conversation about their issue. Effective treatment options are available and most often include a combination of cognitive behavior therapy and pharmacological agents, such as selective serotonin reuptake inhibitors.[34]

12.3.2 Combination Therapeutic Approach

To achieve desired aesthetic results, combining different treatment modalities is often required. Determining the optimal therapies and the order they should be administered is crucial for optimizing patient outcome and satisfaction.[35]

As a first step, it is important to review the patient's skin care routine. Most patients should use a moisturizer

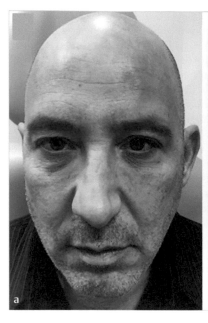
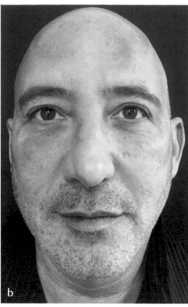

Fig. 12.1 Before and after combinatorial facial approach. **(a)** A man in his 50s presented to the clinic with cheek soft-tissue atrophy, infraorbital hallows, festoons, periorbital lines, prominent naso-labial fold, dynamic rhytids in the forehead, and generalized photoaging. **(b)** Treatments were conducted in two stages over 8 weeks and included two glycolic acid (20%) peels, hyaluronic acid filler to the cheeks, infraorbital area, lips, as well as the nasolabial folds, bilaterally. Neurotoxin injection was performed to the glabella, forehead, and periocular area. After the final treatment, restoration of the medial and lateral cheek fat compartments, relaxation of the frontalis and glabellar complex with correct brow position, and overall improved photodamage was demonstrated.

with proper sun protection factor (SPF) during the daytime and topical retinol at night. In younger patients, hair thinning, or androgenetic alopecia may be the main contributing factor to their perception of aging, and thus, addressing and treating their hair concerns should be conducted before other interventions are pursued. In these patients, utilizing topical and/or oral medications may help prevent further loss and promote growth, respectively. For eligible patients, hair transplantation should be considered, as it improves satisfaction with appearance and visual age considerably.[36] Furthermore, any concurrent hyperpigmentation or other dermatological conditions, such as acne, rosacea, or telangiectasias should be properly addressed. Treatment for hyperpigmentation may be achieved with pigment-specific wavelengths (depending on skin type) with pico-, nano-, or millisecond pulse duration, and for facial redness and telangiectasias treatment with intense pulsed light, pulsed dye laser, or potassium titanyl phosphate laser is effective.[37,38] In men with poikiloderma where dyspigmentation consists of both melanin and prominent blood vessels, the appearance of hyperpigmentation can be significantly reduced by targeting the ectatic vessels alone.[39]

Facial aesthetic procedures including neuromodulation, volume enhancement, chemical peels, energy devices, and lasers are almost always used in combination (▶ Fig. 12.1). Neuromodulator injections should always be conducted in a resting face to properly assess wrinkles and hypertonic muscles. Large studies on the safety and efficacy of combining laser- and light-based treatments, neuromodulator therapy, and dermal fillers on the same day is limited. Injectable fillers complement neuromodulator treatments,[40] and can often be conducted in the same session, though some authors advocate performing

fillers first to avoid manipulating the neuromodulator during injection and to assess the degree of edema after filler placement.[41] Occasionally, letting the neuromodulator take effect over a period of 2 weeks or longer can be of value as the ensuing muscle hypotonia may influence the amount of dermal filler required for optimal results.

When combining neuromodulators and fillers with thermal treatments such as lasers, RF, and ultrasound, there has historically been a concern that thermal treatments may cause rapid degradation of the soft-tissue fillers, potentially impairing their clinical effect. For that reason, thermal treatments are most often administered prior to filler injection if done in the same treatment session.[42] However, the benefit of administering laser before fillers has not been confirmed in clinical trials.[43] When combining different treatment modalities in the same anatomical facial area, one may consider spacing the treatments 1 to 2 weeks apart to allow resolution of side effects and to assess the results to produce gradual augmentation.

Body contouring is another area where combination treatments are routinely used. Even though facial interventions and body contouring can be conducted simultaneously, focusing on one issue at a time is recommended in order to avoid dramatic alteration of appearance. Male patients who desire fat reduction often seek treatment for multiple distinct areas, such as submental and abdominal fat simultaneously. Thus, treatment with either cryolipolysis, laser, RF, or ultrasound[44,45,46] for the abdominal fat in combination with synthetic sodium deoxycholic acid for the submental area may render outcomes superior to that of monotherapy. In addition, a combination of multiple modalities can be used to target a single region. For example, cryolipolysis can be combined with RF treatment to improve fat reduction even further in the flanks.[47]

One of the most critical aspects of performing aesthetic treatments in male patients is to maintain a masculine appearance—unless otherwise desired. There are several procedures that, if performed incorrectly, can result in an unintentional feminized appearance. As such, it is important to discuss what factors are of specific concern to the patient and what they wish to achieve. Important considerations for different procedures discussed in this book are summarized in the following section.

12.4 Procedures

This summary serves to review a few of the fundamental tenets employed for each cosmetic treatment to achieve the best aesthetic outcome and satisfied patients, expanding on the information in the antecedent sections.

12.4.1 Soft-Tissue Augmentation

Facial aging results from a progressive loss of volume due to the redistribution and atrophy of fat, reduction in bone mass and structure, and changes in skin thickness and quality as testosterone levels drop.[48] Soft-tissue fillers play an important role in facial enhancement in men by augmenting male-specific facial features, addressing volume loss, and smoothing out coarse wrinkles (▶ Fig. 12.1, ▶ Fig. 12.2). The sexual dimorphism between musculature, skin thickness, bone structure, and fat distribution must be well understood and is essential for achieving natural results.[49] Men have more prominent facial musculature and a thicker dermis; however, the subcutaneous tissue is thinner overall.[50] The ideal male face highlights prominent supraorbital ridges, a flatter and narrower eyebrow, slightly narrower eyes, heavier eyelids, longer and wider nose, thinner lips, and a larger, squarer jawline[51] (▶ Fig. 12.1, ▶ Fig. 12.2). The lower face in men is traditionally the signature feature of masculinity with a sharper and better-defined square jawline. The male midface is remarkably different from that of a woman with the apex of the male cheek being lower, more medial, and less defined as compared to the female cheek.[52] When using filler to restore volume of the malar eminence, men often do not want the same degree of cheek projection as women. Therefore, rebuilding the cheek must be done subtly to avoid creating a feminized appearance, such as one that is rounder, fuller, and more laterally positioned. In conjunction with addressing the cheek, eliminating infraorbital hollows can produce an energized and refreshed appearance (▶ Fig. 12.1).

12.4.2 Neuromodulation

The goals and expectations of men seeking treatment with neuromodulators differ compared to women. A gender-based approach is key to achieving a more youthful and attractive appearance without compromising the defining features of male anatomy. In the upper face, men have a greater forehead height and width, which can be exacerbated by the presence of androgenetic alopecia.[53] In this region, men prefer softening of these horizontal lines, while still allowing for movement of the forehead. Furthermore, men have a brow shape that is more horizontal and lies lower on the orbital rim.[54] Maintaining brow shape and avoiding arching of the lateral brow can be achieved by placing an injection into the lateral frontalis.[55] The male glabella is wider, projects more anteriorly, and has a deeper furrow than in women, and complete effacement of these lines are desired as compared to

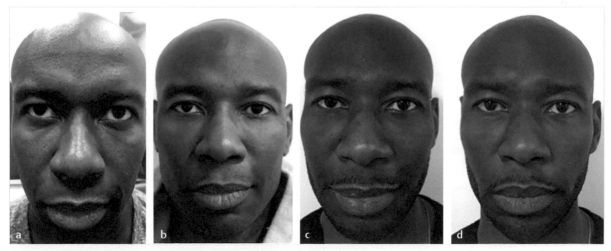

Fig. 12.2 Before and after combinatorial facial approach spanning 5 years demonstrating maintenance therapy. (a) A man in his 30s over a 5-year time period showing maintenance of appearance with regularly spaced pan facial treatments with dermal filler, neurotoxin, and chemical peeling. (b–d) Baseline maintenance over a 5-year period.

other anatomic regions in men.[56] The glabella should be treated in conjunction with the frontalis to prevent feminization of the brow. The orbicularis oculi is broader and extends more laterally in men, with some men having a lower fan pattern of the lateral canthal lines.[10,57–59] These lines indicate masculinity and maturity, so the goal may be only to relax and not immobilize these lines.[60] Men generally do not seek neuromodulator treatment in the mid and lower face, due to a lower incidence of gingival show, fewer rhytids due to highly sebaceous nature of the perioral skin, and preference for a more prominent jawline. On account of the increased facial muscle volume and movement, men require higher units of neuromodulators to achieve the same degree of muscle relaxation as females, and the most common cause of an inadequate result is inadequate dose.[61]

12.4.3 Hair Restoration

Androgenetic alopecia is a common form of hair loss that is characterized by a progressive reduction of terminal hairs involving the anterior, temporal, and vertex scalp in a characteristic pattern. First-line therapies may include topical minoxidil and oral finasteride prior to surgical consideration. Finasteride is an oral inhibitor of dihydrotestosterone (DHT), which competitively inhibits the 5 alpha reductase type 2 enzyme and at a dose of 1 mg a day decreases serum and scalp DHT levels by more than 60%.[62,63] Minoxidil promotes hair growth by increasing the duration of the anagen phase, shortening the telogen phase, and enlarging miniaturized follicles.[64] Once the patient has been medically optimized on the above therapies, hair transplantation can offer a more permanent improvement in hair restoration. Follicular unit transplantation and follicular unit extraction are the current treatments of choice in hair transplantation.[65] However, men can continue to lose hair in areas susceptible to androgenetic alopecia that have not been transplanted, so it is prudent to continue medical treatment to maximize the results of hair transplantation. Platelet-rich plasma (PRP) continues to be evaluated and utilized for the treatment of hair loss with generally positive results; however, larger, more rigorous well-designed studies are necessary to determine the optimal protocol.[66] Other reported treatments for androgenetic alopecia include dutasteride, low-level laser light therapy, camouflaging agents, and scalp micropigmentation or tattooing.

12.4.4 Chemical Peels

Chemical peels are becoming an increasingly popular, noninvasive cosmetic treatment option for men. Chemical peels induce tissue destruction, elimination, and regeneration in a controlled fashion and are commonly classified based on their depth of skin penetration. In men, chemical peels are often used either as monotherapy or in conjunction with other modalities to successfully treat conditions such as acne vulgaris, acne scarring, keratosis pilaris, melasma, actinic keratosis, photodamage, scars, and pseudofolliculitis barbae, or simply for periorbital rejuvenation.[67] Men may require more treatment sessions or higher concentrations than women, due to a greater density of both sebaceous glands and hair follicles.[68] Therefore, some physicians may choose to prime or pretreat with topical retinoids and/or alpha hydroxyl acid to ensure proper depth of penetration of the peeling agent.[69] During treatment, men may be able to better tolerate a more thorough degreasing, greater volume of peeling agents, and more pressure when applying the chemical peeling solution, which may correlate to a deeper and more effective peel.[67] Male patients should refrain from shaving in the postprocedural setting until the treated region has re-epithelialized. Another important consideration is that men may be more concerned about the postprocedural downtime after a chemical peel and should be counseled on the importance of strict photoprotection before and after the peel to minimize background pigmentation.[67]

12.4.5 Lasers, Light, and Energy Devices

Men are seeking treatment with lasers, light-, and energy-based devices to improve the appearance of wrinkles, acne scars, telangiectasias, dyschromia, photodamage, pore size, skin tightening, and overall skin tone.[39] As previously noted, men have increased epidermal and dermal thickness, increased facial muscle mass and movement, increased vascularity, a higher concentration of hair follicles, and more sebaceous glands.[52] When coupled with extrinsic factors such as poor sun protective behaviors, this leads to an increased depth of wrinkles, furrows, and photodamage.[10,70] Therefore, oftentimes higher fluences may need to be used to achieve similar outcomes to their female counterparts. Men overall are more cautious with their treatment plans and more self-conscious about pursuing cosmetic procedures with lengthy downtimes, discomfort, and visually apparent side effects.[39] Nonablative fractional skin resurfacing involves deeper skin penetration with selective thermal damage to the dermis, while largely sparing the epidermis.[71] Ablative fractional modalities involve superficial penetration of the skin with destruction of the epidermis and superficial thermal damage within the dermis, which is achieved with the carbon dioxide and the erbium:yttrium aluminum garnet (Er:YAG) lasers. For facial rejuvenation, ablative lasers are more efficacious than their nonablative counterparts; however, these treatments often require a more prolonged healing process, and with facial erythema may persist for weeks. Historically, men are less likely to wear cosmetic products to conceal discoloration that may occur following laser procedures.[72] The development of newer nonablative fractional lasers with improved side effect profiles may help improve results and decrease downtime. Other special considerations include avoiding more male-specific complications such as iatrogenic alopecia of the beard area, slower wound healing, and increased susceptibility to skin infections.[68,73]

12.4.6 Fat and Cellulite Treatments

Noninvasive or minimally invasive facial and body contouring is becoming increasingly popular to enhance the male physique. The ideal male contour focuses on a well-defined, strong, masculine jawline and developing a V-shaped taper through the upper body.[74] Males tend to focus on the submental chin, jawline, chest, abdomen, and flanks, whereas women additionally are interested in the medial and lateral thighs and posterior upper arms. This is largely due to sexual differences in fat metabolism in which women store more fat in the gluteal–femoral region, whereas men store more fat in the abdominal and chin/neck region.[75] The presence of anabolic hormones in men, such as testosterone, results in less superficial fat compared to women.[76] Noninvasive therapeutic modalities addressing fat reduction and body contouring include cryolipolysis, synthetic sodium deoxycholic acid, laser, RF, HIFEM energy, and ultrasound. Pseudogynecomastia may be very distressing to the male patient and is caused by excess subareolar fat. Standard treatments prior to noninvasive modalities were surgical excision or liposuction. However, currently, cryolipolysis has been demonstrated to be a safe, effective, and well-tolerated nonsurgical treatment of this condition.[77] Noninvasive fat reduction is especially attractive to the male patient since it tends to be less painful and with fewer side effects as compared to liposuction or surgical treatments. One must be cognizant of hair bearing areas, especially when using chemical lipolysis, as alopecia may be an unwanted effect.

12.4.7 Skin Tightening Procedures

Ultrasound, RF, microneedling, and certain laser treatments can be employed to target skin laxity. Similar to fat reduction therapies, men largely seek treatments to enhance their jawline, neck, chest, abdomen, and flanks.[74] Ultrasound and RF also share the dual nature of targeting adipocytes while tightening lax skin depending on the specific device. Benefits of these procedures include gradual results, little to no downtime, minimal discomfort, body-wide application, and less overall potential side effects. However, the results of the treatments are modest compared to surgical alternatives, like facelifts and necklifts. Nonetheless, noninvasive procedures for skin tightening and fat reduction are growing in popularity with almost six times as many performed compared to surgical procedures.[78] RF comes in numerous modalities including monopolar, bipolar, tripolar, multipolar, and

multigenerator. The goal is to turn RF energy into thermal energy, which results in collagen destruction, remodeling, and neocollagenesis. Ultrasound is divided into nonthermal, low-frequency focused ultrasound, and high-frequency, high-intensity ultrasound. Microfocused ultrasound delivers transcutaneous heat that targets deeper subdermal connective tissue in tightly focused zones at consistent programmed depths.[79] Considerations for treating the male patient must address that epidermal and dermal thicknesses are increased, which may account for less dramatic results compared to treating female patients unless settings are adjusted accordingly.

12.4.8 Skin Care

Historically, men centered their skin care regimens around shaving, which continues to be the largest and most developed portion of the male skin care market. As discussed previously in this chapter, there are many physiological differences between male and female skin and the current cosmeceutical market is beginning to target men by addressing their specific skin care needs. Male skin tends to have darker and more red skin tones, more collagen resulting in thicker skin, less subcutaneous fat, and a slower onset of the appearance of aging.[5] Specifically, on the face, males tend to have larger and more numerous sebaceous glands due to the increased amount of terminal hairs.[64] Besides the social perception of increased maturity and masculinity, male facial hair is advantageous in offering a high degree of photoprotection by decreasing the amount of ultraviolet rays reaching the skin surface, which mitigates against aging and the development of actinic keratoses.[65] Shaving, best known for facial hair removal, is also very effective at removing and exfoliating the stratum corneum, making men less likely to seek other methods of exfoliation such as chemical peels or using mechanical devices.[66] Furthermore, male skin produces more sebum and sweat, but has a lower skin pH and sweat evaporation rate as compared to women. Testosterone-driven sebum production in males provides natural skin moisturization, leading to lower rates of topical skin moisturization in males and, in addition, male skin cleansing products tend to be more effective in removing sebum as compared to female products. Skin care regimens for men will continue to evolve and grow as younger men become increasingly interested in skin cleansing, skin moisturizing, photoprotection, and combating facial aging.[67]

12.5 Future Considerations

The number of male patients seeking cosmetic procedures is steadily growing, and younger individuals motivated by age prevention are increasingly being treated as well. Innovative ways of injecting neuromodulators, such as dermal microdeposits, can, in addition to preventing dynamic wrinkles, be utilized to help decrease pore size, oil production, and fine lines.[80] Novel combination therapies, such as combining laser-resurfacing treatments or hair loss treatments with autologous PRP, are being used to boost growth factor stimulation in anticipation of superior outcomes. Furthermore, aesthetic therapies that were once primarily done to the face are expanding to include other body parts as well, for example, arms, legs, and buttocks. Minimally invasive procedures such as laser liposuction are being employed to conduct "high-definition liposuction" to contour around existing muscle groups in various body areas.

There are many exciting trends currently emerging in the aesthetic arena for men. As aesthetic physicians, it is essential to understand how certain cosmetic modifications can alter masculine and feminine features, especially in the face. This is especially important in the transgender population where aesthetic treatments go beyond restoring or augmenting existing features to attempting to masculinize or feminize the individual to match their gender identity.[81] As the aesthetic field expands, more randomized controlled trials with long-term follow-up are needed to assess emerging treatments and treatment combinations to enable physicians to make evidence-based recommendations to our patients.

12.6 Conclusion

The demand for cosmetic procedures among all patients, and specifically male patients, is steadily rising, and enhanced knowledge regarding differences in the anatomy, biochemical behavior of skin, and varying aesthetic ideals between men and women is critical for physicians performing aesthetic procedures. The principal considerations discussed in this book and highlighted in this chapter are critical to achieving the best cosmetic outcomes and satisfied patients. We are amid an exciting era of increasing demand for cosmetic procedures among males, in concert with rapidly expanding portfolio of treatment options. Although once overlooked, tailoring minimally invasive cosmetic procedures to match an individual's gender (or gender identity) is becoming an important objective. Physicians with thorough knowledge of differences between male and female facial structure and physique, and are able to augment, restore, or modify the anatomy to match the patient's desired appearance, can dramatically impact their patient's quality of life.

12.7 Pearls

- A gender-based approach is key to achieving a more youthful and attractive appearance without compromising the defining features of male anatomy.
- The overall skeletal framework of the head is different between men and women, with women having a skull about four-fifths the size of the male skull.[16] Men and

women have different craniofacial shapes; as such, women seek to have a tapered, heart-shaped face with more prominent upper facial features, whereas men desire a more square, chiseled jawline with equally proportioned facial features between the upper and lower face.

- To achieve desired aesthetic results, combining different treatment modalities is often required. Determining the optimal therapies and the order they should be administered is crucial for optimizing patient outcome and satisfaction.
- The male midface is remarkably different from that of a woman with the apex of the male cheek being lower, more medial, and less defined as compared to the female cheek.
- When performing neuromodulation of the frontalis and glabella, men prefer softening of horizontal lines, while still allowing for movement. Furthermore, men have a brow shape that is more horizontal and lies lower on the orbital rim.
- If concerns about BDD arise during a consultation, BDD screening instruments such as "COPS for BDD" can be used to assess the patient.
- Physicians with thorough knowledge of differences between male and female facial structure and physique, and are able to augment, restore, or modify the anatomy to match the patient's desired appearance, can dramatically impact their patient's quality of life.

References

[1] Wieczorek IT, Hibler BP, Rossi AM. Injectable cosmetic procedures for the male patient. J Drugs Dermatol. 2015; 14(9):1043–1051

[2] Singh B, Keaney T, Rossi AM. Male body contouring. J Drugs Dermatol. 2015; 14(9):1052–1059

[3] Escoffier C, de Rigal J, Rochefort A, Vasselet R, Lévêque JL, Agache PG. Age-related mechanical properties of human skin: an in vivo study. J Invest Dermatol. 1989; 93(3):353–357

[4] Van Mulder TJ, de Koeijer M, Theeten H, et al. High frequency ultrasound to assess skin thickness in healthy adults. Vaccine. 2017; 35 (14):1810–1815

[5] Bailey SH, Oni G, Brown SA, et al. The use of non-invasive instruments in characterizing human facial and abdominal skin. Lasers Surg Med. 2012; 44(2):131–142

[6] Laurent A, Mistretta F, Bottigioli D, et al. Echographic measurement of skin thickness in adults by high frequency ultrasound to assess the appropriate microneedle length for intradermal delivery of vaccines. Vaccine. 2007; 25(34):6423–6430

[7] Azzi L, El-Alfy M, Martel C, Labrie F. Gender differences in mouse skin morphology and specific effects of sex steroids and dehydroepiandrosterone. J Invest Dermatol. 2005; 124(1):22–27

[8] Shuster S, Black MM, McVitie E. The influence of age and sex on skin thickness, skin collagen and density. Br J Dermatol. 1975; 93 (6):639–643

[9] Janssen I, Heymsfield SB, Wang ZM, Ross R. Skeletal muscle mass and distribution in 468 men and women aged 18–88 yr. J Appl Physiol (1985). 2000; 89(1):81–88

[10] Weeden JC, Trotman CA, Faraway JJ. Three dimensional analysis of facial movement in normal adults: influence of sex and facial shape. Angle Orthod. 2001; 71(2):132–140

[11] Paganelli A, Mandel VD, Kaleci S, Pellacani G, Rossi E. Favre-Racouchot disease: systematic review and possible therapeutic strategies. J Eur Acad Dermatol Venereol. 2019; 33(1):32–41

[12] Luebberding S, Krueger N, Kerscher M. Skin physiology in men and women: in vivo evaluation of 300 people including TEWL, SC hydration, sebum content and skin surface pH. Int J Cosmet Sci. 2013; 35 (5):477–483

[13] Pochi PE, Strauss JS, Downing DT. Age-related changes in sebaceous gland activity. J Invest Dermatol. 1979; 73(1):108–111

[14] Strauss JS, Kligman AM, Pochi PE. The effect of androgens and estrogens on human sebaceous glands. J Invest Dermatol. 1962; 39:139–155

[15] Guy R, Ridden C, Kealey T. The improved organ maintenance of the human sebaceous gland: modeling in vitro the effects of epidermal growth factor, androgens, estrogens, 13-cis retinoic acid, and phenol red. J Invest Dermatol. 1996; 106(3):454–460

[16] Krogman WM. Sexing skeletal remains. In: The Human Skeleton in Forensic Medicine. Springfield, IL: C.C. Thomas; 1973:112

[17] de Maio M. Ethnic and gender considerations in the use of facial injectables: male patients. Plast Reconstr Surg. 2015; 136(5) Suppl: 40S–43S

[18] Ezure T, Yagi E, Kunizawa N, Hirao T, Amano S. Comparison of sagging at the cheek and lower eyelid between male and female faces. Skin Res Technol. 2011; 17(4):510–515

[19] Kahn DM, Shaw RB , Jr. Aging of the bony orbit: a three-dimensional computed tomographic study. Aesthet Surg J. 2008; 28(3):258–264

[20] Codinha P. Facial soft tissue thicknesses for the Portuguese adult population. Forensic Sci Int. 2009; 184:80.e1–80.e7

[21] American Society for Aesthetic Plastic Surgery. Cosmetic (Aesthetic) Surgery National Data Bank Statistics. New York, NY: American Society for Aesthetic Plastic Surgery; 2019

[22] Cosmetic Surgery National Data Bank Statistics. Aesthet Surg J. 2016; 36 Suppl 1:1–29

[23] Taub A, Bartholomeusz J. Ultrasound evaluation of a single treatment with a temperature controlled multi-frequency monopolar radio frequency device for the improvement of localized adiposity on the abdomen and flanks. J Drugs Dermatol. 2020; 19(1): 28–34

[24] Fritz K, Salavastru C, Gyurova M. Clinical evaluation of simultaneously applied monopolar radiofrequency and targeted pressure energy as a new method for noninvasive treatment of cellulite in postpubertal women. J Cosmet Dermatol. 2018; 17(3):361–364

[25] Kent DE, Jacob CI. Simultaneous changes in abdominal adipose and muscle tissues following treatments by high-intensity focused electromagnetic (HIFEM) technology-based device: computed tomography evaluation. J Drugs Dermatol. 2019; 18(11):1098–1102

[26] Jacob C, Kinney B, Busso M, et al. High intensity focused electromagnetic technology (HIFEM) for non-invasive buttock lifting and toning of gluteal muscles: a multi-center efficacy and safety study. J Drugs Dermatol. 2018; 17(11):1229–1232

[27] U.S. Food and Drug Administration. Re: K190456. Available at: https://www.accessdata.fda.gov/cdrh_docs/pdf19/K190456.pdf. Accessed 02/03/2020

[28] Jagdeo J, Keaney T, Narurkar V, Kolodziejczyk J, Gallagher CJ. Facial treatment preferences among aesthetically oriented men. Dermatol Surg. 2016; 42(10):1155–1163

[29] Koran LM, Abujaoude E, Large MD, Serpe RT. The prevalence of body dysmorphic disorder in the United States adult population. CNS Spectr. 2008; 13(4):316–322

[30] Phillips KA, Castle DJ. Body dysmorphic disorder in men. BMJ. 2001; 323(7320):1015–1016

[31] Gunstad J, Phillips KA. Axis I comorbidity in body dysmorphic disorder. Compr Psychiatry. 2003; 44(4):270–276

[32] Sarwer DB. Awareness and identification of body dysmorphic disorder by aesthetic surgeons: results of a survey of American Society for Aesthetic Plastic Surgery members. Aesthet Surg J. 2002; 22(6): 531–535

[33] Veale D, Ellison N, Werner TG, Dodhia R, Serfaty MA, Clarke A. Development of a cosmetic procedure screening questionnaire (COPS) for body dysmorphic disorder. J Plast Reconstr Aesthet Surg. 2012; 65 (4):530–532

[34] Williams J, Hadjistavropoulos T, Sharpe D. A meta-analysis of psychological and pharmacological treatments for body dysmorphic disorder. Behav Res Ther. 2006; 44(1):99–111

[35] Gold MH. Combination therapy for male cosmetic patients. Dermatol Clin. 2018; 36(1):69–73

[36] Liu F, Miao Y, Li X, et al. The relationship between self-esteem and hair transplantation satisfaction in male androgenetic alopecia patients. J Cosmet Dermatol. 2018

[37] Frucht CS, Ortiz AE. Nonsurgical cosmetic procedures for men: trends and technique considerations. J Clin Aesthet Dermatol. 2016; 9(12): 33–43

[38] Crispin MK, Hruza GJ, Kilmer SL. Lasers and energy-based devices in men. Dermatol Surg. 2017; 43 Suppl 2:S176–S184

[39] Ross EV. Nonablative laser rejuvenation in men. Dermatol Ther. 2007; 20(6):414–429

[40] Coleman KR, Carruthers J. Combination therapy with BOTOX and fillers: the new rejuvnation paradigm. Dermatol Ther. 2006; 19(3): 177–188

[41] Fabi S, Goldman M. Soft tissue augmentation with hyaluronic acid and calcium hydroxylapatite fillers. In: Amir M, Karam MPG, eds. Rejuvenation of the Aging Face. London, UK: JP Medical Ltd; 2015:20

[42] Carruthers J, Burgess C, Day D, et al. Consensus recommendations for combined aesthetic interventions in the face using botulinum toxin, fillers, and energy-based devices. Dermatol Surg. 2016; 42(5):586–597

[43] Fabi SG, Goldman MP, Mills DC, et al. Combining microfocused ultrasound with botulinum toxin and temporary and semi-permanent dermal fillers: safety and current use. Dermatol Surg. 2016; 42 Suppl 2:S168–S176

[44] Hong JY, Ko EJ, Choi SY, et al. Efficacy and safety of high-intensity focused ultrasound for noninvasive abdominal subcutaneous fat reduction. Dermatol Surg. 2020; 46(2):213–219

[45] Coleman WP , III, Coleman W , IV, Weiss RA, Kenkel JM, Ad-El DD, Amir R. A multicenter controlled study to evaluate multiple treatments with nonthermal focused ultrasound for noninvasive fat reduction. Dermatol Surg. 2017; 43(1):50–57

[46] Mazzoni D, Lin MJ, Dubin DP, Khorasani H. Review of non-invasive body contouring devices for fat reduction, skin tightening and muscle definition. Australas J Dermatol. 2019; 60(4):278–283

[47] Few J, Gold M, Sadick N. prospective internally controlled blind reviewed clinical evaluation of cryolipolysis combined with multipolar radiofrequency andvaripulsetechnology for enhanced subject results in circumferential fat reduction and skin laxity of the flanks. J Drugs Dermatol. 2016; 15(11):1354–1358

[48] Donofrio LM. Fat distribution: a morphologic study of the aging face. Dermatol Surg. 2000; 26(12):1107–1112

[49] Rossi AM, Fitzgerald R, Humphrey S. Facial soft tissue augmentation in males: an anatomical and practical approach. Dermatol Surg. 2017; 43 Suppl 2:S131–S139

[50] Sjöström L, Smith U, Krotkiewski M, Björntorp P. Cellularity in different regions of adipose tissue in young men and women. Metabolism. 1972; 21(12):1143–1153

[51] Marquardt SR. Dr. Stephen R. Marquardt on the Golden Decagon and human facial beauty. Interview by Dr. Gottlieb. J Clin Orthod. 2002; 36(6):339–347

[52] Wysong A, Kim D, Joseph T, MacFarlane DF, Tang JY, Gladstone HB. Quantifying soft tissue loss in the aging male face using magnetic resonance imaging. Dermatol Surg. 2014; 40(7):786–793

[53] Whitaker LA, Morales L , Jr, Farkas LG. Aesthetic surgery of the supraorbital ridge and forehead structures. Plast Reconstr Surg. 1986; 78 (1):23–32

[54] Goldstein SM, Katowitz JA. The male eyebrow: a topographic anatomic analysis. Ophthal Plast Reconstr Surg. 2005; 21(4):285–291

[55] Jones IT, Fabi SG. The use of neurotoxins in the male face. Dermatol Clin. 2018; 36(1):29–42

[56] Macdonald MR, Spiegel JH, Raven RB, Kabaker SS, Maas CS. An anatomical approach to glabellar rhytids. Arch Otolaryngol Head Neck Surg. 1998; 124(12):1315–1320

[57] Houstis O, Kiliaridis S. Gender and age differences in facial expressions. Eur J Orthod. 2009; 31(5):459–466

[58] Kane MA, Cox SE, Jones D, Lei X, Gallagher CJ. Heterogeneity of crow's feet line patterns in clinical trial subjects. Dermatol Surg. 2015; 41 (4):447–456

[59] Carruthers A, Bruce S, Cox SE, Kane MA, Lee E, Gallagher CJ. OnabotulinumtoxinA for treatment of moderate to severe crow's feet lines: a review. Aesthet Surg J. 2016; 36(5):591–597

[60] Dayan SH, Ashourian N. Considerations for achieving a natural face in cosmetic procedures. JAMA Facial Plast Surg. 2015; 17(6):395

[61] Flynn TC. Botox in men. Dermatol Ther. 2007; 20(6):407–413

[62] Price VH. Treatment of hair loss. N Engl J Med. 1999; 341(13):964–973

[63] Rittmaster RS. Finasteride. N Engl J Med. 1994; 330(2):120–125

[64] Messenger AG, Rundegren J. Minoxidil: mechanisms of action on hair growth. Br J Dermatol. 2004; 150(2):186–194

[65] Avram M, Rogers N. Contemporary hair transplantation. Dermatol Surg. 2009; 35(11):1705–1719

[66] Gupta AK, Carviel JL. Meta-analysis of efficacy of platelet-rich plasma therapy for androgenetic alopecia. J Dermatolog Treat. 2017; 28(1): 55–58

[67] Reserva J, Champlain A, Soon SL, Tung R. chemical peels: indications and special considerations for the male patient. Dermatol Surg. 2017; 43 Suppl 2:S163–S173

[68] Cohen BE, Bashey S, Wysong A. Literature review of cosmetic procedures in men: approaches and techniques are gender specific. Am J Clin Dermatol. 2017; 18(1):87–96

[69] Landau M. Chemical peels. Clin Dermatol. 2008; 26(2):200–208

[70] Sattler U, Thellier S, Sibaud V, et al. Factors associated with sun protection compliance: results from a nationwide cross-sectional evaluation of 2215 patients from a dermatological consultation. Br J Dermatol. 2014; 170(6):1327–1335

[71] Gold MH. Fractional technology: a review and clinical approaches. J Drugs Dermatol. 2007; 6(8):849–852

[72] Carniol PJ, Gentile RD. Laser facial plastic surgery for men. Facial Plast Surg. 2005; 21(4):304–309

[73] Keaney T. Male aesthetics. Skin Therapy Lett. 2015; 20(2):5–7

[74] Wat H, Wu DC, Goldman MP. Noninvasive body contouring: a male perspective. Dermatol Clin. 2018; 36(1):49–55

[75] Blaak E. Gender differences in fat metabolism. Curr Opin Clin Nutr Metab Care. 2001; 4(6):499–502

[76] Karcher C. Liposuction considerations in men. Dermatol Clin. 2018; 36(1):75–80

[77] Munavalli GS, Panchaprateep R. Cryolipolysis for targeted fat reduction and improved appearance of the enlarged male breast. Dermatol Surg. 2015; 41(9):1043–1051

[78] Juhász M, Marmur E. Energy-based devices in male skin rejuvenation. Dermatol Clin. 2018; 36(1):21–28

[79] MacGregor JL, Tanzi EL. Microfocused ultrasound for skin tightening. Semin Cutan Med Surg. 2013; 32(1):18–25

[80] Bertossi D, Giampaoli G, Lucchese A, et al. The skin rejuvenation associated treatment-Fraxel laser, Microbotox, and low G prime hyaluronic acid: preliminary results. Lasers Med Sci. 2019; 34(7): 1449–1455

[81] Dhingra N, Bonati LM, Wang EB, Chou M, Jagdeo J. Medical and aesthetic procedural dermatology recommendations for transgender patients undergoing transition. J Am Acad Dermatol. 2019; 80(6):1712–1721

Index

Note: Page numbers set **bold** or *italic* indicate headings or figures, respectively.